Practice of Critical Care Pharmacy

Contributors

David Angaran, M.Sc.
Deborah K. Armstrong, Pharm.D.
Jane E. Aumick, R.N.
Henry Blissenbach, Pharm.D.
Joyce B. Comer, Pharm.D.
R Adams Cowley, M.D.
Gary C. Cupit, Pharm.D.
Robert M. Elenbaas, Pharm.D.
Ramón Lavandero, R.N., M.A., M.S.N., C.C.R.N.

Warren E. McConnell, Ph.D.
Donald C. McLeod, M.Sc.
Christine M. Quandt, B.Sc.
Therese S. Richmond, R.N., M.S.N., C.C.R.N.
Susan T. Roberts, R.N.
Philip J. Schneider, M.Sc.
Michael Schobelock, Pharm.D.

Practice of Critical Care Pharmacy

Editors

Thomas C. Majerus, Pharm.D.
The Maryland Institute for
Emergency Medical Services Systems
University of Maryland, Baltimore

Joseph F. Dasta, M.Sc.
College of Pharmacy, College of Medicine
Ohio State University

AN ASPEN PUBLICATION®
Aspen Systems Corporation
1985
Rockville, Maryland
Royal Tunbridge Wells

Library of Congress Cataloging in Publication Data
Main entry under title:

Practice of critical care pharmacy.

"An Aspen publication."
Bibliography: p. 289.
Includes index.
1. Pharmacy. 2. Pharmacy—Vocational guidance. 3. Pharmacy—Study and teaching. 4. Critical care medicine. I. Majerus, Thomas C. II. Dasta, Joseph F. [DNLM: 1. Critical Care—methods. 2. Drug Therapy. 3. Pharmacy. WX 218 P895]
RS92.P63   1985   615.5′8   84-21742
ISBN: 0-89443-571-X

Publisher: John R. Marozsan
Associate Publisher: Jack W. Knowles, Jr.
Editor-in-Chief: Michael Brown
Executive Managing Editor: Margot G. Raphael
Managing Editor: M. Eileen Higgins
Editorial Services: Scott Ballotin
Printing and Manufacturing: Debbie Collins

Copyright © 1985 by Aspen Systems Corporation
All rights reserved.

Aspen Systems Corporation grants permission for photocopying for personal or internal use, or for the personal or internal use of specific clients registered with the Copyright Clearance Center (CCC). This consent is given on the condition that the copier pay a $1.00 fee plus $.12 per page for each photocopy through the CCC for photocopying beyond that permitted by the U.S. Copyright Law. The fee should be paid directly to the CCC, 21 Congress St., Salem, Massachusetts 01970.
0-89443-571-X/85 $1.00 + .12.

This consent does not extend to other kinds of copying, such as copying for general distribution, for advertising or promotional purposes, for creating new collective works, or for resale. For information, address Aspen Systems Corporation, 1600 Research Boulevard, Rockville, Maryland 20850.

Library of Congress Catalog Card Number: 84-21742
ISBN: 0-89443-571-X

Printed in the United States of America

1 2 3 4 5

To

Son Brandon
Daughter Natalie
my parents
Gilbert and Elizabeth

Thomas C. Majerus

Wife Desma
Daughter Dana
my mother Ann
and the memory of my father Frank

Joseph F. Dasta

> 4 Feb 85
>
> To Dr. John Siegel —
> with respect and
> kindest regards.
>
> *Majerus*

Table of Contents

Foreword xiii

Preface xv

PART I—EMERGING ROLES 1

Chapter 1—**Introduction to Critical Care** 3
Joseph F. Dasta

    What Constitutes Critical Care? 3
    Development of Critical Care 4
    Drugs and Critical Care 4
    Drug-Related Research in Critical Care 6
    Pharmacy and Critical Care 7
    Summary 9

Chapter 2—**The Justification of Critical Care Pharmacy Positions in Hospitals** 13
Henry Blissenbach

    Identifying the Need 13
    Gaining the Necessary Support 15
    Writing the Proposal 17
    Preparing the Budget 19
    Determining the Qualification of Applicants 21
    Implementing the Program 22
    Evaluating the Program 23
    Summary 26

Chapter 3—The Expansion of Clinical Pharmacy Education to Critical Care Pharmacy Training 29
Donald C. McLeod

Evolution of Clinical Pharmacy Education 29
Doctor of Pharmacy Programs 39
Postgraduate Training in Critical Care Pharmacy 44
Summary 48
Appendix 3–A 50

Chapter 4—The Fellowship Program in Critical Care Pharmacy... 59
Warren E. McConnell

Identifying the Need 59
Defining the Terms 60
Developing the Fellowship 60
Protocol and Guidelines 60
Evaluating Preceptors and Fellows 61
Appendix 4–A 67
Appendix 4–B 69

Chapter 5—Nurses: The Pivotal Element in Critical Care Pharmacy 77
Ramón Lavandero and Therese S. Richmond

What is Nursing? 77
Education and Credentialing in Nursing 80
The Nurse's Role in Drug Therapy 83
Learning about Drugs 84
Frequently Asked Drug Questions 87
Critical Care Nurse-Pharmacist Collaboration 90
Appendix 5–A 95
Appendix 5–B 98

Chapter 6—Critical Care Nursing Education in a Neurotrauma Center—A Learning Contract 101
Jane E. Aumick and Susan T. Roberts

Critical Care Nursing Education 101
Critical Care Nursing and Pharmacology 103
Appendix 6–A 106
Appendix 6–B 116
Appendix 6–C 118
Appendix 6–D 119

	Appendix 6–E	121
	Appendix 6–F	122

PART II—PRESENT AND FUTURE ROLES 125

Chapter 7—The Pharmacist in Surgical Intensive Care and Anesthesiology 127
Deborah K. Armstrong, Joseph F. Dasta, Michael Schobelock, and Philip J. Schneider

Description of the SICU Area	128
Administrative Considerations—Drug Distribution Control	129
Program Description	135
Appendix 7–A	152
Appendix 7–B	155

Chapter 8—The Pharmacist in Neurosurgery Intensive Care 163
Christine M. Quandt

Neurosurgery Intensive Care Environment	163
Admission—Discharge Guidelines	164
Neurologic Assessment	164
Specialized CNS Monitoring	165
Pharmacist's Role	169
Summary	181

Chapter 9—The Pharmacist in Coronary Care and Cardiovascular Surgery Intensive Care 187
David Angaran

Demographics of the Units	188
Drug Records and Data Collection	189
Drug Distribution Systems	189
Justification, Organization, and Implementation of the System	198
Description of Activities	201
Summary	206

Chapter 10—The Pharmacist in Medical Intensive Care 207
Joyce B. Comer

Demographics	207
Position Development	208

Service Development 211
Research 217
Conclusion 218

Chapter 11—The Pharmacist in Pediatric and Neonatal Intensive Care **219**
Gary C. Cupit

Historical Perspective 219
Neonatal Intensive Care Unit 219
Pediatric Intensive Care Unit 230
Summary 237
Appendix 11–A 239

Chapter 12—The Pharmacist in Emergency Medicine **243**
Robert M. Elenbaas

Emergency Medicine 243
Emergency Medicine at Truman Medical Center 245
Clinical Pharmacy within Emergency Medicine 245
General Implementation of Program 253
Conclusions 257

Chapter 13—The Pharmacist in the Trauma Center **259**
Thomas C. Majerus

Trauma Center Environment 259
Organization of Emergency Medical Services System 260
Echelons of Care 261
Prehospital Care 261
Clinical Side of the System 263
The Clinical Pharmacist 264
Pharmacokinetic Applications 264
Nutrition Support 272
Drug Distribution 273
Therapeutic Monitoring 274
Drug Interactions in the Trauma Patient 275
Trauma Patients in a Nontrauma Hospital 276
Research 277
Teaching 277
Service Justification 278
General Considerations 278

　　　　　　　Commencing Critical Care Pharmacy Services 279
　　　　　　　Summary 282

Epilogue—　The Future of Critical Care Pharmacy **285**
　　　　　　Thomas C. Majerus

Appendix A—A Critical Care Bibliography **289**
　　　　　　Joseph F. Dasta

Index **301**

Foreword

The crisis in medicine today continues to be the delivery of emergency care. A revolutionary systems approach to the treatment of shock and traumatic injuries began in Maryland in 1960, and this program evolved into the establishment of the Maryland Institute for Emergency Medical Services Systems (MIEMSS).

Part of our mission as a public institution is to make available specialized patient care. The first responsibility is to save life and to prevent disability. To meet this objective, we must recognize that the overall care of the severely ill or injured patient is beyond the capabilities and the experience of any individual physician. Thus a holistic approach to treatment is mandatory, and it requires the cooperative efforts of a multidisciplinary team of specialists at the attending level.

Until eight years ago, pharmacy support at MIEMSS consisted only of filling physician orders. Dr. Majerus then introduced the Institute to the concept of clinical pharmacy, a field new to MIEMSS. Services that were introduced included pharmacokinetic manipulation of drug dosing, a logical approach to hyperalimentation (which is totally different for the critically ill patient), an orderly approach to fluid and electrolyte balance, and a refreshing and objective outlook toward drug-induced problems in the critically ill and traumatized patient.

In this book, Dr. Majerus and Mr. Dasta have provided pharmacists and nurses with a valuable resource for the implementation of intensive and critical care pharmacy services. By viewing the important role of the pharmacist, one can easily see how critical care pharmacy has evolved to complement the medical and nursing management of the critically ill and injured patient. This book describes their program, which has been developed in a wide variety of intensive care and emergency settings, and also provides an honest appreciation of the role of the critical care nurse. Dr. Majerus, as a teacher, willingly and refreshingly shares his experiences and knowledge with all specialties and professions by crossing professional boundaries.

I am sure the reader of this book will find that it demonstrates the tremendous benefit of a critical care pharmacy in the treatment of critically ill and injured patients. Dr. Majerus shows that sophisticated pharmacologic support of these patients is crucial to their recovery. Through his devotion and the application of clinical pharmacology concepts, Dr. Majerus has further developed our concept of holistic care in the treatment of these unfortunate victims.

R Adams Cowley, M.D.
Director, MIEMSS

Preface

Although there are several textbooks on critical care medicine and therapeutics, there is no comprehensive textbook addressing the practice of pharmacy in critical care. This book primarily is a compilation of information about specific critical care practice and educational efforts by the leaders in the pharmacy profession who have practiced in critical care for several years.

The purpose of this book is to stimulate interest in critical care pharmacy and to provide guidance to students, practitioners, administrators, and educators wishing to devote their time, resources, or talents to critical care pharmacy practice. For the student with a special interest area or the practitioner entering this discipline, this book, written by established practitioners, provides information on the scientific basis of critical care therapeutics; an overview of critical care seen by pharmacists, physicians, and nurses; and descriptions of successful role models in various critical care areas. The pharmacy administrator with a desire to implement critical care pharmacy services can use information in the chapter on justifying critical care positions and can extract segments of the chapters dealing with specific practice areas such as the way their positions were approved and the impact of these services on patient care. Also, the educator should be able to appreciate the potential role of pharmacy in critical care practice and, it is hoped, would incorporate aspects of critical care therapeutics into advanced training programs. Finally, the nonpharmacist should readily see the role of pharmacy in the pharmacologic care of critically ill patients and should expect similar involvement by pharmacists in their critical care unit.

As the chapters were being reviewed by the editors, it became apparent that they were reading descriptions of "pockets" of highly specialized and developed pharmacy practice sites. As critical care medicine expands, pharmacists, clearly, must meet the pharmacologic challenge of these critically ill patients. The handful of pharmacy educators and practitioners who participated in this book cannot possibly meet this need alone. It is hoped, therefore, that readers of this book who are dedicated to developing and providing pharmacy services in critical care will take this information and will apply it in daily practice. It is further hoped that those who hold key positions in hospitals and colleges of pharmacy will foresee the possibility of widespread growth and development in critical care pharmacy, and that this book will stimulate allocation of resources to make that potential a reality.

Thomas C. Majerus
Joseph F. Dasta
December 1984

Part I
Emerging Roles

Chapter 1
Introduction to Critical Care

Joseph F. Dasta

WHAT CONSTITUTES CRITICAL CARE?

The *American Heritage Dictionary* defines critical care as "of or pertaining to a crisis." The mere mention of critical care to a nonmedical person evokes emotions of fear, dread, suffering, and death. Even some health care professionals have an aversion to entering the critical care unit. The door usually has a sign stating "authorized personnel only" or "immediate family members only." Upon entering the unit, one hears the rhythmical sound of the ventilator and the piercing shrill of an alarm. Despite this unusual environment, many dedicated health care professionals (including pharmacists) practice in this area. The challenge is to correct acute problems, to resuscitate patients, to relieve pain, and to extend human life while minimizing the hazards of treatment.

A Consensus Development Conference held at the National Institutes of Health (NIH) on March 7–9, 1983, defined critical care medicine:[1]

> Critical care medicine (CCM) is a multidisciplinary and multiprofessional medical/nursing field concerned with patients who have sustained or are at risk of sustaining acutely life-threatening single or multiple organ system failure due to disease or injury. These conditions necessitate prolonged minute-to-minute therapy or observation in an intensive care unit (ICU) which is capable of providing a high level of intensive therapy in terms of quality and immediacy.

The critical (intensive) care unit is an area in the hospital designed to provide surveillance and support of vital functions and therapy for patients with acute, multiple organ failure.[2] Peter Safar, who is considered to be the father of critical care, has suggested that the term *reanimation* be used to describe the resuscitation efforts given to critically ill or injured patients at the scene, during transportation, or in the hospital.[3] In the broadest form, critical care has no boundaries inasmuch as this discipline can be practiced in parking lots, shopping centers, and modern shock-trauma units. Furthermore, because the problems of critically ill patients are varied, the discipline of critical care crosses traditional departmental and specialty lines.[4] The clinician caring for these patients must, therefore, be versatile in physiology, biochemistry, biomedical engineering, computer technology, hemodynamic monitoring, pharmacology, toxicology, and therapeutics.[5]

DEVELOPMENT OF CRITICAL CARE

After World War II, special nursing and monitoring units soon developed in hospitals. The first units in the hospital designed for "special care" were developed in the 1950s to care for victims of poliomyelitis.[3] By 1960, ten percent of the facilities of community hospitals included intensive care units.[6] Over the last 25 years, rapid scientific and technological advances have led to the development of sophisticated critical care units, including coronary, medical, surgical, neurosurgical, thoracic, burn, neonatal, and pediatric intensive care units. Recently, these units have expanded to shock-trauma units. It is estimated that nearly 4000 hospitals in the United States currently have special care units with approximately 45,000 acute care beds.[6,7] There is a projected need for 2½ times this number of beds.[6]

The national cost of patient care in critical care units has been estimated to be in excess of 15% of total hospital costs—between $10 billion and $20 billion per year.[1] The average daily cost for a patient in the critical care ward of one hospital was $1,250.[7] Hospital charges are reported to average about $20,000 per patient for a typical critical-care-unit bill. If everyone who is presently eligible for critical care received all indicated therapy, the cost of this care could consume the entire gross national product.[8] In light of these enormous costs, research must be directed to the evaluation of tangible benefits to patients and hospitals.[1] A recent study showed that the one-year mortality rate of seriously ill patients admitted to one acute care ward did not change from 1973 to 1978; however, the quality of life at one year had improved.[9] Epidemiological data suggest that the decline in neonatal mortality is, in part, related to the development of neonatal intensive care units.[10] Although this information is promising, further work is needed to quantitate the influence of critical care on not only mortality but also the quality of life.[11]

DRUGS AND CRITICAL CARE

Treatment of a critically ill or injured patient often involves intubation, placement of various catheters, and dependence on various life-support machines;

however, drugs play an equally important role in overall patient care. The complexity of patient status coupled with the pharmacology, pharmacokinetics, and pharmacodynamics of drugs used in these patients makes the prescribing and monitoring of drugs difficult, even for the experienced clinician. The importance of the subject of drugs is evidenced by the recent publication of a 799-page textbook devoted to drugs and the critically ill patient.[12]

The critically ill patient with multiple systems disease frequently receives a variety of drugs—antibiotics, vasoactive compounds, antiarrhythmics, bronchodilators, and anticonvulsants—to treat life-threatening disorders, while continuing to receive many of the drugs taken at home. Patients admitted to critical care units receive an average of 7 to 17 drugs per patient, and most of these drugs are administered intravenously.[13,14] The chance of drug interactions and adverse drug reactions increases as the number of administered drugs increases. Once the therapeutic endpoint of a drug has been achieved, discontinuation of the drug should be considered. It is, therefore, important to perform daily "pharmacologic housekeeping" in these patients to minimize the number of drugs received.

Drugs given to critically ill patients often have narrow therapeutic indices and are usually given in maximal doses. Because of tenuous patient status, slight underdosing or overdosing can be disastrous. Simply choosing the correct drug is not sufficient; special consideration must be given to the dosage, the dosage form, the route and rate of administration, and the effect of the disease on drug disposition. Unfortunately, little is known about the pharmacokinetics of drugs in critically ill or injured patients. The patient with multiple organ system dysfunction, major burns, shock, trauma, and surgery may have altered absorption, metabolism, plasma protein binding, distribution, and elimination of certain drugs.[15] Inasmuch as critically ill patients may be hemodynamically unstable, the effect of their disease on drug disposition may change rapidly. Therefore, close monitoring and frequent assessment of drug concentrations and response are needed. Patients must be evaluated in a total context, including their attachment to various life-support systems. For example, the ventilator with positive end-expiratory pressure can reduce liver blood flow and impair the hepatic clearance of drugs whose metabolism is flow-dependent.[16] In one study, creatinine clearance increased from an average of 70 mL/min to 82 mL/min in respiratory failure patients when their ventilator mode was changed from controlled mechanical ventilation to intermittent mandatory ventilation.[17]

An important, and frequently overlooked, aspect of drugs is drug incompatibility and the drug delivery system. Observing patients closely may reveal that the nurse is adding multiple drugs in the same volume control system, or is infusing several drugs through the same intravenous line. A chemical degradation resulting in an inactive compound administered to the patient can be viewed as a lack of response or a worsening disease state. The response of the physician in this case may be to prescribe other drugs or change patient prognosis.

Delivery of drugs by the intravenous route may not guarantee complete bioavailability. Insulin, diazepam, and nitroglycerin adsorb to intravenous bags and tubing made of polyvinyl chloride plastic;[18,19] nitroglycerin adsorbs also to pulmonary artery catheters.[20] The rate and extent of drug loss to these devices often change with time, depending upon drug concentration, temperature, flow rate, and length of tubing. Similarly, the use of mini-bags to administer the aminoglycosides is associated with a variable rate and extent of drug delivery.[21] Understanding this problem can be helpful in explaining unpredictable aminoglycoside serum concentrations. Intravenous chloramphenicol sodium succinate, although completely available from the delivery system, is incompletely converted to free chloramphenicol in the blood; the average bioavailability in one study was only 69%.[22] Drugs, however, are not the only substances affected by the delivery system. A recent study evaluated the effect of various intravenous delivery systems on the development of hemolysis and the osmotic fragility of infused red blood cells.[23] The results of the study revealed that the piston-type pump can be used to infuse whole blood or packed red blood cells, whereas the diaphragm-type pump is suitable for administering whole blood only. Further studies are needed to evaluate the delivery of drugs or other substances administered intravenously to patients.

In fluid-restricted patients, it may be necessary to increase the concentration of drugs given intravenously. To compensate for the concentration change, a reduction in flow rate is needed. The drug in its original concentration is in the fluid of the remaining intravenous line and the central venous or pulmonary artery catheter. The reduced flow rate results in a considerably lower dosage because of the amount of time needed to clear this fluid from the lines.[24] Depending upon the flow rate, the time required to purge this solution in one study ranged from 28 seconds to over 300 seconds.[25] During this time, the patient's blood pressure or cardiovascular status may change, and additional drugs may be given to correct this perceived problem.

DRUG-RELATED RESEARCH IN CRITICAL CARE

The process of caring for the critically ill generates many unanswered therapeutic questions. The published research on drug therapy in critically ill patients is small. Pharmacokinetics and pharmacodynamic response to drugs in critical illness have not been extensively evaluated in the case of most drugs.

There are many reasons for this paucity of information. Only a few persons practicing in critical care have interest and experience in conducting drug-related research. This is, in part, due to the relative newness of the discipline. Also, conducting clinical investigations in critical care is extremely difficult because the strict control of variables external to the study is often not possible. Patients frequently have multiple organ systems involvement, and many diagnostic and therapeutic interventions are being continually performed. The constantly changing physiologic parameters of the patient make studies requiring a static environment virtually impossible. In addition, there are ethical considerations to be taken into account when performing drug studies on potentially dying patients. Despite these obstacles, the critically ill patient provides the researcher with numerous opportunities for data collection. For example, most patients have a central venous or pulmonary artery catheter in place, and many have arterial catheters for blood pressure monitoring. These catheters permit multiple blood sampling and obviate the need for venipuncture. There is also substantial physiologic information routinely collected about these patients—including blood pressure, heart rate, electrocardiogram, central venous or pulmonary artery pressures, cardiac output, urine output, numerous blood chemistries, arterial blood gases, gastric pH, and intracranial pressure.

Cost containment methods must be viewed as a major research topic. In the preface to the 1984 textbook of the Society of Critical Care Medicine (SCCM), the editors state that one of the immediate needs in the field of critical care is the development of strategies to assess the cost-effectiveness of specific therapeutic approaches.[8] Studies should be conducted to evaluate various aspects of drug therapy. Examples include empiric antibiotic therapy, the impact of pharmacokinetic drug level monitoring on morbidity and mortality, colloids versus crystalloids, the duration of antibiotic prophylaxis, and the role of H_2-receptors in stress ulcer prevention. Furthermore, distributive pharmacy services must be cost-justified, and clinical activities must be cost-effective as well as beneficial to patient care.

PHARMACY AND CRITICAL CARE

Pharmacists have a unique opportunity to use their knowledge of drugs in the management of critically ill patients. The complexity of total patient care, the rapid growth of information, and the polypharmacy nature of the environment make the pharmacist a key provider of drug-related information and advice. Depending upon the level of clinical involvement, manpower needs vary. If one highly trained clinical pharmacist is needed for 20 to 30 critical care beds, approximately 2,000 clinicians would be needed for the estimated 45,000 acute care beds in U.S. hospitals. To meet basic needs, these persons need to spend at least 75% of their time in the critical care ward. In smaller community hospitals, however, a pharmacist may need to spend less time in critical care while devoting time and effort to other responsibilities throughout the hospital. In major teaching hospitals, the patient-to-pharmacist ratio may even be lower because of the need for teaching time throughout the day. Unfortunately, these estimates do not consider evening and weekend shifts, which are particularly important in critical care.

Despite the potential for significant pharmacist involvement, development of pharmaceutical services to critical care areas has been slow. Broad-based collaborative relations between pharmacists and critical care physicians have not occurred. At the recent NIH conference on critical care, the pharmacist was not mentioned as a necessary member of the critical care team.[1] It was noted that pharmacists may be "peripherally" involved—along with nurses aides, unit clerks, and the clergy. The editor of *JAMA* has stated that the pharmacist is the most appropriately trained person at the interface between drugs and people.[26] It is paradoxical that a person with the training and the experience of a clinical pharmacist is not viewed by physicians as a primary member of the critical care team.[27]

A possible reason for pharmacy's slow entry into the critical care scene is the lack of adequate training sites in critical care at the Pharm.D. or the post-Pharm.D. levels. Although this has been the situation historically, pharmacy educators are beginning to recognize critical care as a specialty, and programs are being developed to train critical care practitioners and researchers. Critically ill patients require special needs that are difficult for traditional unit-dose systems to accommodate. As a result, the critical care areas are often the last to be serviced by modern pharmacy systems. Both clinical and distributional services of pharmacists have, therefore, been lacking in relation to the global need of hospitals.

There have been reports describing and evaluating critical care pharmacy services. One of the first accounts was a letter-to-the-editor in the *New England Journal of Medicine*, which described the pharmacist as a member of the cardiopulmonary resuscitation (CPR) team.[28] Subsequent papers have further described the activities of the CPR pharmacist as preparing medications, recording pertinent information, calculating doses, and providing therapeutic and pharmaceutical information during a cardiac arrest.[29,30] In one study, various health care professionals viewed the pharmacist as a valuable and necessary member of the CPR team.[30]

Emergency medicine is one area in which pharmacists have documented the need for their services. The first substantive report appeared in 1977 in which Elenbaas and coworkers described the emergency medicine program at Truman Medical Center.[31] Their role in clinical practice, education, and research is presented and includes an evaluation of the services provided. Of particular interest in their survey was the observation that physicians and nurses not only rated the pharmacist's contribution to patient care highly but that they supported charging a fee for these clinical pharmacy activities. Other papers have been published that describe the involvement of pharmacists in emergency medicine at a university medical center, government hospital, and a community health center.[32-34] Majerus described clinical pharmacy services in a unique clinical setting—the trauma center.[35] Pharmacokinetic dosing, toxicology consultations, nutrition support, and pharmacotherapeutics can be provided by a knowledgeable clinical pharmacist practicing in the trauma center.

A recent development in critical care pharmacy is the combination of clinical and distributive services in the operating room and anesthesiology.[36,37] Drug distribution requirements in the operating room include providing drugs quickly, controlling narcotics, and decreasing lost charges.[38,39] One study has shown that $12,000 annually was saved after the implementation of an operating room pharmacy.[40] Clinically, the pharmacist is available for consultation on questions relating to intraoperative antibiotics, theophylline therapy, and drug management of patients with shock and life-threatening arrhythmias.

A description and an evaluation of two critical care pharmacy satellites have been recently published.[41,42] The first satellite served 82 beds (including 14 intensive care, 14 coronary care, 10 hemodialysis, and 44 cardiac rehabilitation beds), 16 hours per day, seven days per week. The implementation of this system, in addition to providing clinical services, resulted in a 50% reduction in the percentage of floor-stock drugs used. This reduction corresponded to the floor-stock inventory of each unit, which decreased from $607 to $105. Drug order turn-around time decreased from 103 to 65 minutes. An annual reduction in lost charges of $14,136 was also documented. The second paper described the development of a 24-hour satellite pharmacy servicing 8 to 10 medical and 6 coronary intensive care beds.[42] Drug distribution, clinical services, and research activities were also described.

The literature on critical care pharmacy is small compared with other areas, but there have been recent developments. A specialty column "Critical Care Therapeutics" appeared in May 1982 in the journal *Drug Intelligence and Clinical Pharmacy*.[5] This column represents a forum in which current problems and practices relating to the drug therapy of critically ill patients can be expressed. Although this is the only column in the pharmacy literature relating to critical care, two sections in internal medicine journals have recently been instituted. The section "Emergency Medicine and Critical Care" was announced in the August 26, 1983, issue of *JAMA*[43] and "Critical Care Medicine" appeared in the July 1983 issue of the *Archives of Internal Medicine*.[44] More directly, the Society of Critical Care Medicine publishes the journal *Critical Care Medicine*; the official publication of the American Association of Critical Care Nurses is *Heart & Lung*. It is clear that physicians, nurses, and pharmacists have recognized the importance of critical care to their respective disciplines and have provided proper avenues of publishing pertinent information.

SUMMARY

Critical care is a new and growing field. The potential for practice, teaching, service, and research by pharmacists is enormous. Caution is needed, however; the potential exists for developing critical care "burnout."[45] The daily stress and the constant surroundings of death and suffering can affect the mind and soul of clinicians working in this environment. The critical care pharmacist is a special breed of practitioner, however, who must cope with the stress and persevere. It is hoped that the material presented in this text will stimulate young practitioners to pursue critical care practice and will provide administrators with guidelines to develop and to implement critical care pharmacy programs in their hospitals.

REFERENCES

1. NIH consensus development conference on critical care medicine. *Crit Care Med* 1983;11:466–469.

2. Weil MH, Shubin H, Boycks EC: A crisis in the delivery of care to the critically ill and injured. *Chest* 1972;62:616–620.

3. Safar P: Reanimatology—the science of resuscitation. *Crit Care Med* 1982;10:134–136.

4. Shapiro BA: Critical care medicine. *JAMA* 1982;247:2945.

5. Dasta JF: Critical care therapeutics: A frontier for clinical pharmacy. *Drug Intell Clin Pharm* 1982;16:398–399.

6. Angaran DM: Critical care pharmacy, in McLeod DC, Miller WA (eds): *The Practice of Pharmacy, Institutional and Ambulatory*. Cincinnati, Harvey Whitney Books, 1981, pp 171–181.

7. Gregory GA: Who should receive intensive care? *Crit Care Med* 1983;11:767–768.

8. Shoemaker WC, Thompson WL, Holbrook PR (eds): *Textbook of Critical Care*. Philadelphia, WB Saunders, 1984, p xv.

9. Cullen DJ, Keene R, Waternaux C, et al: Results, charges, and benefits of intensive care for critically ill patients:Update 1983. *Crit Care Med* 1984;12:102–106.

10. Paneth N, Kiely JL, Wallenstein S, et al: Newborn intensive care and neonatal mortality in low-birth weight infants:A population study. *N Engl J Med* 1982;307:149–152.

11. Robin ED: A critical look at critical care. *Crit Care Med* 1983;11:144–148.

12. Chernow B, Lake CR: *The Pharmacologic Approach to the Critically Ill Patient*. Baltimore, Williams & Wilkins, 1983.

13. Buchanan N, Cane RD: Drug utilization in a general intensive care unit. *Intensive Care Med* 1978;4:75–77.

14. Campos RA, Herraez FXV, Marcos RJ, et al: Drug use in an intensive care unit and its relation to survival. *Intensive Care Med* 1980;6:163–168.

15. Dasta JF: Pharmacokinetics of drugs in critically ill patients. *Syva Monitor* 1982;11:1–9.

16. Bonnet F, Richard C, Glaser P, et al: Changes in hepatic flow induced by continuous positive pressure ventilation in critically ill patients. *Crit Care Med* 1982;10:703–705.

17. Steinhoff H, Falke K, Schwarzhoff W: Enhanced renal function associated with intermittent mandatory ventilation in acute respiratory failure. *Intensive Care Med* 1982;8:69–74.

18. Baaske DM, Amann AH, Wagenknecht DM, et al: Nitroglycerin compatibility with intravenous fluid filters, containers, and administration sets. *Am J Hosp Pharm* 1980;37:201–205.

19. Mason NA, Cline S, Hyneck MI, et al: Factors affecting diazepam infusion:Solubility, administration-set composition, and flow rate. *Am J Hosp Pharm* 1981;38:1449–1454.

20. Jacobi J, Dasta JF, Reilley TE, et al: Loss of nitroglycerin to pulmonary artery delivery systems. *Am J Hosp Pharm* 1983;40:1980–1982.

21. Armistead JA, Nahata MC: Effect of variables associated with intermittent gentamicin infusions on pharmacokinetic predictions. *Clin Pharm* 1983;2:153–156.

22. Nahata MC, Powell DA: Bioavailability and clearance of chloramphenicol after intravenous chloramphenicol succinate. *Clin Pharmacol Ther* 1981;30:368–372.

23. Gibson JS, Leff RD, Roberts RJ: Effects of intravenous delivery systems on infused red blood cells. *Am J Hosp Pharm* 1984;41:468–472.

24. Spigelman AD, Angaran DM: Volume of infusion controller and delayed vasopressor effect. *Ann Intern Med* 1983;99:415–416.

25. Kahn JK, Kirsh MM: The infusion delivery time of the flow-directed pulmonary artery catheter:Clinical implications. *Heart Lung* 1983;12:630–632.

26. Lundberg GD: The clinical pharmacist. *JAMA* 1983;249:1193.

27. Dasta JF: Progress in critical care pharmacy. *Drug Intell Clin Pharm* 1984;18:156–157.

28. Elenbaas R: Pharmacist on resuscitation team. *N Engl J Med* 1972;287:151.

29. Schwerman E, Schwartau N, Thompson CO, et al: The pharmacist as a member of the cardiopulmonary resuscitation team. *Drug Intell Clin Pharm* 1973;7:299–308.

30. Ludwig DJ, Abramowitz PW: The pharmacist as a member of the CPR team: Evaluation by other health professionals. *Drug Intell Clin Pharm* 1983;17:463–465.

31. Elenbaas RM, Waeckerle JF, McNabney WK: The clinical pharmacist in emergency medicine. *Am J Hosp Pharm* 1977;34:843–846.

32. Carmichael JM, Hak SH, Edgman SM, et al: Emergency-room services for a community health center. *Am J Hosp Pharm* 1981;38:79–83.

33. High JL, Gill AW, Silvernale DJ: Clinical pharmacy in an emergency medicine setting. *Contemp Pharm Pract* 1981;4:227–230.

34. Culbertson V, Anderson RJ: Pharmacist involvement in emergency room services. *Contemp Pharm Pract* 1981;4:167–176.

35. Majerus TC: Shock-trauma:Clinical pharmacy in emergency medicine. *Top Hosp Pharm Manag* 1982;2:87–93.

36. Moritani D, Stein ZLG: Operating room pharmacy:A new specialty. *US Pharm* 1981;6:H2–H6.

37. Evans DM, Guenther AM, Keith TD, et al: Pharmacy practice in an operating room complex. *Am J Hosp Pharm* 1979;36:1342–1347.

38. McAllister JC, Murray J, Skolaut MW, et al: A new look at pharmacy services in the operating suite and recovery room. *Contemp Pharm Pract* 1980;3:6–10.

39. Powell PJ, Maland L, Bair JN, et al: Implementing an operating room pharmacy satellite. *Am J Hosp Pharm* 1983;40:1192–1198.

40. Hague B, Maland L, Powell PJ, et al: The anesthesiology operating room pharmacy. *Anesthesiology* 1983;59:A478.

41. Caldwell RD, Tuck BA: Justification and operation of a critical-care satellite pharmacy. *Am J Hosp Pharm* 1983;40:2141–2145.

42. Hall K, Guay M: The implementation of comprehensive critical care pharmacy services through the development of a 24-hour satellite pharmacy. *Can J Hosp Pharm* 1982;35:184–188.

43. Rinke CM: Emergency medicine and critical care:JAMA's new section. *JAMA* 1983;250:1073.

44. Weil MH, Rackow EC: Critical care medicine:Caveat emptor. *Arch Intern Med* 1983;143:1391–1392.

45. Orlowski JP: Critical problem of critical care burnout. *Crit Care Med* 1982;10:200.

Chapter 2
The Justification of Critical Care Pharmacy Positions in Hospitals

Henry Blissenbach

Human nature is such that we hesitate to involve ourselves in areas, situations, or activities with which we are not familiar. Unless pharmacy practice includes the critical care units, pharmacists tend to stay away. After all, the signs around the entrances to critical care units—"restricted," "limited," "immediate family only"—imply that pharmacists are not welcome; they should stay out. Wrongly, pharmacists correlate this misunderstanding of those signs with "not needed."

During the past years, critical care units have been in an untouchable position. Quality assurance, for example, was an activity applied to other units of the hospital. Very little was done in most institutions to analyze critically the quality of care in the critical care unit. In fact, the exact role of these units varied from hospital to hospital even though the objective of the critical care unit is clear: to maximize life by using aggressive medical therapies. Because all who benefit from the availability of a critical care unit have certain expectations of that unit, the pharmacist (despite any uneasiness in dealing with the critically ill patient) must answer the need for assurance of quality in the use of sophisticated pharmacologic intervention on the critical care units.

IDENTIFYING THE NEED

In order to establish a clinical pharmacy service in the critical care unit, pharmacists need to prove that patient care will be significantly improved. Documentation of need is best done from the perspective of the persons involved.

The Patient's Need

The main benefactor of pharmacy services—the patient—is often overlooked. They trust the health care system and believe that certain things, such as the following, are true:

- The medications ordered for them are necessary and rational.
- The medications are not only effective but harmless.
- The medications they receive are, in fact, ordered by their physician.

Polypharmacy is a routine occurrence in the critical care unit.[1] Campos and associates pointed out the large number of different drugs used per patient—as many as seventeen.[2] Abrahamson and associates noted that 15% of all reported incidents and resulting from human error involved medications.[3] The patients (and their families) deserve assurance that medications are used appropriately.

The Physician's Need

If physicians who care for patients in critical care units were asked how they could utilize the pharmacist, their answers might be surprising. The critically ill patient presents a different challenge for the physician. In addition to a concern about the quality of life, there is a concern about the quantity of life. The critically ill patient is at a high risk of death, and so barriers are broken, egos are lessened, and a cooperative team effort becomes important. Most physicians, in fact, seek out the pharmacist's advice, but they request advice only if it is readily available.

Studies have demonstrated the impact of erroneous decisions made by physicians for patients in the critical care unit. Robin[4] points out that every patient care decision made by the physician has the potential for both benefit and harm and that all patient interventions require some form of risk-benefit analysis. Many erroneous decisions could be prevented. The medications, their combinations, the maximum doses used—all these factors increase the risk of harm to the patient. Because the critical care physician realizes this, he welcomes input in order to reduce the risk of drug toxicity. The pharmacist is the person with the skills to provide this input.

The Critical Care Nurse's Need

Many years ago, nursing personnel assumed responsibility for medication in the critical care units. They accepted it, although they felt uncomfortable with it. Now pharmacists are attempting to invade their "turf." Nurses have functioned without pharmacists for years; why should they need them now?

Nurses need pharmacists now for the sake of better patient care. Times have changed; medications, attitudes, and responsibilities have changed. Nurses in the critical care unit receive sophisticated advanced training that allows them to assume many primary care functions. They no longer have the time to perform those functions they perceive to belong to others (such as medications). Furthermore, the rapid changes in advanced technology on the critical care unit require these nurses continually to increase their knowledge base in critical care nursing. Little time is left to learn about increasingly sophisticated medications.

What is the pharmacist's responsibility to the critical care nurse? These nurses usually administer the medications, and, more importantly, they are responsible for observing the results. They titrate the dosage of potent drugs according to certain monitoring criteria. The nurse is the one health care provider who maintains constant contact with the critically ill patient. As Waisbren[5] points out, the critical care physician needs to spend very little time on the critical care unit because, with proper monitoring and staffing, there are few critically ill patients who need a physician in constant attendance. They do, however, need the nurse, and nurses need to know how medications affect this monitoring of their patients. The pharmacists are the specialist source for such information.

The Hospital's Need

It appears that in the future one of the areas of most rapid growth in hospital admissions will be critical care.[6] The population is living longer, and, as persons become critically ill, medicine continues to find ways to keep patients alive. Yet, as this demand continues to rise and the expenditure required increases as well, the third-party payers are demanding specific criteria to assure the quality of care. The hospital has a responsibility to the patient to ensure that the service is of such a quality that patients get better and that the services are reasonable and affordable.

We can speculate on the impact that improper medication monitoring has on both the morbidity and the mortality of the patient. With the increased emphasis on prospective payments based on the diagnosis, not on length of stay, hospital administrators need to be assured that all potential risks against a longer hospital course beyond the "normal" length of stay have been averted.

When we look, then, at the recipients of a clinical pharmacy service to the critical care unit, we see that the documentation of need for clinical pharmacist services is feasible. Furthermore, care of the critically ill patient requires both technology and personnel. Civetta[7] states that in critical care medicine we must look beyond technology. It is the human resource that provides us with the tools to monitor, to regulate, and to recommend on an individual basis. Successfully saving the lives of critically ill and injured patients in a cost-effective manner requires the cooperative effort of the entire health care team. Skills in therapeutics, pharmacokinetics, and pharmacology make the pharmacist a much needed member of the critical-care-unit team.

GAINING THE NECESSARY SUPPORT

The ability to gain the support necessary to establish clinical pharmacy services in the critical care unit is directly related to the sophistication of the present services, the power base of the pharmacy within the medical staff, and the relationship of pharmacy with nursing. Less than optimal services or adversary relationships have to be dealt with during the planning process for the new service. Nevertheless, attempting to establish a new distribution method or attempting to patch political fences can delay the process of establishing critical care pharmacy services.

Medical Staff Support

The Pharmacy and Therapeutics (P&T) Committee is the pharmacy department's liaison to the medical staff to gain physician approval for programs and projects. The success of prior programs needs to be evaluated through the P&T Committee. Will a proposal meet with resistance, or, with proper justification, will it be approved? Before bringing a proposal to the committee, the key physicians on the committee must be made aware of the plans. In fact, for a project as important as the establishment of pharmacy services in the critical care unit, the value of a subcommittee should be considered. This subcommittee should include the chairman of the P&T Committee, other influential committee members, the medical director of the unit, and other physicians who are primary users of the critical care unit. With the endorsement of this subcommittee, the P&T Committee will undoubtedly approve the project.

Nursing Staff Support

Generally, there are three strata of nursing personnel whose support is needed: the critical care nurses, the head nurses, and the nursing administration. Again, the situation within the institution must be assessed. Where does the sphere of influence originate within the nursing staff? In some hospitals, the decisions are made unilaterally by the nursing administration. Others use a team concept. Whatever the method, be sure that nursing personnel at all levels are involved in the planning process. Ideally, a subcommittee that includes nursing personnel should be formed, probably as a subcommittee of the pharmacy-nursing committee. There, the pharmacy department can identify and alleviate the concerns nursing personnel may have about "turf invasion." Be sure that representation on this subcommittee is appropriate—from the staff level to the administrative level. The staff nurses have the concerns; the nursing administration makes the decision. More than likely, however, the decision will be based on the staff nurses' enthusiasm for the project. The wise pharmacy administrator, then, asks some of the critical care nurses to review the proposal and to comment on it. Their reaction will provide ideas to plan a strategy for nursing.

Administrative Support

Do not forget administrative support. It is crucial that the administrator be continually aware of our intentions, our purposes, and our plan. A severe setback to the plans could occur if the administration feels it has been ignored in the planning process. Gaining the support of the medical staff and the nursing personnel should provide the needed administrative endorsement.

In summary, gaining the necessary support from nursing and medical staff is best accomplished through the formal committee mechanism (Table 2–1). Nursing support is an important element in gaining physician acceptance. The medical staff seldom approves another department's program if nursing personnel oppose it.

WRITING THE PROPOSAL

Before any formal committee involvement occurs, a written proposal should be prepared. It may be only in a rough draft form, but it provides a proposal with which to start. This proposal should address the distribution system and the clinical program. The format of the proposal could be similar to the following:

- background
- literature review
- other supporting data
- goals and objectives
- college of pharmacy teaching responsibilities
- distribution system

Table 2–1 Committee Support Process

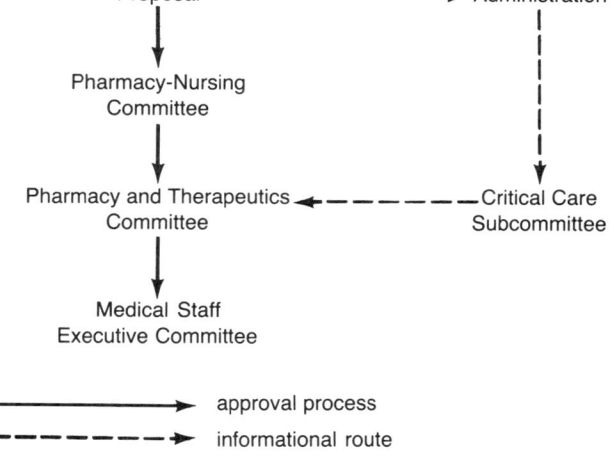

- staffing requirements
- cost containment

Background. Outline the current extent of pharmacy services to the critical care unit; identify problems with the current service. This narrative should identify the reasons the current level of service is inadequate. Detailed information should be pertinent to the proposed changes; that is, do not describe technicians' functions when no changes are expected.

Literature Review. A search of the literature to find published descriptions of pharmacy services to critical care units is in order. These articles should describe the impact of clinical pharmacists on the care of the critically ill patient. Take key sentences from these articles and put them into a report format, such as "Berger and associates have described how drug errors decreased by 65% after the change in pharmacy services to the critical care unit." Be sure that these quotations are referenced so that followup is feasible. This is not an area to limit one's words. Ideally, the reader of the proposal should get the impression that there is sufficient support for your proposal in the literature and that any hospital without these more sophisticated services does not meet even the standards reported in the literature.

Other Supporting Data. Any evidence of Joint Commission on Accreditation of Hospitals (JCAH) recommendations and requirements; any evidence of medical staff desire; any impact on the ability to ensure compliance with legal influences (i.e., State Boards, local and federal laws and regulations); and any information that can help to assure compliance with these data need to be included.

Goals and Objectives. These goals and objectives should be realistic. Do not address only what you desire to do, but what you can realistically do. Helpful in this respect are studies that show the likelihood of success with various clinical pharmacy functions.[8] One must determine the services desired and then measure the likelihood of successfully providing these services in terms of staff capabilities, hospital politics, and budget restraints. For example, if a medication administration service is desired, but no personnel increases are being given to any department, it would be foolish to include increased staffing as a goal—at least in the original proposal.

Also, carefully list goals and objectives by priority. Determine the top priorities and list them first. The lesser priorities should be given less attention in the proposal. Thus, you must decide whether providing drug information or therapeutic monitoring, decreasing hospital stay on the critical care unit, providing education, and so forth are necessary to the success of your service. Often, medical staff committees approve most, but not all, of a proposal. Hence, be prepared to cut back slightly on the proposal, and these cutbacks should be the lowest priority functions.

It is also important to include a statement of how these proposed changes in services are conducive to achieving the goals and objectives of the hospital. Each institution has a mission statement of some kind and has written goals and objectives, both short and long range. Typically, the continuous improvement of patient care at an economically feasible rate is the underlying theme. The proposal to establish clinical pharmacy services on the critical care unit should contribute to implementation of the hospital's mission statement.

College of Pharmacy Teaching Responsibilities. Affiliation with a college of pharmacy teaching program can be a help or a hindrance to a hospital; which one it is depends on the type of the hospital. Even in the most conservative private hospitals, however, students have been accepted and utilized in a most positive way. If there is a teaching commitment on the part of the pharmacy department, the proposal should outline the impact the proposed new service will have on the educational arrangement. What will the students do? Who is responsible? Will they provide any service?

Distribution System. A change in service usually means changes in the current distribution system. The ideal distribution system involves decentralization of the pharmacist and, if necessary, the pharmacy. The decentralized pharmacy or satellite allows the pharmacist to enter the patient care area to distribute medications from a unit satellite. This arrangement provides a mechanism to get pharmacists into the critical care unit, but it can also provide a "hiding place" for the pharmacist who continues an attachment to the distribution function.

An option is the decentralized pharmacist system, which maintains the distribution activities in a central location. This system allows the pharmacist more time for clinical activities, less distribution time, and continual visibility on the unit. It also requires increased staffing—which needs to be addressed in the proposal. Describe in the proposal the distribution system needed.

Staffing Requirements. Changes in services usually involve changes in staffing. As priorities are identified, a realistic approximation of staffing can occur. To try to "slip" through a proposal for increased services without addressing staffing changes is generally not a good idea. The administration needs to approve staffing changes, and these should be evident in the proposal.

Cost Containment. The ability of these new services to affect diagnosis related groups (DRGs) and prospective payment is a critical problem in today's hospital economics. This concern is addressed in the next section.

PREPARING THE BUDGET

The budget or the costs involved in the implementation of any proposal are tremendously important. Most of the available data suggest that the majority of hospital costs are for personnel and the minority of costs are for materials. In this era of DRGs and general cost-containment efforts, any proposal requesting an increase in personnel costs has to be well documented. With this in mind, the following guidelines can be used for budgeting clinical services to the critical care units.

Understand the impact that government and private insurers continue to have on the overall cost of health care in general and pharmacy services in particular. Prepare the budget statement with these factors in mind, and emphasize the way the new clinical services can decrease both length and cost of patient stay—

- by decreasing drug costs through active formulary input and providing the capability for recommending therapeutic alternatives to the physician while present on the unit;
- by therapeutically monitoring patients' medications to minimize pharmacologic failures;
- by suggesting alternative therapy that would have higher probability for a rapid patient recovery;
- by assuring that unnecessary medications are discontinued promptly;
- by auditing medication use to identify inappropriate prescribers and then intervening;
- by reducing the vast drug inventories usually found in the critical care areas as floor stock.

The budget request should be consistent with the hospital's goals and objectives. The budget must reflect the hospital's future direction and should specifically identify how, in fact, each proposed service change directly affects one of the hospital's objectives. Determine your hospital's case-mix.

Furthermore, the need to increase the number of pharmacists to cover the critical care units versus the need to modify the present distribution system and to do the work with the current staff must be evaluated. If increasing the staff is the intent of the proposal, the budget should reflect the salaries plus benefits of the new pharmacists. The number of persons needed depends on the planned services. If the proposal provides for these new services with only the current pharmacist staff, however, the budget should reflect the costs associated with changes needed in the current pharmacy services. The proposal would have determined the changes needed to enable the current staff to carry out this new role, and those changes would probably be made in the distribution system. The current method of drug distribution, of course, would determine whether the changes would be minor or major.

It is hard to get approval for any request that has associated increased costs to the hospital. The best approach is to direct the budget request at prospective payment concepts. The focus of attention for these cost-decreasing, third-party-payer incentive programs is then on the entire institution, not on the individual departments. Hence, any program that affects the "bottom line" of the entire hospital's cost data would be favorably reviewed. Clinical pharmacy services in the critical care unit may well show an increase in the cost of pharmacy services, but it would necessarily show a decrease in the cost of medical care (or a decreased length of stay) in the institution.

DETERMINING THE QUALIFICATIONS OF APPLICANTS

You have now gained the necessary approval for changing the scope of pharmacy services to include a clinical service to the critical care units. How do you select your critical care pharmacists? The choice of pharmacists must be made by determining those characteristics necessary for success in this new endeavor and by applying these characteristics to interested members of the staff. If none of the staff fulfill these criteria, outside pharmacists must be hired.

Knowledge Base. The most important ingredient in a successful clinical endeavor probably is therapeutic knowledge. Even though some pharmacists have experience as clinical pharmacists or are a product of a school with a strong clinical program, the gap in the knowledge base between individual pharmacists can be quite wide. Pharmacists should be expected to function as independent clinicians. If persons with advanced clinical knowledge are not currently on the staff, the staff must be trained or pharmacists with advanced training must be employed. To have an impact on the care of the patient, the pharmacist must be a drug expert, must understand the patient's disease, and must correlate this knowledge with treatment. Several programs have developed critical care pharmacy residencies in which persons can gain extensive experience in caring for critically ill patients. These persons should be viable candidates for this type of position.

Past Performance. When evaluating the current staff, one must determine whether the pharmacist(s) under consideration are actually capable of delivering the proposed service. Successful service can be achieved only by the use of pharmacists whose past performances almost guarantee a successful service. The pharmacist must be committed to the service and to patient care. He or she must also have shown the ability to work well with other health professionals, such as nurses and physicians. Personal presentation, not knowledge, often leaves the most lasting impression on nurses and physicians. Pharmacists who have served on multidisciplinary committees, who have been on medical staff committees (such as the P&T Committee), and who have been visible to some extent in the patient care areas of the hospital are likely candidates for the position. Pharmacists who previously have been less than adequate in central pharmacy roles should not be considered.

Motivation. If the clinical pharmacist is unmotivated, the chances of developing a credible service are slim. However, all of the textbook recommendations for motivating pharmacists are of no avail when the individual pharmacist has little or no personal motivation. Clinical services need pharmacists who want to become better people, want to grow professionally, want to be more productive. They need persons who are willing to continue to learn as they practice and who are motivated to go that "extra step" when needed. An effective clinical service cannot tolerate the "clock-watching" mentality; rather, it demands that persons often put in extra time or time-on-their-own in order to ensure the proper therapy for patients in their units. Motivation, then, is essential.

IMPLEMENTING THE PROGRAM

When implementing the clinical pharmacy service to the critical care unit, do not jeopardize the current drug distribution system; if anything, enhance it. Hence, the first approach to implementation is to make whatever distribution system changes are necessary. At this point, decide whether the distribution system should be centralized or decentralized and whether the pharmacy or pharmacist should be decentralized.

Next, determine which interested parties need to be notified that a different service is about to be offered. Notification would be important to the nursing staff. The extent of the inservices to the nursing staff is directly proportional to the changes made in the distribution system. Minor changes demand minor attention; major changes, however, may need in-depth sessions. The medical staff usually is less interested in distribution changes, unless they directly affect them (such as a change on the Medication Administration Record). If the medical-staff-committee planning-approach outlined previously has worked, the executive committee of the medical staff should already have approved the service and the medical staff should already be aware of the change. Any further "flag-waving" may cause unnecessary interference with getting the service implemented; however, if the medical staff has been insisting on this service, reinforcement of the commitment to implement it may be wise.

Implementation of the program also recognizes that pharmacists need to understand the expectations of the position. They must be cognizant of the goals and objectives and of their role in accomplishing them. The pharmacists need to know that management will provide the necessary support for them to accomplish those objectives. Pharmacists also need to be clinically prepared. They must have an understanding of the nursing unit and the specific functions of personnel: Who makes up the patient care team? What are the functions of monitors, intravenous (IV) lines and ventilators? Who is in the decision-making role? Who carries out the orders? What are the politics of the unit? Are there any unwritten rules? What about cliques—are they prevalent? Before pharmacists are sent into the critical care unit, they must be prepared and must be assured that there are no hidden "surprises" that cannot be handled. A specific job description should be prepared, which should include a listing of the expected functions and how they will be judged.

To ensure that pharmacists are able to find drug information efficiently and quickly, they must have a library on or in an area adjacent to the unit. Ideally, a small office directly off of the critical care unit usually works best. There, the pharmacist can review drug information without interruption. Private articles and notes for easy and rapid access also can be stored there. This means that you may have to budget for some additional equipment (desk, chair, file cabinet, shelves) and some textbooks, journals, and so forth to provide the clinical work area necessary.

EVALUATING THE PROGRAM

After implementation comes evaluation. The evaluation of the service should include three important areas: (1) impact on the patient, (2) feedback to the clinical pharmacist, and (3) cost-savings data.

Impact on Patient Care

To determine the impact of clinical pharmacy service on patient care, a documentation of the services provided is needed. The services have already been stated in the objectives; the evaluation simply determines whether the objectives are being met.

In the past, persons involved with clinical services have found this documentation difficult to provide. There are three primary reasons for this situation. First, inasmuch as clinical pharmacy services are relatively new and generally have not been provided in the past, the personnel who should inform pharmacists of problems (i.e., nurses and physicians) really do not do this because they do not know what a clinical pharmacy service should be. Unlike the drug distribution system, no objective guidelines exist to allow for "complaints." Secondly, pharmacists have not been accustomed to documenting services in the patient's chart. Historically, the chart has been the private property of the nurse and the physician. Today, that has changed: respiratory therapists, physical and occupational therapists, clinical nutritionists, and others all write in the patient's chart. Often pharmacists still hesitate to write in the chart; yet, the only permanent record of the patient's hospital care is in the chart. Thirdly, documentation of daily activities has not been expected of pharmacists in the past; traditional pharmacy services have been measured in terms of the number of doses dispensed. As a result, pharmacists too frequently ignore documenting drug information questions, therapeutic interventions, and other clinical functions. These services have been looked at as "part of the job," but they have not ordinarily been substantiated.

Apparently, to be able to document an impact on patient care, pharmacists need to change some habits. Time will change the impression that a clinical pharmacy service is simply an extra service provided by the pharmacy department and that when it is not adequate, that is all right. The time will come when nurses and physicians complain whenever a clinical service provided by the pharmacist is ignored or missed. Clinical services that are established in institutions and on critical care units will become the standard for hospitals. Over time, these services formerly considered something "nice to have" will become expectations. In the meantime, during the implementation phase, when the medical and nursing staff are informed of the new service, ask for their help in monitoring the service. Be sure they understand the objectives, and that when these are not reached, they are to bring it to the pharmacist's attention—complain.

That habit of not entering documentation in the patient's chart must also be changed. Ask any pharmacist why it is not done and several reasons are given—the politics of the institution dictate that we do not, or we think it is illegal, or we do not know how to do it. The main reason, however, is the standard response: "We've never done it before, why start now?" In order to do any kind of auditing of pharmacy service, permanent documentation of each intervention in the care of the patient is necessary. Times have changed those concerns physicians had about who should write in charts. They are now used to other health care providers entering information. If the pharmacist's input in the patient's care is of enough magnitude that it affects the outcome, it should certainly be documented. The difficulty with the question of documentation is not so much a problem of deciding the importance of what should be documented; rather, it is the habit of charting. Ideally, all input in the care of the patient by pharmacists should be documented. Yet, when entering information in the chart, pharmacists need to be cognizant of the political and legal implications to them and to the physician. Unquestionably, clinicians need to develop the habit of documenting the significant therapeutic information provided in the patient's chart. Where to chart this information (i.e., the patient's progress notes or the physician's progress notes, etc.) depends on the institution.

The third habit is a difficult one to change. Pharmacists need to develop a mechanism to document their clinical activities. They need to show that their interventions into the care of the patient caused a change in the outcome of that patient. This problem is difficult and, heretofore, unresolved. At the minimum, the service hours associated with the clinical aspects of pharmacy service must be tabulated. Information is needed about how much time is spent performing these clinical functions. Several pharmacy departments have developed mechanisms for recording these statistics.[9] Some of these require assignment of an average time for each function and tabulation of the number of times each function is performed. Whatever the method used, a mechanism needs to be developed.

Feedback to the Clinical Pharmacist

When pharmacists are prepared to assume this clinical role in the critical care unit, they should be made aware of expectations of them. They need, however, continued feedback and reinforcement about whether they are progressing satisfactorily and whether the objectives of the service are being met. Any information about the critical care unit service should be discussed with the pharmacists covering those units.

Of equal importance is a demonstration that others notice and appreciate the effort pharmacists put forth. There are times when the frustrations and complaints become seemingly intolerable. The feeling that nobody notices or cares about an outstanding effort is disheartening. The supervisory staff needs to continue to provide the positive reinforcement necessary to ensure continuation of outstanding clinical performance. All persons need to be told that they are appreciated.

Cost-Savings Data

Besides documentation of the service's impact on patient care, the pharmacist needs to provide cost figures showing that clinical pharmacy service decreases the overall costs to the hospital for care of the patient. There are three effective ways for pharmacy to do this: (1) show a decrease in inventory cost; (2) show a decrease in the cost of drug therapy per case; and (3) show that by utilizing appropriate therapies, the length of patient stay is decreased.

The best mechanism to decrease inventory costs is through effective formulary utilization. The clinical skills and subsequent presence of the pharmacist on the critical care unit—in conjunction with in-depth knowledge of the patient's medical condition—certainly allow for formulary maintenance. The critical care pharmacist is present at the time the order is written, and so he can intervene with formulary directives while the physician is still on the unit. In general, only a select group of medications is used on the critical care unit. By formulary development and then maintenance, pharmacists should be able to show a decrease in the inventory costs of critical care drugs.

Decreasing the overall cost of therapy on a per-case basis requires the calculation of the average cost of each disease or problem treated on the critical care unit. By getting a listing of the case-mix and then auditing the costs (on the average) of the medications used, medication costs can be determined. The next step is to evaluate each of these medications and to determine whether a less expensive regimen could be used without sacrificing the quality of patient care. This evaluation includes not only the cost of the drugs but the costs of the accessories needed to give these medications. For example, the pharmacist should evaluate whether an expensive antibiotic given once a day may be really cheaper, in the final analysis, than the less expensive antibiotic given several times a day. (Remember that items such as IV solutions, infusion control devices, special tubings, and so forth—all necessary for certain medications—increase the total cost of patient care.) Clinical pharmacy service on the critical care unit should be able to individualize therapy in order to take advantage of these optional regimens. Pharmacists should be able to show a decrease, then, in the average costs of each case-mix.

The ability of a hospital to provide patients with care that moves them out of the hospital sooner is the emphasis demanded by Prospective Payment Systems (PPS). By use of DRGs, pharmacists have the information available to tell them how much the hospitals are reimbursed for various diseases and procedures. When they can show that clinical input on the critical care unit actually decreases length of stay in these expensive areas, clinical pharmacy service will be cost-effective. The mechanism to do this involves constant therapeutic monitoring that is specifically directed at the reasons for medication-related lengthening of stay. These reasons could include identification of the correct drug to treat the illness sooner in the hospital stay; early identification of an adverse drug reaction, the subsequent stopping of the offending drug, and the starting of a different one; and evaluation of dosages by establishing (by determination of serum levels or by estimates of serum levels) whether the amount of a drug is effective for the particular problem. Interestingly, with the PPS, continuous audits by the fiscal department are available. The hospital can know whether its patients are having abnormally long hospital stays or whether the length of stay is consistent with the PPS. The pharmacist is able to look at the data on patients treated in the critical care unit and judge whether they have too long a length of stay and, importantly, whether the pharmacist could intervene in the medication regimen of patients to decrease this length of stay.

SUMMARY

Pharmacists should be able to establish and to provide a credible, beneficial, and challenging clinical pharmacy service in the critical care units if some important concepts are followed:

- A need must exist on the part of the recipients (patients, physicians, nurses, and hospitals) for a clinical component to the pharmacy service.
- A strategy must be used from the beginning to gather support for the clinical pharmacy program. That strategy involves a multidisciplinary effort in the approval process.

- A proposal should be written and available at the first discussion meeting. This all-inclusive proposal should be designed in such a way that, after reading the proposal, the reader feels that a clinical pharmacy service to the critical care unit is nearly a standard of practice and that, if their institution does not have this service, they are behind the times.
- This proposal must accurately reflect the clinical services the pharmacy can realistically provide and that which is necessary to provide it.
- This new service should identify with the mission statement of the hospital and reflect the hospital's goals and objectives.
- Pharmacists who have the knowledge base, the communications skills, and the motivation to function in the patient care area should be chosen. Hence, pharmacists would be chosen from the existing staff or hired from outside.
- Implementation of the service requires communication with all the health care providers who would be affected, including pharmacists.
- An ongoing evaluation is a necessary ingredient to the clinical pharmacy service and includes documentation of the endeavors, as well as cost-related data and cost-benefit data.

REFERENCES

1. Dasta J: Critical care therapeutics: A frontier for clinical pharmacy. *Drug Intell Clin Pharm* 1982;16:398–399.

2. Campos RA, Herraez FXV, et al: Drug use in an intensive care unit and its relation to survival. *Intensive Care Med* 1980;6:163–168.

3. Abrahamson NS, Wald KS, et al: Adverse occurrences in intensive care units. *JAMA* 1980;224:1582–1584.

4. Robin E: A critical look at critical care. *Crit Care Med* 1983;11:144–148.

5. Waisbren B: Realities of critical care medicine—present and future. *J Med Soc NJ* 1980;77:803–806.

6. Thompson WL: Critical care tomorrow: Economics and challenges. *Crit Care Med* 1982;10:561–568.

7. Civetta J: Beyond technology: Intensive care in the 1980s. *Crit Care Med* 1981;9:763–767.

8. Kelly W, Seaver D: Strategic planning for clinical services. *Am J Hosp Pharm* 1981;38:1786–1788.

9. Toohey JB, Herrick JD, Trautman RT: Adaptation of a workload measurement system. *Am J Hosp Pharm* 1982;39:999–1004.

Chapter 3

The Expansion of Clinical Pharmacy Education to Critical Care Pharmacy Training

Donald C. McLeod

Early chronicles of clinical pharmacy have noted that practice development has clearly led the way for educational reform.[1] Patient medication profiles, for example, were not promulgated by educators, but by a lone voice in the wilderness of practice. Eugene White, a community practitioner in a backroads town of Virginia, persisted in a one-man crusade extolling the patient care need for and the professionalism of a patient-oriented pharmacy record system.[2] His work is now in the lexicon of every college of pharmacy.

Practitioners and residents in hospital pharmacy began the clinical pharmacy movement in the mid-1960s. Within a few years, the wisdom of this direction was so obvious that federal capitation funds were made available to every college of pharmacy in the United States so that at least rudimentary clinical training would be available to all students. Clinical pharmacy practice and education have come a long way in the last two decades. Nevertheless, much remains to be done, and part of this challenge involves the practice of pharmacists in critical care units of hospitals. The purpose of this chapter is to review the development of clinical pharmacy education and relate its progress to training in clinical care.

EVOLUTION OF CLINICAL PHARMACY EDUCATION

The Pharmaceutical Survey of 1948

The Pharmaceutical Survey of 1948, directed by Dr. Edward C. Elliott, analyzed the profession of pharmacy and made many recommendations for improving its ability to provide health care services in a time of rapid development of new drugs and industrialization of drug production. The findings and recommendations of the Pharmaceutical Survey of 1948[3] state:

The degree that should be conferred upon graduates in pharmacy has been a subject of some discussion in recent years. The degree of Bachelor of Science in Pharmacy, now generally awarded to graduates, is in keeping with degrees conferred for the completion of other four-year professional programs, such as chemistry, bacteriology, agriculture, and engineering. No other degree could be justified at present for the completion of professional training that is on the baccalaureate level.

The bachelor's degree does not, however, confer the status that is desired by pharmacists, particularly those who work in rather intimate professional association with physicians, dentists, and members of other health professions who hold professional doctor's degree. A professional doctor's degree has come to be regarded by many as a needed asset for the pharmacist.

A six-year program for pharmaceutical education and training, consisting of two years of general education and basic science training in a college of arts and sciences and four years of professional education in a school of pharmacy, would have much merit. It would overcome the deficiencies indicated previously for shorter programs, and it would provide adequate training for the profession of pharmacy. Moreover, it would provide enlarged opportunity for the diversification of training which the profession needs.

A six-year program is in accordance with trends in American education. Education for nearly all the health professions except nursing now requires this amount of time. As was pointed out earlier, there is a tendency to prolong the period of general education through fourteen years of schooling, that is, through the community college or the sophomore year of the four-year college of arts and sciences. Professional education adapts itself to this tendency by beginning the specialized training at or after the fifteenth year of schooling.

A six-year program would provide ample time for a student to secure the desired education in the foundational and cultural subjects; it would provide sufficient time for teaching the pharmacy and allied courses in their proper sequence; it would provide the flexibility necessary to meet the individual professional and personal interests and needs of students; and, finally, it would enable schools of pharmacy to confer a professional doctor's degree that would be generally recognized.

The American Association of Colleges of Pharmacy, at its annual meeting in San Francisco in August 1948, after hearing reports by the director of the survey and the assistant director in charge of curriculum studies, the report by its Committee on Curriculum and a report by its Committee on a Professional Degree in Pharmacy adopted a resolution commending the survey for the preparation of the outlines of areas of study in the curriculum, approving in principle the proposed optional six-year program, authorizing the member-schools to offer the degree of Doctor of Pharmacy for completion of the six-year program, and directing that provision be made for changes in the constitution and bylaws of the association insofar as may be necessary to authorize the new program and degree.[3]

Early Doctor of Pharmacy Programs

The University of Southern California in the early 1950s and the University of California at San Francisco in the early 1960s were the first colleges of pharmacy to develop six-year doctor of pharmacy (Pharm.D.) programs. These two programs predated current clinical pharmacy practice concepts, and, although responding to the professional development apparently envisioned by the Survey of 1948, did not introduce a significant clinical component into their curricula until the latter half of the 1960s.

Some other colleges followed an alternate route of adding one to two years onto the B.S. in pharmacy curriculum (mandated nationally to be at least five years in duration in the early 1960s). This was an optional program for a student and was similar in concept to the M.S. programs in hospital pharmacy. The University of Michigan developed the first of these programs. These programs were generally two years in duration and contained a year of additional academic courses followed by a year of clinical clerkship or residency training. In the mid-1960s, the University of Kentucky developed a rigorous three-year Pharm.D. program in the post-baccalaureate mode.

Roots of Contemporary Clinical Pharmacy Practice

Hospital Pharmacy Practice

Clinical pharmacy practice is directed toward promoting and ensuring for patients the safe and rational use of drugs. Successful application of this practice concept requires that the clinical pharmacist practice in an integrated way with physicians, nurses, and others concerned with drug use. The clinical pharmacy movement clearly had its roots in hospital pharmacy practice. Francke[4] has shed some light on the germination of clinical pharmacy as follows:

> Using the term clinical in a very broad sense, formal training for clinical practice in hospital pharmacy developed quite apart from the colleges of pharmacy. Whitney at Michigan in the 1930s and Clarke at The New York Hospital in the 1940s were pioneers in this field. I recall the great frustration and disappointment expressed by Mr. Whitney because he

could not interest either the dean or the faculty of the college in the prospect of using the tremendous interdisciplinary teaching facilities of a great university hospital for the education and training of undergraduate pharmacy students. This situation began to change in the late 1940s when Flack at Jefferson Hospital in Philadelphia, Purdum at Johns Hopkins and myself at Michigan developed programs which combined residencies and advanced degrees. However, these programs affected only a few graduate students and had almost no effect on the instruction of undergraduate students.

Within the hospital, pharmacists served on key administrative committees and formally discussed therapeutics with physicians on the pharmacy and therapeutics committee. The primary focus was certainly on patient care rather than on gross commercialism so rampant in "retail pharmacy."

Unit-Dose Services and Drug Information

The 1960s ushered in two developments in hospital pharmacy that were to hasten the development of clinical pharmacy: the development of unit-dose drug distribution systems and pharmacy-based drug information systems.

Studies in the early 1960s documenting high incidences of hospital medication errors led to experimentation with pharmacist-directed unit-dose drug distribution systems. To execute these new systems of drug control, the pharmacist had to interact with the nurse and the physician within the patient care area. The medical chart was suddenly open to the pharmacist, and the need to understand laboratory tests, medical jargon, and diagnostic terms became overwhelming. Many young pharmacists quickly realized the ill-preparation they had received academically to participate in direct patient care.

Along with unit-dose systems, the idea of the pharmacist providing an unbiased and patient-oriented drug information service was advanced by Walton and Burkholder at the University of Kentucky and by others.[5] Whereas unit-dose services were a baptism by fire, drug information services provided an academic and literary means of advancing rational drug therapy. Suddenly, pharmacists were developing newsletters of drug information not dependent on the support of a drug company, but financed by hospital funds to promote rational drug therapeutics. As many pharmacists would learn, the pen is indeed mightier than the sword, particularly in an intellectual marketplace.

Biopharmaceutics and Pharmacokinetics

Although the origin of clinical pharmacy has its main roots in hospital pharmacy, at least one academic development, as described by Levy,[6] helped to show that clinical pharmacy's contribution is based in the pharmaceutical sciences:

I am convinced that the introduction of biopharmaceutics and pharmacokinetics into the curriculum and research activities of schools of pharmacy was largely responsible for the subsequent development of clinical pharmacy. These two disciplines focused students' (and faculty members') attention on the drug product as a therapeutic modality rather than as a physical object and provided pharmacists with much of the knowledge base and intellectual qualifications that make them functional and valuable members of the modern health care team. The development of these disciplines is also largely responsible for the integration of pharmaceutical scientists (here defined narrowly as individuals trained by and/or teaching and doing research in departments of pharmaceutics or pharmacy) into the front ranks of the health sciences. Last, but certainly not least, biopharmaceutics and pharmacokinetics, together with pharmacology and therapeutics, constitute most of the intellectual basis of clinical pharmacy.

I have traced these developments to make the point that a significant change in the orientation of academic pharmaceutical research and (consequently) in the undergraduate pharmaceutical curriculum (i.e., the introduction of physical chemistry applied to pharmaceutical systems and its subsequent extension to clinical aspects in the form of biopharmaceutics) had a profound effect on the evolving nature of pharmacy practice. It matters little, in this respect, whether one believes that clinical pharmacy will constitute most or only some of pharmacy practice in the future. The point is that the content and orientation of the academic curriculum in pharmacy can have a pronounced, almost dramatic, influence on the nature of professional practice and therefore on pharmacy's future.

Interdisciplinary Support

Equally important to the conceptual changes in the thinking of hospital pharmacists and some pharmaceutical educators, interdisciplinary involvement of other health professionals was vital to clinical pharmacy success. The Pharmacy-Medicine-Nursing Conference on Health Education at the University of Michigan in 1967 was pivotal from a broad public relations viewpoint.

W.N. Hubbard, Jr., M.D., dean of the University of Michigan College of Medicine, reminded the audience of the definition and obligations of a professional:[7]

> The definition of a professional has been the subject of a good deal of lighthearted and also serious discussion. For my own purposes I would suggest that a professional is a person identified by society to serve on

their behalf an essential role. The professional is brought forth by society for its purposes. He does not arise *de novo* and he is not self-justifying. The professional must ask himself a question beyond that of all other educated men, what is my societal role? And for those in this room the answer comes clearly, it is to foster the health of the people.

Each of the health professions is beginning to recognize that its own self-justification and enhancement, no matter how selflessly conceived, can turn into an egotistical self-indulgence unless it is tested constantly against the bench mark of whether it directly enhances the health of the people. Enhance; not merely be relevant to it or participate in the general effort, but to have a positive, demonstrative, enhancing effect on the health of the people. This is the fundamental nature of the necessary revolution in the health professions that must precede increased effectiveness and efficiency of health services.

At this same conference at the University of Michigan, Dr. Donald Brodie spoke of the need for changes in pharmacy education:[8]

The gap between the termination of our present curriculum and the bedside is a new frontier—a new dimension—in pharmacy education. To bridge this gap, educationally-speaking, the development of a clinical component in pharmaceutical education will be required. The clue to the development of the clinical component lies in the fact that in the environment of the bedside the pharmacist functions as a biologist, because here the language of communication is the language of biology.

The scientific core of the clinical component will be an uninterrupted sequence of courses in the biological sciences, from general biology or zoology to pharmacology. What professional courses will be required cannot be specified but, certainly, the subject matter areas should include a knowledge of the diseased state and the patient's condition, the relationship of laboratory tests and clinical diagnosis to drug therapy, hospital procedure and routine, an orientation in medicine, a discriminating evaluation in the use of drugs, and clinical pharmacology. Much of this subject matter must, of necessity, be taught by medical clinicians.

One of the most difficult factors in the evolvement of this clinical component is the manner in which clinical training for pharmacy students can be developed. Medical students are in continual dialogue both with their peers and with their physician preceptors, and thereby acquire skill in the oral application of their knowledge to clinical situations while students. The development and presentation of medical cases and going on rounds with physicians facilitates this skill. Presently, the pharmacy student gets practically no experience in the spontaneous exchange of the information that he has acquired. The future of pharmacy and pharmaceutical education will be related to the effectiveness with which the clinical component in pharmaceutical education can be developed. The need is apparent, the cost is great, the reward is high.

Residency Training

Residency training in hospital and clinical pharmacy has paid tremendous dividends for pharmacy practice. Again, practice led the way over education. The following is an interesting prologue to the first formal accreditation of hospital pharmacy residencies by the American Society of Hospital Pharmacists (ASHP) in 1963:[9]

> At the 1957 ASHP Annual Meeting the Society and the American Association of Colleges of Pharmacy (AACP) held a debate on a resolution passed by the AACP which stated: "Resolved, that training in hospital pharmacy, not complemented with or accompanied by further academic training, is not in the best interest of the future developments of hospital pharmacy and the profession." Archambault and Francke upheld the negative side for the Society; Deans Tice and Zopf were protagonists, and the stimulating debate ended in a draw.

About 2,000 pharmacists have completed residency training in the United States, and most leaders in hospital and clinical pharmacy are former residents of these innovative programs. With residency training, leading institutional pharmacists had gained a method, long successful in medicine, whereby practitioners could directly build the future of practice without waiting on endless debates in colleges of pharmacy. Colleges of pharmacy, at least leading ones, are now responding to these practitioner demands by jointly aiding some residency training and providing needed academic preparation by Pharm.D. programs.

Specialization in Pharmacy

The health care and drug control functions provided by pharmacists are now sufficiently diverse and call on special skills and training. As a result, functional specialization is a reality in contemporary pharmacy practice.

Medicine As an Analogy

To appreciate specialization in pharmacy, one must consider the broad spectrum of the process in medicine, the profession to which pharmacy must most closely relate in the health care process. Pharmacy should not blindly emulate medicine in specialization, but should study it for important guidance.

Schondelmeyer and Kirking[10] have described major issues and events surrounding the development of specialization in medicine. The prime factors leading to specialization were scientific and technological change resulting in a body of knowledge and skills so vast that a physician could not be competent in all medical areas. Specialization had to be profitable to exist, and it became profitable only when specialists had sufficient medically valid knowledge to attract and to treat patients whom the general practitioner was unable to treat. The early specialists in the mid-1800s were viewed as competing with the general practitioner and were largely scorned by the American Medical Association (AMA). In the late 1800s, thousands of physicians from the United States received specialty training in highly advanced German and other European medical centers; a consequence was increased distance between generalists and specialists. Nevertheless, the profitability and prestige of specialization were dominant factors in its increasing importance within American medicine.

In the period from 1864 to 1902, many specialty medical societies were formed in the United States; these are listed in Table 3-1.[10] Specialists claimed that the ineptitude of the AMA forced them to turn to independent national societies. One past president of the AMA stated that the specialty societies were founded by physicians who had no time to spare for entertainment, excursions, medico-politico wrangling, and other pastimes of the association. Specialists became powerful forces in the profession, controlling elite medical societies, dominating medical faculties and hospital staffs, and serving wealthy and powerful clients.

There are now 23 medical specialty boards in the United States, which set standards and certify physicians as competent in a specific specialty. These

Table 3-1 National Specialty Medical Societies, 1864–1902

Organization	Date of Founding
American Ophthalmological Society	1864
American Otological Society	1868
American Neurological Society	1875
American Dermatological Association	1876
American Gynecological Society	1876
American Laryngological Association	1879
American Surgical Association	1880
American Association of Genito-Urinary Surgeons	1886
American Orthopedic Association	1887
American Pediatric Society	1888
American Laryngological, Rhinological, and Otological Society	1895
American Academy of Ophthalmology and Otolaryngology	1896
American Gastroenterological Association	1897
American Proctological Society	1899
American Urological Association	1902

boards, and the year of their respective incorporation, are shown in Table 3-2.

Within critical care medicine, there is now the Society of Critical Care Medicine (SCCM), founded in 1970 by a group of internists, pediatricians, anesthesiologists, and surgeons who felt that critical care medicine warranted status as a subspecialty of primary boards.[11] In 1974, a recommendation by SCCM to the American Board of Medical Specialties (ABMS) to implement such a subspecialty board was rejected.

Subsequently, the Joint Committee on Critical Care Medicine (JCCCM) has been formed by the American Board of Anesthesiology, the American Board of Pediatrics, the American Board of Surgery and the American Board of Internal Medicine (ABIM). Dissent exists within this group, and currently the ABIM is separately petitioning the ABMS for a subspecialty board.[11] Nevertheless, it appears that a board in critical care medicine will result or perhaps differing boards sponsored by the ABIM and the other members of the JCCCM. The delays and dissent reflect the often tortuous route to the full creation of a medical specialty or subspecialty.

Table 3-2 Medical Specialty Boards

Board	Year of Incorporation
American Board of Ophthalmology	1917
American Board of Otolaryngology	1924
American Board of Obstetrics and Gynecology	1930
American Board of Dermatology	1932
American Board of Pediatrics	1933
American Board of Radiology	1934
American Board of Psychiatry and Neurology	1934
American Board of Orthopedic Surgery	1934
American Board of Colon and Rectal Surgery	1935
American Board of Urology	1935
American Board of Pathology	1936
American Board of Internal Medicine	1936
American Board of Surgery	1937
American Board of Anesthesiology	1938
American Board of Plastic Surgery	1939
American Board of Neurological Surgery	1940
American Board of Physical Medicine and Rehabilitation	1947
American Board of Preventive Medicine	1948
American Board of Thoracic Surgery	1950
American Board of Family Practice	1969
American Board of Nuclear Medicine	1971
American Board of Allergy and Immunology	1971
American Board of Emergency Medicine	1976*

Note: *Formed after compilation of the 1977-1978 Annual Report.

Specialization Process

As a profession, pharmacy is only now beginning to address the need for official specialization. Based on practice demands, job descriptions, market demand, and post-graduate training programs, the most obvious practice-related possibilities are hospital pharmacy administration, clinical pharmacy, and nuclear pharmacy. However, the picture is not simple.

In 1974, the American Pharmaceutical Association (APhA) created the Board of Pharmaceutical Specialties (BPS). One basic purpose of the BPS is to judge petitions by practitioner groups who may be seeking specialty recognition. Early pronouncements by the BPS and APhA stated that a specialty could not be based on location of practice (i.e., hospital or community pharmacy) or on administrative responsibilities (presumably hospital pharmacy administration). The BPS has listed seven general criteria that must largely be met for a group of practitioners to hope to qualify as a pharmacy specialty (Exhibit 3–1).[12]

The immediate effect of these early pronouncements and criteria was to disqualify the overwhelming majority of pharmacists from becoming specialists. To date, only nuclear pharmacy has petitioned the BPS; this petition was successful, and a board in nuclear pharmacy has been implemented.[13]

The American College of Clinical Pharmacy (ACCP) has begun development of a petition on behalf of general clinical pharmacy, feeling that recognition in more narrow areas, such as pediatrics, nutrition, psychiatry, and critical care, should

---

Exhibit 3–1 Criteria for the Recognition of Specialties in Pharmacy Practice

A. Significant and clear health demand must exist to provide the necessary public reason for certification.
B. Specifically trained practitioners must be needed in the area to fulfill pharmacy's responsibility to the public health and welfare.
C. The area of specialization shall include a reasonable number of persons who devote most of their practice time to the specialty area.
D. Specialized knowledge of the pharmaceutical sciences, which have their basis in the biological, physical, and behavioral sciences, must be required.
E. The area of specialization shall represent an identifiable and distinct field of practice that calls for special knowledge and skills acquired by education and training or experience beyond basic pharmaceutical education and training.
F. Schools of pharmacy or other organizations shall offer recognized education and training programs to those persons seeking advanced knowledge and skills in the area.
G. There must be transmission of knowledge through teaching clinics and the professional literature immediately related to the specialty.

Source: Board of Pharmaceutical Specialties: *Petitioners' Guide for Specialty Recognition.* Washington, D.C., American Pharmaceutical Association.

follow the general recognition.[14] The ASHP has backed special interest groups (SIGs) within the ASHP and is planning a fellowship designation to be recommended by the various 14 groups.[15] The section of clinical practice of the APhA's Academy of Pharmacy Practice, in an APhA poll, has overwhelmingly backed the position that clinical pharmacy is not a specialty (unpublished data). The ACCP is the only group with rigorous standards for membership, and its position probably closely reflects the view of the more highly trained Pharm.D. graduates with clinical residency training. At any rate, pharmacy is now wrestling with a process begun 120 years ago in medicine.

Clinical Pharmacy

Although clinical pharmacy concepts are now widely promoted in the profession, most practitioners, and even current B.S. graduates in pharmacy, do not have sufficient clinical skills to be considered specialists. The great majority of competent clinical pharmacists are Pharm.D. graduates, many of whom have completed advanced clinical residencies in general clinical pharmacy or in more specific therapeutic areas.

There is no formal specialization; however, most leading institutions are specifying the Pharm.D. degree and residency experience, or the equivalent, for clinical pharmacy positions. It seems inevitable that specialty recognition of clinical pharmacy or subspecialties within the discipline will be achieved. Physicians who have practiced with competent clinical pharmacists seem to have less difficulty with the concept of pharmacy specialization than do most pharmacists, pharmacy educators, and Association politicos.

DOCTOR OF PHARMACY PROGRAMS

The development of the early Pharm.D. programs has been previously described. Pharm.D. practitioners constitute the great majority of advanced clinical practitioners in pharmacy, and these programs have been very important in the maturation of pharmacy.

Rationale for the Doctorate Degree

The established health science professions that have a clearly identifiable advanced body of scientific knowledge upon which their practices are based have seen fit to bestow the clinical doctorate degree upon graduates of their university programs. This is true for medicine, dentistry, optometry, and podiatry.

Clinical pharmacy is fundamentally directed toward ensuring rational patient drug therapy. To accomplish this end, the clinical pharmacist is consulted by physicians, consults with patients, and makes critical pharmacotherapeutic recommendations. To succeed in this endeavor, the clinical pharmacist must understand the theory of medicine as well as major aspects of pharmacy and therapeutics.

The clinical pharmacist, to be maximally effective, needs education and training commensurate with other clinical doctorate practitioners, and current Pharm.D. programs are conceived on this basis. The doctorate degree is also entirely appropriate to foster the collegial teamwork and interprofessional respect needed for the success of pharmacy in the clinical setting. Accompanied by appropriate performance, the clinical doctorate will enhance the respect and ultimate opportunities afforded the profession by the public and by those within the other health care professions.

Curriculum and Program Structure

Accreditation Standards

The Accreditation Standards and Guidelines for Professional Degree Programs of Colleges and Schools of Pharmacy, adopted in 1981, addresses requirements for B.S. and Pharm.D. programs in pharmacy.[16]

The standards state:

Standard No. 5. The Doctor of Pharmacy Curriculum

A doctor of pharmacy program should provide a core curriculum that is enriched with knowledge and clinical practice experiences significantly beyond those provided in the baccalaureate program. The curriculum should also provide selective or elective instruction to provide students with the opportunity to obtain more in depth education and training in differentiated areas of pharmacy practice requiring advanced clinical practice knowledge and skills. The curriculum should produce pharmacy practitioners who are professionally more mature in clinical pharmacy practice than those in baccalaureate programs. Differentiation should be primarily based upon scope, depth, and proficiency differences in knowledge or skills rather than in location or practice.

Guidelines:

1. Doctor of Pharmacy curricula, in contrast to baccalaureate curricula, should include instruction to provide students with in depth knowledge in the following areas:
    a) pharmaceutical sciences—especially biopharmaceutics and pharmacokinetics

b) biomedical sciences—pathology, biostatistics, research design
c) social and behavioral sciences—especially patient communications and education
d) clinical sciences and clinical practice—disease processes and diagnosis, clinical pharmacy practice, drug therapeutics, drug literature evaluation, clinical toxicology, clinical pharmacokinetics
2. Traditional methods of providing biomedical and clinical science instruction using lecture and laboratory methods cannot provide adequate understanding of systemic disease processes and diagnoses. Therefore, to supplement teaching in these areas, students should work with patients, participate in patient care rounds, and attend clinical case conferences in various patient settings to develop understanding of disease processes, diagnosis, and overall patient management.
3. Disease states and therapeutics must be studied from a broad view, including social, behavioral, and psychological aspects of patient care.
4. The quantity and nature of the clinical experience component are important elements differentiating doctor of pharmacy from baccalaureate curricula. Although both a clinical clerkship and externship are required in each curriculum, greater clerkship time is required in doctor of pharmacy curricula. Required clerkships should provide students with the opportunity for significant exposure to disease problems and drug therapy associated with all age groups. Students should have experience in the following settings:
a) inpatient clerkships
b) clerkships in outpatient organized health care settings (i.e., outpatient clinics associated with hospitals, family practice centers, health maintenance organizations, etc.)
c) a clerkship in a drug information center
d) adequate specialized clerkships, (e.g., nutritional support, mental health, clinical pharmacokinetics, cardiology, nephrology, long term care, geriatrics, etc.) available on a selective or elective basis to produce pharmacy practitioners with greater scope, depth, and proficiency in clinical pharmacy practice
5. Clerkship experience should include the application of clinical pharmacokinetics principles in developing dosage regimens for inpatients and outpatients.

6. Clerkships should be provided only in inpatient or outpatient environments where pharmacy practitioners have access to complete patient data base and where an interdisciplinary team approach exists for the provision of health care. Community pharmacies meeting these minimum criteria can be used as clerkship sites.
7. The clinical components of the doctoral program should have as a minimum goal 1500 clock hours of clerkship and externship experience in not less than one academic year. At least 1300 of the required clock hours should be clerkship hours, emphasizing clinical rather than distributive pharmacy practice functions.
8. Clerkships should require a major time commitment of the student to assure a continuity of professional services and learning experience. Therefore, the majority of the clerkship component should occur during the student's final academic year on a full-time basis.
9. Clerkships should be constructed to allow students to develop clinical judgment skills and self confidence, to assess therapeutic problems, and to make appropriate decisions.
10. Elective or selective instruction should be available in differentiated areas of pharmacy practice (e.g., mental health, pediatrics, family medicine, internal medicine, geriatrics, etc.), requiring advanced clinical pharmacy knowledge and skills.

Program Structures

Two basic types of Pharm.D. programs are prevalent in the United States. The first is the minimum six-year program which awards the Pharm.D. as the entry level practice degree. This program requires two years of general college followed by four years of pharmaceutical education. The last academic year is usually composed of at least eight months of clinical clerkships analogous to medical student clerkships. The second type of program is developed in the graduate school mode and is an elective two-year program following the five-year B.S. in pharmacy curriculum. Keen competition exists for places in these programs, and graduates are generally highly motivated and professionally quite mature.

Curricular Content

The Pharm.D. curriculum at the University of California at San Francisco (UCSF) is presented here as an example of typical program content.[17] This program has a long history and has been viewed as the pace-setting, first-degree Pharm.D. program. After this analysis, a brief discussion of alternate courses and postbaccalaureate, two-year Pharm.D. programs will be presented.

The four-year professional curriculum at UCSF, which follows at least two years of general college, is outlined in Table 3–3. Hours shown are quarter hours (3 quarter hours = 2 semester hours). Basic courses in essential biomedical sciences (e.g., biochemistry, physiology, and pathology) are included. The pharmaceutical component is far more developed than that of any medical school

Table 3–3 Curriculum Content of Pharm.D. Program at the University of California at San Francisco

Year	Quarter Hours
First Year	
Organic chemistry	13
Physical chemistry	7
Biopharmaceutics-physical pharmacy	11
Clinical pharmacy orientation	2
Nonprescription drug products	3
Pharmacy law	2
Histology	3
Gross anatomy	3
Second Year	
Pharmaceutical chemistry	8
Biochemistry	9
Physiology	12½
Pharmacology-toxicology	5
Pharmacokinetics	3½
Microbiology	5
Immunology	1½
Prescription practice	4
Third Year	
Pharmaceutical chemistry	5
Clinical pharmacy (therapeutics)	20½
Drug information service	½
Pathology	3
Pharmacology-toxicology	7
Parasitology	4
Public health programs	2
Clinical toxicology	2
Nutrition	3
Fourth Year	
Inpatient clinical clerkship	18
Ambulatory clerkship	13
Elective clerkship	9

Note: Electives are not shown; 190 quarter hours are required for the degree.

curriculum and includes extensive coursework in pharmaceutical chemistry, biopharmaceutics, pharmacokinetics, pharmacology-toxicology and clinical pharmacy (therapeutics).

Elective or required courses taken in many programs may include advanced clinical pharmacokinetics, biostatistics, drug assay methodology, physical assessment, drug literature evaluation, and hospital pharmacy administration.

The primary combined curriculum difference in the graduate-type, two-year Pharm.D. graduate programs at schools other than UCSF is as follows:

- more clerkship experience (approximately 15 or more months rather than 8 or 9 months)
- more extensive pathophysiology
- more elective possibilities as noted above

Program Availability

There are currently 72 accredited colleges of pharmacy in the United States. Quite a few of these colleges are not part of a health science center or medical campus and do not offer the Pharm.D. degree. A few colleges that are part of health science centers have not had leaders with the wisdom or the ability to develop the clinical doctorate program. Exhibits 3–2 and 3–3 list those colleges currently offering the first-degree Pharm.D. and those with the elective graduate-type program.[18]

POSTGRADUATE TRAINING IN CRITICAL CARE PHARMACY

Just as the graduating medical student is not prepared to handle most specialty practice problems, the graduating Pharm.D. student has not sufficient experience to practice competently in difficult areas, such as critical care. Early practitioners

Exhibit 3–2 List of Colleges of Pharmacy Offering Six-Year First-Degree Doctor of Pharmacy Programs

University of California at San Francisco
University of Southern California
Mercer University
University of Illinois at Chicago
University of Michigan
University of Nebraska
University of Tennessee

Exhibit 3–3 List of Colleges of Pharmacy Offering the B.S. in Pharmacy and the Pharm.D. Degrees

---

Auburn University
University of Arizona
University of Arkansas for Medical Sciences
University of the Pacific
Florida Agriculture and Mechanical University
University of Florida
University of Georgia
Purdue University
University of Iowa
University of Kentucky
University of Maryland
Massachusetts College of Pharmacy
Northeastern University
Wayne State University
University of Minnesota
Creighton University
St. John's University
State University of New York at Buffalo
University of North Carolina at Chapel Hill
Ohio State University
University of Cincinnati
Duquesne University
Philadelphia College of Pharmacy and Science
Medical University of South Carolina
University of Rhode Island
University of Texas at Austin
University of Utah
Virginia Commonwealth University
University of Tennessee
University of Washington

---

were simply put into critical care and gradually developed competency in the area. Some Pharm.D. programs do not even yet have required or elective rotations in critical care.

Medical Curriculum in Critical Care Medicine

Before a discussion of the need and structure of clinical pharmacy training in critical care, examination of expectations of medical practitioners in the area may be instructional.

The SCCM has published the core curriculum to be used in training residents in critical care medicine and has described needed skills.[11] These are produced in

Appendix 3–A. It is obvious that many items in the core curriculum for physicians are not needed by clinical pharmacists who may practice in critical care. The curriculum does, however, impress one with the depth and scope of the medical area. It is apparent that a nonphysician pharmacotherapy adviser in critical care must have very special training and experience.

Critical Care Pharmacy Residency at Ohio State University

When the Pharm.D. program and faculty development were planned at Ohio State in the late 1970s, critical care was designated as a high priority area of practice and teaching. Hospital care was becoming increasingly specialized and had a tertiary care nature. In addition, it was felt that if a Pharm.D. graduate could handle the major therapeutic problems in critical care, then general problems in the hospital should be rather routine. Dasta and McLeod described the first critical care pharmacy residency, developed at Ohio State.[19] Since the inception of this program, six post-Pharm.D. residents have been trained (1981 to 1984).

This residency, now described as a pharmacy residency in cardiovascular and critical care pharmacy, is a 12- to 24-month program containing the rotations listed in Exhibit 3-4. A study group is now working on standards for accreditation of critical care pharmacy residencies by the ASHP.[20]

Exhibit 3–4 Advanced Residency in Critical Care Pharmacy at Ohio State University

The advanced residency in critical care pharmacy consists of a 12-month program involving training and application of pharmacotherapeutics and pharmacokinetics to various areas of critical care medicine. Areas of practice include the following:

- coronary intensive care
- cardiology
- thoracic surgery
- peripheral vascular surgery
- general surgical intensive care
- thoracic and neurosurgical intensive care
- medical intensive care
- burn intensive care
- nutritional support
- emergency medicine
- neonatal intensive care
- adult internal medicine subspecialties

Fellowships in Critical Care Pharmacy

Fellowships in various areas of clinical pharmacy are recognized generally to occur after appropriate residency experience and to be devoted largely to clinical research and further career development. The ASHP Critical Care Pharmacy Fellowship is discussed further in Chapter 4.

Role of Colleges of Pharmacy

Except for no more than a dozen individual clinical pharmacy faculty members who have pioneered in critical care pharmacy, colleges of pharmacy have been relatively silent in recognizing clinical and manpower needs in the area. It is easy to rally a college committee to study the use of handheld calculators on examinations, but fundamental health care priorities may be unrecognized or, worse, ignored.

At a very minimum, every college offering the Pharm.D. degree should have a viable clerkship in critical care medicine. This clerkship should be required of each student. The college also must aid and encourage the university hospital pharmacy department to employ practitioners who can complement what a single faculty member can provide. A nucleus of at least two to three practitioner-educators is needed to sustain service, teaching, and research in the teaching hospital's critical care units.

Several leading colleges of pharmacy have committed considerable financial resources to post-Pharm.D. residency training. If competent practitioners in critical care are to be generally available, residencies must be developed. Colleges should play a part in leading the way, although most residencies have previously been conceived and implemented by hospital pharmacists. Certainly a legitimate role of the college is to promote research in the area of critical care by its faculty and students.

Role of Leading Hospitals

As in medicine, a few dozen teaching hospitals determine many of the possibilities for pharmacy. If clinical pharmacy is worth having, it should be as effective and efficient as possible; however, it will be effective only if well-trained clinicians are available, employed, and fully engaged in their respective areas of expertise. Leading hospitals, therefore, must help to subspecialize clinical pharmacy into major therapeutic areas to allow the maturation of the discipline and its contribution to pharmacotherapy.

Hospital pharmacy departments must also support residency training in critical care. Hospitals, not colleges of pharmacy, have led the way in residency training and should continue to do so. Two residents can generally be supported by one pharmacist's salary. The imaginative director of pharmacy can blend the practice contribution of residents and their training needs into a cost-effective program, particularly with post-Pharm.D. residents who are very mature professionally.

This concept of residency training is highly important to the continued success of clinical pharmacy in health care.

SUMMARY

This chapter has traced the development of clinical philosophies and capabilities in pharmacy and has suggested developmental needs in pharmacy education to meet patient care needs in critical care medicine.

Lest clinical pharmacy be written off as too little too late, an organized profession must soon emerge that responds not only to mandates but to opportunities. Risks must be taken and setbacks experienced in the broad sweep of progress. A small segment of the profession—clinical pharmacy—has not hesitated to take risks based on reasonable opportunities. Only half of the colleges of pharmacy have responded in the last 20 years to clinical pharmacy by evolving early Pharm.D. programs or developing new ones. It could easily be asked whether there is a mandate. It is not a surprise that an area such as critical care has been largely underestimated and overlooked as an important practice area. Important areas such as psychiatry have been developed well by only four or five colleges of pharmacy.

Allies in the cause of clinical pharmacy development, whether they be pharmacists, physicians, educators, or health care administrators, must become more articulate and united. The idea of a single human can become the heritage of all mankind. This potential must be recognized and pursued by individual clinical practitioners if clinical pharmacy is to be further developed, and if critical care pharmacy, in particular, is to be commonplace. It is to be hoped that clinical pharmacy will be recognized as an essential component of critical care medicine. This goal will be accomplished only if clinical pharmacy educators and practitioners provide the leadership and direction.

REFERENCES

1. McLeod DC: Clinical pharmacy: The past, present and future. *Am J Hosp Pharm* 1976;33:29–38.

2. White EV: The office practice of family pharmacy, in McLeod DC, Miller WA (eds): *The Practice of Pharmacy*. Cincinnati, Harvey Whitney Books, 1981, pp 216–234.

3. Findings and recommendations of the pharmaceutical survey of 1948. Washington, DC, American Council on Education.

4. Francke DE: Contributions of residency training to institutional pharmacy practice. *Am J Hosp Pharm* 1967;24:192–203.

5. Walton CA: The problem of communicating clinical drug information—A challenge and a hope for professional pharmacy. *Am J Hosp Pharm* 1965;22:458–463.

6. Levy G: Preparing for pharmacy's future. *Am J Pharm Educ* 1983;47:332–334.

7. Hubbard WN Jr: Emerging patterns of education and practice in the health professions—medicine. *Pharmacy-Medicine-Nursing Conference on Health Education,* Ann Arbor, Michigan, February 16–18, 1967, pp 5–9.

8. Brodie DC: Emerging patterns of education and practice in the health professions—pharmacy. *Pharmacy-Medicine-Nursing Conference on Health Education,* Ann Arbor, Michigan, February 16–18, 1967, pp 23–36.

9. American Society of Hospital Pharmacists: Report of New York Convention. *Bull Am Soc Hosp Pharm* 1957;14:328.

10. Schondelmeyer SW, Kirking DM: Perspectives on medical specialization. *Drug Intell Clin Pharm* 1980;14:30–36.

11. Grenvik A, Leonard JJ, Arens JF, et al: Critical care medicine—certification as a multidisciplinary subspecialty. *Crit Care Med* 1981;9:117–125.

12. Board of Pharmaceutical Specialties: *Petitioners' Guide for Specialty Recognition.* Washington, DC, American Pharmaceutical Association.

13. Pharmacy's first specialty. *Am Pharm* 1982;NS22:612–615.

14. Kelly KL: Task force on credentialing in clinical pharmacy. *Drug Intell Clin Pharm* 1980;14:824.

15. SIG News. *ASHP Newsletter* 1981;14:(March) 5.

16. Miller WA: Chair report for the task force on Pharm.D. accreditation standards. *Am J Pharm Educ* 1981;45:377–384.

17. *Catalogue.* College of Pharmacy, University of California at San Francisco, 1982–83.

18. U.S. Colleges of Pharmacy. *Am J Pharm Educ* 1984;48:115–116.

19. Dasta JF, McLeod DC: The design of a critical care residency, Poster presentation, *American Association of Colleges of Pharmacy Annual Meeting,* Scottsdale, Arizona, AACP, June 29, 1981.

20. *ASHP Supplemental Standard and Learning Objectives for Specialized Residency Training in Critical Care Pharmacy Practice, Working Draft,* March 1984.

Appendix 3–A

Core Curriculum for Critical Care Medicine Certification

Whereas the following core curriculum, including the list of skills, represents the ideal objectives of the critical care medicine (CCM) physician's knowledge and skills, specific programs may concentrate on either the pediatric or the adult aspects of CCM, although the principles of pediatric and adult CCM are the same—i.e., to optimize the patient's physiological response in critical, life-threatening situations caused by injury and disease.

The core curriculum listed below is not meant to be exhaustive; it refers to conditions and managements of which the CCM physician should have specific knowledge and experience, particularly in relation to critical illness. The tabulation should not be misinterpreted as listing conditions requiring admission to a critical care unit.

Core Curriculum

A. Resuscitation
   1. Basic and advanced cardiopulmonary resuscitation certification of the American Heart Association
   2. Central nervous system resuscitation
B. Cardiovascular physiology, pathology, pathophysiology, and therapy
   1. Shock
      a) Hypovolemic
      b) Cardiogenic
      c) Traumatic
      d) Septic
   2. Myocardial infarction and its complications
   3. Cardiac arrhythmias and conduction disturbances—pacemakers
   4. Pulmonary embolism
   5. Pulmonary edema—cardiogenic, as well as noncardiogenic
   6. Cardiac tamponade and other acute pericardial diseases

Source: Grenvik A, Leonard JJ, Arens JF, et al: Critical care medicine—certification as a multidisciplinary subspecialty. *Crit Care Med* 1981;9:117–125.

7. Acute valvular disorders
8. Acute aortic or peripheral vascular disorders, including A-V fistulae
9. Acute complications of cardiomyopathies and myocarditis
10. Management of early postcardiac surgery patients
11. Vasopressor or vasodilator therapy and cardio-assist devices
12. Current concepts of Starling's Law of the heart and capillary circulation to include calculations and interpretation of hemodynamic parameters
13. Hemodynamic effects caused by ventilatory assist devices
14. Congenital lesions
15. Persistent fetal circulation

C. Respiratory physiology, pathology, pathophysiology, and therapy
   1. Acute respiratory failure
      a) Hypoxic—adult respiratory distress syndrome
      b) Hypercapnic
      c) Neurological; mechanical
   2. Status asthmaticus
   3. Smoke inhalation; airway burns
   4. Aspiration; chemical pneumonitis; drowning
   5. Flail chest; barotrauma
   6. Bronchopulmonary infections
   7. Upper airway obstruction
   8. Pulmonary function tests
      a) Pulmonary mechanics
      b) Respiratory adequacy—e.g., blood gases
   9. Oxygen therapy
   10. Hyperbaric oxygen
   11. Mechanical ventilation
      a) Pressure and volume ventilators
      b) Positive end-expiratory pressure, intermittent mandatory ventilation, continuous positive airway pressure, high frequency ventilation, etc.
      c) Indications
      d) Hazards
   12. Airway maintenance
      a) Endotracheal intubation
      b) Tracheostomy
      c) Long-term intubation vs. tracheostomy
         • Advantages
         • Disadvantages
   13. Bronchiolitis
   14. Hyaline membrane disease
   15. Croup, epiglottis

D. Renal physiology, pathology, pathophysiology, and therapy
   1. Renal failure
      a) Prerenal
      b) Renal
      c) Postrenal
   2. Derangements secondary to alterations in osmolality and electrolytes
   3. Acute acid-base disorders
   4. Principles of hemodialysis and of peritoneal dialysis

E. CNS physiology, pathology, pathophysiology, and therapy
   1. Coma
      a) Metabolic
      b) Traumatic
      c) Infectious
      d) Mass lesions
      e) Vascular-anoxic-ischemic

f) Overdose
   (1) Barbiturates
   (2) Narcotics
   (3) Tranquilizers
   (4) Organophosphates
   (5) "Street" drugs
   (6) Salicylate, acetaminophen
   (7) Petroleum distillates
   (8) Heavy metals
2. Hydrocephalus
3. Congenital malformations
4. Psychiatric emergencies

F. Metabolic and endocrine effects of critical illness
  1. Colloid osmotic pressure
  2. Alimentation
     a) Enteral
     b) Lipid IV
     c) Hypertonic-glucose, amino acid solutions IV
  3. Endocrine
     a) Thyroid storm
     b) Myxedema coma
     c) Adrenal crisis (Addison)
     d) Disorders of antidiuretic hormone metabolism
     e) Diabetes mellitus
        (1) Ketotic and nonketotic hyperosmolar coma
        (2) Hypoglycemia
     f) Pheochromocytoma

G. Infectious disease physiology, pathology, pathophysiology, and therapy
  1. Antibiotics
     a) Aminoglycosides
     b) Antifungal agents
     c) Antituberculosis agents
     d) Penicillins and others
     e) Antiviral agents
     f) Agents for parasitic infections
  2. Infection control for Special Care Units
  3. Anaerobic infections
  4. Systemic sepsis
  5. Tetanus
  6. Hospital acquired and opportunistic infections in the critically ill
  7. Adverse reactions secondary to antimicrobial agents

- H. Hematological disorders secondary to acute illness
    1. Acute defects in hemostasis
        a) Thrombocytopenia
        b) Disseminated intravascular coagulation
        c) Primary fibrinolysis
    2. Anticoagulation, fibrinolytic therapy
    3. Principles of blood component therapy
        a) Platelet transfusion
        b) Packed red cells (including frozen red cells)
        c) Fresh frozen plasma
        d) Specific coagulation factor concentrates
        e) Albumin, plasma protein fraction
        f) Stroma free, hemoglobin
        g) White blood cell transfusion
    4. Acute hemolytic disorders
    5. Acute syndromes associated with neoplastic disease or antineoplastic therapy
    6. Acute disorders of the immune-suppressed patient
    7. Neonatal bleeding disorders
    8. Sickle cell crisis
- I. Gastrointestinal-genitourinary-obstetric-gynecological acute disorders
    1. Acute pancreatitis with shock
    2. Upper gastrointestinal bleeding, including variceal bleeding
    3. Lower gastrointestinal bleeding
    4. Acute hepatic failure
    5. Mesenteric infarction
    6. Toxic megacolon
    7. Acute perforations of the gastrointestinal tract
    8. Ruptured esophagus
    9. Acute inflammatory diseases of the intestine
    10. Acute vascular disorders of the intestine
    11. Obstructive uropathy—acute urinary retention
    12. Urinary tract bleeding
    13. Toxemia of pregnancy
    14. Hydatidiform mole
- J. Trauma, burns
    1. Management of multisystem trauma
    2. CNS trauma (brain and spinal cord)
    3. Skeletal trauma, including the spine
    4. Chest trauma
        a) Blunt
        b) Penetrating
        c) Cardiac
    5. Abdominal trauma—blunt/penetrating
    6. Crush injury
    7. Burns
- K. Monitoring, bioengineering, biostatistics
    1. Prognostic indices and severity scores
    2. Principles of electrocardiographic monitoring, measurement of skin temperature or resistance, transcutaneous measurements
    3. Invasive hemodynamic monitoring
        a) Transduction—principles of strain gauge transducers
        b) Signal conditioners, calibration, gain, adjustment
        c) Display techniques
        d) Principles—arterial, central venous and pulmonary artery pressure monitoring
        e) Assessment of cardiac function and derived hemodynamic parameters
    4. Noninvasive hemodynamic monitoring—e.g., systolic time intervals
    5. Electrical safety
    6. Thermoregulation

7. Brain monitoring (intracranial pressure, cerebral blood flow, cerebral metabolic rate, EEG)
8. Respiratory monitoring (airway pressure, intrathoracic pressure, tidal volume, dead space-tidal volume ratio, compliance resistance)
9. Metabolic monitoring (oxygen consumption, carbon dioxide production, respiratory quotient)

L. Life-threatening pediatric conditions
   1. Tracheo-esophageal fistula
   2. Esophageal atresia
   3. Diaphragmatic hernia
   4. Omphalocele
   5. Gastroschisis
   6. Necrotizing enterocolitis
   7. Hyperbilirubinemia
   8. Neonatal seizure
   9. Bronchiolitis
   10. Hyaline membrane disease
   11. Croup, epiglottis
   12. Congenital malformations
   13. Bleeding diathesis
   14. Sickle cell crisis
   15. Reye's syndrome
   N.B. Some of these conditions are also listed under organ disease classifications.

M. Administrative and management principles and techniques
   1. Guidelines for training physicians in critical care medicine
   2. Organization and staffing critical care units
   3. Joint Commission standards for special care units, JCAH
   4. Medical record keeping in special care units
      a) Problem-oriented record approach
      b) System structures record approach
      c) Manual versus mechanical (computer) record generation
      d) Organization of physician, nursing, technical, and laboratory records within special care units
   5. Priorities in the care of the critically ill or injured

N. Pharmacokinetics and dynamics; drug metabolism and excretion in critical illness
   1. Uptake
   2. Metabolism
   3. Excretion

O. Ethical and legal aspects in Critical Care
   Medicine
   1. Death and dying
   2. Ordinary versus extraordinary life
      support mechanisms
   3. Organ transplantation
   4. Standards of treatment for handicapped
      and mentally retarded
   5. The rights of patients/the right to
      refuse treatment

Appropriate experience in a critical care fellowship should include management of patients in the following categories:

- patients in a surgical intensive care unit
- patients in a medical intensive care unit
- patients in a pediatric intensive care unit

It should be recognized that some hospitals have one ICU that includes categories of each of the previously mentioned patients. Experience in the management of a variety of critically ill patients is more important than is the locale of the patients.

Appropriate rotations may include but need not be confined to the following:

- neonatal ICU
- neurosurgical intensive care
- cardiac catheterization laboratory
- pulmonary function laboratory
- respiratory therapy
- burn unit
- dialysis unit
- coronary care unit
- shock-trauma unit

Critical Care Medicine Skills

The critical care specialist must possess fundamental knowledge of, and the technical skills required for, performing certain critical procedures. These procedures have such potential life-saving importance in the care of critically ill patients that they must be available on a continuous basis. Also, the critical care specialist must be knowledgeable in the procedures that are extremely valuable in routine caring for the critically ill patient. He must appreciate the indications, contraindications, complications, pitfalls, and uses of these procedures.

A. Airway
   1. Maintenance of open airway in nonintubated, unconscious, paralyzed patients
   2. Intubation (oral, nasotracheal, esophageal obturator airway, cricothyrotomy, transtracheal catheterization, tracheostomy)
B. Breathing ventilation
   1. Ventilation by bag and mask
   2. Indications, applications, techniques, criteria, and physiological effects of positive end-expiratory pressure; intermittent positive pressure breathing, intermittent mandatory ventilation, continuous positive airway pressure, etc.
   3. Use of intermittent positive pressure breathing therapy, bronchodilators, humidifiers, ventilatory modes
   4. Suction techniques
   5. Chest physiotherapy
   6. Fiberoptic laryngotracheobronchoscopy
   7. Weaning techniques
   8. Management of pneumothorax (needle, chest tube insertion, different drainage systems)
   9. Monitoring airway and intrathoracic pressures
   10. Operation of mechanical ventilators
   11. Measurement of endotracheal tube cuff pressures
   12. Interpretation of sputum cultures by smear
   13. Performance of bedside pulmonary function tests
   14. Application of appropriate oxygen therapy
C. Circulation
   1. Arterial puncture and blood sampling
   2. Insertion of central venous, arterial, and pulmonary artery catheters
   3. Pericardiocentesis
   4. Management of arterial and venous air embolization
   5. Transvenous pacemaker insertion
   6. Cardiac output determinations by Cardio-Green and thermodilution techniques
   7. Use of computers and calculators to determine various derived parameters, e.g., systemic and pulmonary vascular resistance
   8. Obtain 12-lead ECG
   9. Dynamic ECG interpretation
   10. Infusion of epinephrine, dopamine, dobutamine, Isuprel, nitroprusside, and other vasoactive drugs
   11. Recognizing complications of vasodilator therapy
   12. Use of infusion pumps for vasoactive drugs
   13. Cardioversion
   14. Application and regulation of intra-aortic assist devices
   15. Understanding use of extracorporeal membrane oxygenation
   16. Recognition and evaluation of hypertension
D. Central nervous system
   1. Lumbar puncture
   2. Management of intracranial pressure monitors
   3. Monitoring of modified EEG
   4. Application of hypothermia
E. Renal
   1. Sodium and potassium balance
   2. Calculation and interpretation of creatinine clearance

3. Interpretation of urine electrolyte analysis
   4. Evaluation of oliguria
   5. Differentiating prerenal, renal, and postrenal failure
F. Gastrointestinal tract
   1. Insertion of transesophageal devices, e.g., Sengstaken-Blakemore tubes
   2. Prevention and management of upper gastrointestinal bleeding
G. Hematology
   1. Utilization of blood component therapy
   2. Management of massive transfusions
   3. Autotransfusion
   4. Proper ordering and interpretation of coagulation studies
H. Infection
   1. ICU sterility techniques and precautions
   2. Sampling, staining, interpretation, etc. of blood, sputum, urine, drainage fluid samples
I. Metabolism-nutrition
   1. Tube feeding
   2. Total parenteral nutrition
   3. Monitoring and assessment of metabolism and nutrition
   4. Maintenance of temperature homeostasis
J. Monitoring-bioengineering
   1. Utilization, zeroing, calibration of transducers
   2. Use of amplifiers and recorders
   3. Trouble shooting equipment
   4. Correcting basic electrical safety hazards
K. Trauma
   1. Temporary immobilization of fractures
   2. G-suit application
   3. Use of special beds, e.g., circle electric bed, roto bed
L. ICU laboratory
   1. Blood gas analysis
   2. Calculation of oxygen content, intrapulmonary shunt, alveolar-arterial gradients
   3. Recognition and therapy of respiratory and metabolic acidosis and alkalosis

Chapter 4
The Fellowship Program in Critical Care Pharmacy

Warren E. McConnell

IDENTIFYING THE NEED

Clinical fellowships in differentiated areas of pharmacy practice are relatively recent innovations in the profession. A national survey of postgraduate pharmacy fellowships, conducted in 1981 by Karl, Powell, and Cyr, turned up a total of 58 specialty fellowships in 19 different topic areas.[1] Two-thirds of these fellowships had been in existence three years or less; the oldest program had been conducted less than nine years. Although none of the programs identified in the survey was designated as a critical care fellowship, there were 2 in primary care and 1 in emergency medicine. Unfortunately, the survey instrument did not define *fellowships*, to differentiate them from *residencies*; therefore, it is quite likely that some—if not many—of the programs identified as fellowships were, in fact, conducted as residencies.

The Research and Education Foundation of the American Society of Hospital Pharmacists (ASHP) launched its first fellowships (in oncology pharmacy) in 1978. At that time the Foundation's Board of Directors adopted a statement setting forth the philosophy and objectives for the fellowship program (Appendix 4–A). The statement focuses on the research emphasis that characterizes fellowships and describes five broad research objectives. The document differentiates between fellowships and residencies, pointing out that the latter are more structured and are conducted according to clearly-defined standards, whereas fellowships are purposely flexible in order to accommodate the individual needs and interests of participants. Since its adoption, the Philosophy and Objectives statement has guided the development of all ASHP Research and Education Foundation fellowship programs.

DEFINING THE TERMS

The need for a clear distinction between residencies and fellowships led the Commission on Credentialing of the ASHP to develop the following definitions:[2]

> A pharmacy residency is a structured, directed, postgraduate training program in a defined area of pharmacy practice. Residencies exist primarily to train practitioners and managers of professional practice activities. Within a given residency program, there is considerable consistency in content for each resident.
>
> A pharmacy fellowship is a directed, but highly individualized program which emphasizes research. The focus of a pharmacy fellowship is to develop the participant's (the fellow's) ability to conduct research in his area of specialization.

These definitions were subsequently approved by the ASHP Board of Directors (in 1981) and by the ASHP Research and Education Foundation Board of Directors (in 1982).

DEVELOPING THE FELLOWSHIP

The Fellowship in Critical Care Pharmacy conducted by the ASHP Research and Education Foundation was initiated in 1981 through a grant from the IVAC Corporation, manufacturer of parenteral infusion devices. One fellowship is available each year. The first fellow completed the one-year program in June 1983. The application requirements and selection procedures have undergone two major revisions since the program was started. These have been evolutionary changes intended to assure the recruitment and selection of the best qualified fellows, preceptors, and training sites. Greater emphasis is now given to the selection of fellows who are already well-oriented to critical care pharmacy practice and who can devote most of their fellowship year to involvement in research activities. In other words, the requirements and procedures are designed to assure, insofar as possible, that the program is conducted as a fellowship rather than as a residency.

PROTOCOL AND GUIDELINES

The *Protocol and Guidelines* for the Fellowship in Critical Care Pharmacy (Appendix 4–B) provides a brief description of the fellowship, outlines its objectives, states the qualifications for the fellowship applicant, the preceptor, and the institution, and describes the application procedures for fellowship candidates and preceptors. It also describes the selection procedures and criteria, as well as how the program is conducted and administered.

The *Protocol and Guidelines* were developed by the Foundation in cooperation with selected members of the ASHP Special Interest Groups (SIGs) on Adult Clinical Pharmacy Practice, Intravenous Therapy Practice, and Pediatric Pharmacy Practice. Members of these SIGs continue to serve as advisors to the Foundation on all professional aspects of the fellowship program.

The ASHP Research and Education Foundation sponsors one 12-month Fellowship in Critical Care Pharmacy each year, beginning in July. The application deadline for candidates and preceptors is January 15. Candidates are required to submit with their application a letter of support from the preceptor of each program to which they apply. The support letter commits the preceptor to accept the applicant if he or she receives a fellowship appointment. This means that the candidate and the supporting preceptor must meet to discuss the fellowship program and the proposed research, preferably at the site where the fellowship will be conducted, before submitting applications to the Foundation.

EVALUATING PRECEPTORS AND FELLOWS

After the January 15 application deadline, a five-member selection panel reviews all applications to select the fellow and the preceptor at the institution where the fellowship will be conducted. Fellowship applications are evaluated in combination with the preceptor-institution application for each program to which the candidate has applied. The qualifications of the fellowship applicant and the respective supporting preceptor and institution are considered in the selection process.

In evaluating fellowship applicants, the selection panel places heavy emphasis on the candidate's motivation and ability to undertake a fellowship program that is predominantly a research experience. This emphasis is the reason for requiring an advanced degree (Pharm.D. or M.S.) and completion of an ASHP-accredited pharmacy residency as prerequisites for fellowship applicants. The fellowship is not intended to be used to orient a pharmacist to critical care pharmacy practice; a residency serves this purpose.

In evaluating preceptor applicants and their institutions, the selection panel looks closely at the preceptor's research background and experience. The best evidence of this qualification is the preceptor's record of research publications. The selection panel also carefully considers the institution's resources to support research and the level of administrative and interdisciplinary support for the fellowship, as evidenced by the letters of agreement submitted with the preceptor-institution application. The application form for fellowship candidates is depicted in Exhibit 4–1; the form for preceptors, in Exhibit 4–2.

Exhibit 4–1 Fellowship Application

ASHP Research and Education Foundation

Fellowship in Critical Care Pharmacy

Funded by the IVAC Corporation. Offered in cooperation with the ASHP SIGs on ADULT CLINICAL PHARMACY PRACTICE, INTRAVENOUS THERAPY, and PEDIATRIC PHARMACY PRACTICE

> Please type or print all information.

Name (First, Middle, Last) _____

*Birthplace _____ *Social Security No. _____

Current address (residence) _____

_____ Residence telephone (___) _____

Business address _____

_____ Business telephone (___) _____

Permanent address (where mail will always reach you) _____

Education

List colleges and universities attended with dates of attendance and degrees earned.

College or University	Dates (Years)	Degree/Major

Residency Training

Institution	Preceptor	Dates (Years)

Professional Experience

List, in reverse chronological order (most recent first), your experience record in pharmacy practice. Include research experience, if applicable.

_____
_____
_____
_____

*Required for tax purposes.

Source: ASHP Research and Education Foundation.

Fellowship Program in Critical Care Pharmacy 63

Exhibit 4–1 continued

List any other experience, skills or qualifications you believe would qualify you for the fellowship.
_____
_____

Publications
List publication citations.
_____
_____
_____

Health
Are you aware of any conditions which would preclude your fulfilling the work requirements of the fellowship?

Yes _____ . No _____ . If yes, please describe _____
_____

Additional Application Documents Required
Note: The following items of information are to be appended to this form:
1. A statement, not to exceed 1000 words, describing your career goals, why the fellowship will help in achieving these goals, and what, if any, experience or training you have had in the specialty practice area of this fellowship.
2. A letter supporting your application written by the principal preceptor for each fellowship site you have listed below.
3. Separate statements not to exceed 500 words each describing the proposed research project you have discussed with each preceptor supporting your application.

Fellowship Sites

Institution	City/State	Preceptor
_____	_____	_____
_____	_____	_____

Letters of Reference
Provide (below) the names of two health professionals from whom you will request letters of reference attesting to your practice abilities and aptitudes. (Letters should be submitted directly to the ASHP Research and Education Foundation.)

1. _____
2. _____

I understand I am not eligible to apply for an ASHP Research and Education Foundation fellowship offered at an institution where I have served a residency or had significant practice experience.

_____   _____
Signature   Date

Mail original plus six (6) copies of completed application and attachments to:

ASHP Research and Education Foundation
4630 Montgomery Avenue
Bethesda, MD 20814

Exhibit 4–2 Preceptor-Institution Application

ASHP Research and Education Foundation

Fellowship in Critical Care Pharmacy
Funded by the IVAC Corporation

Offered in cooperation with the ASHP SIGs on
Adult Clinical Pharmacy Practice, Intravenous Therapy Practice, and Pediatric Pharmacy Practice

To be completed by the principal preceptor.
Please type or print all information.

Name _____ Earned degrees _____
    First   M.I.   Last

Hospital/Institution _____

Current position title _____ Yrs. in this position _____

Title of person to whom you report _____

Current academic title (if any) _____

Name of college _____

Percentage of time you spend in the following activities:

    Critical care services   _____ %   Administration   _____ %

    Teaching   _____ %   Other (_____)   _____ %

    Research   _____ %   TOTAL = 100%

Your business address _____

_____ Business telephone (___) _____

Home address _____

_____ Home telephone (___) _____

INSTITUTIONAL INFORMATION

Classification (by control):
☐ Nongovernment, not-for-profit   ☐ Government, non-federal
☐ Investor-owned, for profit   ☐ Government, federal

Type (by service):
☐ General medical/surgical
☐ Specialty (_____)

Beds and Utilization:
Licensed bed capacity (number) _____

Acute care beds, adult _____   Acute care beds, pediatric _____   Intensive care beds _____

Pharmaceutical Services:

Director of pharmaceutical services _____ Yrs. in this position _____

Clinical services routinely provided by pharmaceutical services department staff: _____

_____

_____

_____

Source: ASHP Research and Education Foundation.

Exhibit 4-2 continued

ADDITIONAL APPLICATION DOCUMENTS REQUIRED

NOTE: The following items of information are to be appended to this form, each clearly labeled as indicated (Exhibit A, Exhibit B, etc.). Note also that Exhibits B and C must be separate from, and in addition to, Exhibit A, even though there is redundancy.

Exhibit A - Curriculum vitae of principal preceptor

Exhibit B - Description of principal preceptor's research involvement in the area of critical care pharmacy

Exhibit C - A list of publication citations reporting principal preceptor's research activities. (Only citations of publications in nationally recognized refereed professional journals should be listed.)

Exhibit D - Description of the research resources of the institution and the pharmaceutical services department, including current level of research funding, staff qualifications, and interdisciplinary relationships.

Exhibit E - A statement of not more than one (1) single-spaced page describing briefly the research project proposed for the fellow, including the anticipated role the fellow will play, what the fellow may be expected to learn, and whether the research project will result in a publishable or presentable paper.

Exhibit F - A statement of not more than one (1) single-spaced page describing the education and training program to be offered to the fellow, in addition to the research involvement.

Exhibit G - Curriculum vitae of physician co-preceptor (if one is being designated).

LETTERS OF AGREEMENT

Provide the names of the individuals (indicated below) you are requesting to submit to the Foundation letters of agreement indicating their support, in principle, of the fellowship program, their willingness to participate in it, and their agreement to use of the institution and respective departments as the site for the fellowship program:

Chief hospital administrative officer _____

Chief of critical care medicine service _____

Director of pharmaceutical services _____

CO-PRECEPTOR

If a physician co-preceptor is being designated for this fellowship program, provide that individual's name and title:

Co-Preceptor _____

Title _____

AGREEMENT

I agree to serve as the principal preceptor and chairman of the advisory committee to any fellow applicant in whose behalf I submit a letter of support, should that applicant receive a fellowship appointment, and to accept the duties and responsibilities required for the term of the fellowship.

I am a member of the ASHP SIG on _____

_____   _____
Signature   Date

Mail original plus six (6) copies of completed application and exhibits to:

ASHP RESEARCH AND EDUCATION FOUNDATION
4630 Montgomery Avenue
Bethesda, MD 20814

Further information and application forms may be obtained by writing to the ASHP Research and Education Foundation, 4630 Montgomery Avenue, Bethesda, Maryland 20814.

REFERENCES

1. Karl AF, Powell SH, Cyr DA: Postgraduate pharmacy fellowships. *Drug Intell Clin Pharm* 1981;15:981–985.

2. Commission on Credentialing: *Statement of Definition of Pharmacy Fellowship and Residency.* Bethesda, Maryland, American Society of Hospital Pharmacists, 1981.

Appendix 4-A

Philosophy and Objectives of the Fellowship Program

The ASHP Research and Education Foundation, organized in 1968 to encourage and support the advancement of institutional pharmacy practice, is establishing a number of postgraduate fellowship programs. These fellowships are directed, highly individualized training programs emphasizing research. The focus of the fellowship is to develop the participant's (the fellow's) ability to conduct research in his/her area of specialization. The broad research objectives for the fellowship programs include:

1. The development of clinical scientists who can bridge the gap between the knowledge base and the art of practice in evolving specialized practice areas;
2. The study of unmet drug service needs of patients, physicians, nurses, and institutions and the development of experimental programs to meet one or more of these unmet needs;
3. The investigation of the knowledge requirements in the behavioral, social, economic, and managerial sciences for pharmacists in all areas of institutional practice;
4. The investigation of techniques and systems to improve the effectiveness and efficiency of management and operation of hospital pharmacy services;
5. The refinement of advanced knowledge and skills of selected pharmacists in specialized areas of practice.

The ASHP Research and Education Foundation fellowships have no uniform definition. The fellowships differ from residencies in that residencies are more structured and are conducted according to clearly defined standards. The fellowships, on the other hand, are purposely flexible in order to accommodate the individual needs and interests of participants. Furthermore, more residencies

---

Source: ASHP Research and Education Foundation.

accept entry level practitioners as trainees and are often affiliated with an academic degree component, whereas the fellowships are intended as midcareer development programs for persons who have completed residencies or advanced academic degrees, or who have been involved for a significant period of time in a specialized area of practice.

Although the ASHP Research and Education Foundation fellowships are independent of academic degree programs, they are typically offered through broad-based academic health centers, specialized health care institutions, and national associations. The fellowships are offered for finite periods of time, usually one year, determined in advance. Although the primary objective of any individual fellowship has been predetermined, the orientation in each program is to the educational and developmental needs and interests of the participant. Program assignments are usually generated by the fellow in accordance with personal interests and goals as well as institutional and organizational objectives.

Most ASHP Research and Education Foundation fellowships strongly emphasize the research element, that is, a purposeful, critical search for facts, methods, or principles, based upon a perceived need for new knowledge or for solution to a recognized problem, or a search for ways to do things better. Only through such emphasis on research can there be reasonable assurance that the profession, as well as individual participants, will derive maximum benefit from the fellowship programs.

Appendix 4–B

Protocol and Guidelines for Fellowship in Critical Care Pharmacy

A. DESCRIPTION

The ASHP Research and Education Foundation Fellowship in Critical Care Pharmacy is funded by IVAC Corporation, of La Jolla, California, and offered in cooperation with the ASHP SIGs on Adult Clinical Pharmacy Practice, Intravenous Therapy Practice, and Pediatric Pharmacy Practice. The fellowship program is administered by the ASHP Research and Education Foundation (hereinafter known as the Foundation), 4630 Montgomery Avenue, Bethesda, Maryland 20814.

The 12-month fellowship will begin on or about July 1 of each year. The fellowship is intended to encourage and to assist qualified pharmacists to develop research capabilities and to refine practice competencies in the area of critical care pharmacy. The fellowship is conducted as an educational program with primary emphasis on research. It provides formalized research training and advanced clinical practice experience well beyond that ordinarily available in the pharmacist's own practice environment.

B. OBJECTIVES

The major objective of the Fellowship in Critical Care Pharmacy is to develop the fellow's competencies in the scientific research process, including writing research proposals, conducting research, evaluating results, and reporting the research. The research training and experience involves clinical studies relating to the use of drugs in the care and management of critically ill or injured patients.

Source: ASHP Research and Education Foundation. Funded by IVAC Corporation, Inc. Offered in cooperation with the ASHP SIGs on Adult Clinical Pharmacy Practice, Intravenous Therapy Practice, and Pediatric Pharmacy Practice.

A minor objective of the fellowship is to refine the pharmacist's competencies in providing clinical services for critically ill or injured patients.

C. QUALIFICATIONS OF THE FELLOWSHIP APPLICANT

1. The fellowship applicant will be a graduate of a school or college of pharmacy accredited by the American Council on Pharmaceutical Education.
2. The applicant will have a Master of Science in Pharmacy or Pharm.D. degree and will have completed an ASHP-accredited residency program or will have had equivalent clinical experience.
3. The applicant will be eligible for licensure to practice in the state where the fellowship program will be conducted.
4. The applicant will demonstrate possession of basic knowledge and skills in the following areas by citing academic courses completed or by describing residency or work experiences completed:
   a. Physiology, pharmacology, pharmacokinetics, and pathophysiology of disease
   b. Management of critical illness involving major organ systems (including, but not limited to, cardiovascular, pulmonary, renal, metabolic-endocrine-nutritional, neurological-neurosurgical)
   c. Bedside monitoring methods and procedures
5. The applicant will have demonstrated involvement in, or a confirmed interest in, critical care pharmacy, as evidenced by membership in one of the ASHP SIGs, by previous practice experience, or by letters of recommendation.

D. QUALIFICATIONS OF THE PARTICIPATING INSTITUTION

1. The participating institution will be a general medical and surgical hospital with organized resources for the routine care and management of critically ill or injured patients.
2. The institution will have ongoing, formalized education, training, and research programs in critical care medicine.
3. The pharmaceutical services department of the participating institution will meet the requirements of the *ASHP Minimum Standard for Pharmacies in Institutions*.
4. Pharmacists in the pharmaceutical services department will be regularly employed in providing clinical services to inpatients and will participate in the clinical teaching and research programs of the institution.
5. No institution will be eligible as a fellowship site more often than every third year.

E. QUALIFICATIONS OF THE PRINCIPAL PRECEPTOR

1. The principal preceptor will be a clinical pharmacist regularly involved in the care and management of critically ill or injured patients in the medical, surgical, coronary, and pediatric intensive care services of the institution.
2. The principal preceptor will have been involved for a significant period of time in practice, teaching, and research programs related to the management of critically ill patients, as evidenced by published papers in the professional literature.
3. The principal preceptor will be a member of the ASHP SIG on Adult Clinical Pharmacy Practice, Intravenous Therapy Practice, or Pediatric Pharmacy Practice, or another specialized pharmacy practice interest group.
4. A physician practicing in critical care medicine may be designated as co-preceptor to the fellow.

F. APPLICATION PROCEDURE—FELLOWSHIP APPLICANTS

1. Fellowship applicants will obtain application forms and instructions from the Foundation.
2. Each application will include the following items:
   a. A completed "Fellowship Application" form
   b. A statement of not more than 1,000 words describing the applicant's career goals, why the fellowship will help in achieving these goals, and what (if any) experience or training in critical care practice the applicant has had
   c. A letter from a clinical pharmacist qualified to serve as principal preceptor for the fellowship, expressing willingness to assume responsibility for training the applicant, if selected for the fellowship, and addressed to the applicant and signed by the writer (NOTE: This letter is evidence to the Foundation that the applicant and the potential preceptor have mutually discussed the proposed education, training, and research program for the fellowship, preferably at the site where the fellowship will be conducted, and have mutually agreed to each other's acceptability.)
   d. A statement of no more than 500 words describing a proposed research project that the applicant and supporting preceptor (clinical pharmacist submitting letter in F.2.c. above) have mutually discussed and which the applicant would pursue during the fellowship year
   e. A curriculum vitae (personal résumé) giving professional and educational experience, background and achievements, as well as other personal information.
3. The applicant will request letters of reference from two health care professionals who can attest to the applicant's professional practice abilities and

aptitudes. The letters should be submitted directly to the Foundation by the writers.
4. Applicants may apply to more than one institution, but separate supporting letters and statements of proposed research projects (items *F.2.c.* or *d.* above) must be submitted for each institution to which application is being made.
5. Completed applications (*original and six copies of all items*) must be mailed (postmarked) no later than January 15.

G. APPLICATION PROCEDURE—PRECEPTOR APPLICANTS

1. Preceptor applicants will obtain application forms and instructions from the Foundation.
2. Each application will include the following items:
   a. A completed "Preceptor-Institution Application" form
   b. A curriculum vitae of principal preceptor giving educational and experience background and other personal information. (NOTE: If a physician co-preceptor is designated, his/her curriculum vitae also should be submitted.)
   c. A description of principal preceptor's research involvement in the area of critical care pharmacy practice
   d. A list of publication citations reporting principal preceptor's research activities. (Only citations of publications in nationally recognized refereed professional journals are to be listed.)
   e. A statement of no more than one single-spaced page describing the research program proposed for the applicant, including the anticipated role the applicant will play, what may be learned by the applicant, and whether or not the research will encompass a project that will result in a publishable or presentable paper. (NOTE: If different research projects have been discussed with different applicants, a separate statement should be submitted for each.)
   f. A brief statement of the research resources of the institution and the pharmacy department, including current research funding, staff qualifications, and interdisciplinary relationships
   g. A statement of no more than one single-spaced page describing the education and training program that will be offered to the applicant, in addition to the research involvement
3. The following persons at the participating institution will submit to the Foundation letters of agreement indicating their support, in principle, of the fellowship program, their willingness to participate in it, and their agreement to use of the institution and the respective departments as the site for the fellowship:

a. the chief hospital administrative officer
b. the chief of critical care medicine service, or his designee
c. the director of pharmaceutical services
4. A preceptor may support the application of more than one fellowship candidate, but no more than one fellow will be assigned concurrently to a given preceptor. (NOTE: The preceptor's letter expressing willingness to assume responsibility for training the applicant, submitted on the applicant's behalf, is a commitment to accept the applicant if he/she receives a fellowship appointment, and is evidence to the Foundation that the applicant and preceptor have mutually discussed the proposed education, training, and research program for the fellowship, preferably at the site where the fellowship will be conducted.)
5. Completed applications *(original and six copies of all items)* must be mailed (postmarked) no later than January 15.

H. SELECTION PROCEDURE

1. Each fellowship award is competitive. Selection will be made by a panel appointed by the Foundation Board of Directors; decisions of the selection panel will be final and without appeal.
2. Selection will be based on information provided in the applications submitted to the Foundation by fellowship applicants and by the respective preceptors supporting their candidacy.
3. The qualifications of both the fellowship applicant and the respective supporting preceptor and institution will be considered in the selection process.
4. Selection criteria for fellowship applicants will include but not be limited to educational and experience backgrounds, professional qualifications, performance record, stated career goals, merit of proposed research project, letters of reference.
5. Selection criteria for preceptors-institutions will include but not be limited to past and present level of involvement in clinical practice, research, and teaching; merit of the research, educational, and training programs proposed for the fellowship; available facilities and financial resources; level of administrative and interdisciplinary support for the fellowship program.
6. The Foundation will notify all fellowship and preceptor applicants of the outcome of their applications on or about March 1.

I. CONDUCT AND ADMINISTRATION OF THE FELLOWSHIP

1. The selected fellow is expected to enroll in one of the ASHP SIGs related to critical care practice.

2. An advisory committee of at least three members will be appointed to assist the fellow. The committee membership should include the preceptor, as chairman, the chief of critical care medicine or his designee, and another person representing either the pharmaceutical or medical services.
3. The preceptor will assist the fellow in selecting the advisory committee members.
4. The preceptor will notify the Foundation of the committee appointments.
5. The advisory committee will meet with the fellow at least every three months.
6. The preceptor will verify to the Foundation the successful completion of the fellowship program by the fellow who must submit to the Foundation Board of Directors a summary of accomplishments during the 12-month program and an objective evaluation of the experience.
7. The fellowship is awarded to an individual applicant, with the funds administered by the institution where the fellowship is conducted.
8. The funds are to be used solely for the fellow's stipend, travel allowance, and fringe benefits ("honorarium"). No portion of the stipend or travel allowance is to be used for administrative purposes.
9. If for any reason the fellow does not complete the one-year program, any unexpended portion of the stipend and/or travel allowance is to be returned to the ASHP Research and Education Foundation.

J. SELECTION PANEL

1. The selection panel will have responsibility for evaluating applications and selecting eligible fellow candidates and the respective training institutions and preceptors.
2. The selection panel will be appointed by the Foundation Board of Directors, pursuant to recommendations from the ASHP SIGs on Intravenous Therapy Practice, Adult Clinical Pharmacy Practice, and Pediatric Pharmacy Practice.
3. The selection panel will consist of not more than five members, all of whom will be clinical pharmacists practicing in the area of critical care pharmacy.
4. Panel members will be appointed for one-year terms and are eligible for reappointment at the discretion of the Foundation Board of Directors.

K. PROMOTION

The ASHP Research and Education Foundation, in cooperation with the ASHP SIGs on Adult Clinical Pharmacy Practice, Intravenous Therapy Practice, and

Pediatric Pharmacy Practice, will be responsible for promotion of the fellowship program.

L. FUNDING

The fellowship program will be funded by the IVAC Corporation, La Jolla, California. One fellowship will be available annually, with the appointment beginning in July of each year. The selection panel and Foundation Board of Directors will review the fellowship program annually.

Chapter 5

Nurses: The Pivotal Element in Critical Care Pharmacy

Ramón Lavandero and Therese S. Richmond

Nurses are the pivotal element in the effective use of drugs to treat critically ill persons. As members of an interdisciplinary health care team, critical care nurses collaborate with other professionals in providing effective drug therapy. Physicians select and prescribe the drugs. Pharmacists dispense those drugs and offer recommendations based on a patient's total drug profile. Critical care nurses administer the prescribed drugs. In addition, they carefully assess the patient beforehand and, afterwards, evaluate the effectiveness of the therapy, helping the patient and the family to learn about the drugs and their use as part of a comprehensive treatment plan. This chapter describes the role of critical care nurses as interdisciplinary team members and emphasizes their responsibilities in drug therapy.

Two categories of nurses are licensed in the United States: registered nurses (RN)—also called professional nurses—and licensed practical/vocational nurses (LPN/LVN). LPN/LVNs complete a one-year vocational program that focuses on meeting basic physical and hygienic needs of the patient. They are licensed after completing an examination that is different from the RN examination. Some hospitals assign LPN/LVNs to critical care units, but they are given a very limited scope of responsibility. In recent years, the Joint Commission on Accreditation of Hospitals (JCAH) has discouraged assigning LPN/LVNs to critical care units. Throughout this chapter, the terms *nurse, registered* or *professional nurse*, and *critical care nurse* refer only to RNs.

WHAT IS NURSING?

Definitions of nursing come in many flavors, but all share a common ingredient—their focus on providing care that promotes the well-being of the people who receive that care. The variety of definitions demonstrates the creativity that has shaped the development of modern nursing. Florence Nightingale's work in the mid-19th century marked the beginning of modern nursing. Nightingale's dictum that nurses are responsible for putting "the patient in the best condition for nature to act upon him" is still hailed as one of the most precise and succinct definitions of nursing.[1] A sample of other definitions of nursing is shown in Exhibit 5–1.

The variety of possible approaches to nursing practice shows that the profession has remarkable potential for flexibility in adapting to changing health care needs. This variety also accentuates the inherent tension between diversity and conformity that can typify a dynamic and evolving profession. Diversity is essential if the profession is to continue maturing and to avoid stagnation. Nevertheless, a certain degree of conformity is needed to enable the profession to maintain a common mien that is easily recognizable to nurses and non-nurses alike.

The American Nurses' Association (ANA), the major professional nursing organization in the United States, sought to lessen the tension by commissioning a

Exhibit 5–1 Some Definitions of Nursing

> The unique function of the nurse is to assist the individual, sick or well, in the performance of those activities contributing to health, or its recovery (or to peaceful death) that he would perform unaided if he had the necessary strength, will or knowledge. And to do this in such a way as to help him gain independence as rapidly as possible.
>
> Virginia Henderson[2]
>
> [Nursing is] an interpersonal process that aids patients to meet their present needs so that more mature ones can emerge and be met.
>
> Hildegard E. Peplau[3]
>
> The goal of nursing is to assist a person (1) whose behavior is commensurate with social demands, (2) who is able to modify his behavior in ways that support biologic imperatives, (3) who is able to benefit to the fullest extent during illness from the physician's knowledge and skill, and (4) whose behavior does not give evidence of unnecessary trauma as a consequence of illness.
>
> Dorothy E. Johnson[4]
>
> Nursing as a learned profession is both a science and an art. A science may be defined as an organized body of abstract knowledge arrived at by scientific research and logical analysis. The art of nursing is the utilization of the science of nursing for human betterment, and its fulfillment is a lifetime endeavor . . . the science of nursing seeks to study the nature and direction of unitary human development integral with the environment and to evolve the descriptive, explanatory, and predictive principles basic to knowledgeable practice in nursing. No other science or learned profession deals with unitary man as a synergistic phenomenon whose behaviors cannot be predicted by knowledge of the parts.
>
> Martha E. Rogers[5]

special task force charged with defining the nature and the scope of general and specialized nursing practice. The results of the task force's deliberations were published as the 1980 document titled *Nursing: A Social Policy Statement*, which defines nursing as "the diagnosis and treatment of human responses to actual or potential health problems."[6] The American Association of Critical Care Nurses (AACN) maintained conformity by defining critical care nursing as "that specialty within nursing which deals with human responses to life threatening problems."[7] AACN is the professional organization representing critical care nurses in the United States. A profile of the association is presented in Appendix 5–A.

Scope of Critical Care Nursing Practice

AACN has defined the scope of critical care nursing practice in terms of three essential components: (1) the critically ill patient, (2) the critical care nurse, and (3) the critical care environment.[8(pp5-6)] The *critically ill patient* is one who has real or potential life-threatening health problems. These problems require continuous observation and intervention so that complications can be prevented and health restored. The patient's family or significant others are included in this definition.

AACN identifies the *critical care nurse* as an RN who is "committed to ensuring that all critically ill patients receive optimal care."[8(p5)] That nurse's practice should be based on four characteristics: (1) individual professional accountability; (2) thorough knowledge of the interrelatedness of body systems and the dynamic nature of the life process; (3) recognition and appreciation of the wholeness, uniqueness, and significant social and environmental relationships of a person—that is, a holistic perspective; and (4) an appreciation of interdisciplinary collaboration among all health team members. The critical care nurse is expected to participate in ongoing educational activities in order to acquire and to maintain advanced knowledge of physiologic, psychosocial, and therapeutic aspects of critical care. The critical care nurse's clinical practice should use the nursing process as its framework. This problem solving approach consists of four phases: (1) assessment, (2) planning, (3) intervention, and (4) evaluation.

The *critical care environment* or critical care unit is a geographically designated area of a hospital that has been designed to provide care for critically ill patients. This care is usually provided in separate patient care areas, but it may take place in any setting that meets the structure standards established by AACN.

Legal Basis for Nursing

Any discussion of the definition of nursing must take place in the context of the legal definition of nursing. This definition, stated in each state's nurse practice act, specifies the legal boundaries of a nurse's practice. Nurse practice acts are broadly stated descriptions of functions that may be carried out by a registered nurse.

Practice acts generally do not include lists of specific activities, which would make them quite limiting. Consequently, a growing concern for practicing nurses is the clinical situation in which a nurse's actions may violate a state's medical or pharmacy practice acts. This problem is a particular concern for those in expanded roles, such as nurse practitioners and nurse midwives.

During the past ten years, most states have modified their nurse practice acts to reflect more closely the profession's evolution. Many states have done this by issuing administrative statutes that govern expanded activities performed by nurses. Others have followed New York State's initiative by writing entirely new practice acts.[9]

EDUCATION AND CREDENTIALING IN NURSING

Diploma, associate, and baccalaureate degree programs prepare registered nurses for direct patient care. Graduates of all three programs take the same national examination for licensure as do registered nurses, but the programs differ in focus, location, and length.

Diploma programs prepare RNs to practice in hospitals. Accordingly, diploma programs are hospital-based, although they may affiliate with colleges in which students take basic science and a few liberal arts courses. Diploma programs originally offered a 36-month course of studies open only to full-time unmarried students who lived in dormitories at the hospital. Programs now vary in length from 24 months to 3 academic years. Students no longer are required to be unmarried or to live in school dormitories. Some schools offer a part-time course of studies as well. Graduates receive a diploma issued by the school and may receive academic credit for any courses taken through a college affiliation.

Associate degree (ADN) programs prepare RNs to practice in hospitals, but their course of studies combines clinical nursing courses with some courses in basic sciences and other general education areas in order to meet the requirements for an associate degree. ADN programs are based primarily at community and junior colleges, although some are associated with four-year institutions. The full-time course of studies usually can be completed in two academic years.

Baccalaureate degree (BNS) programs prepare nurses to practice in a variety of roles and health care settings. Students take prerequisite courses in the basic sciences and liberal arts, along with nursing courses that satisfy the requirements of an upper division major. BSN programs are affiliated with colleges and universities, offering a course of studies that usually takes four full-time academic years to complete. Some schools offer only an upper division curriculum, which permits students to complete prerequisite courses at an accredited institution of their choice. These programs appeal especially to non-nurse college graduates and other adult learners with considerable college work behind them. Graduates of baccalaureate degree nursing programs receive a bachelor's degree, usually designated as a BSN. Non-nurse college graduates also may seek admission to basic educational programs that confer either a master's degree (MSN) or a professional doctorate (ND) upon graduation. Yale University and Pace University offer this type of MSN program; Case-Western Reserve University offers the ND program.

Entry into Practice Controversy

Predictably, three major entry routes leading to identical licensure have caused some confusion among nurses and non-nurses alike. Each type of program offers a course of studies designed to prepare its graduates for particular types of nursing practice, often in differing settings. However, nurses take the same examination upon graduation and are licensed as RNs on the basis of the same cut-offs for passing. Armed with identical licenses, these nurses are theoretically eligible for the same positions, leaving it up to employers to differentiate among the qualifications of graduates from the various types of programs.

Entry into practice, as it is called, continues to be a major source of discord among nurses across the nation. The American Nurses' Association issued a 1965 position paper titled "Educational Preparation for Nurse Practitioners and Assistants to Nurses—A Position Paper" proposing that all education for nurses in the United States take place in academic institutions. The paper also proposed two categories of nurses: (1) professional nurses, who would be prepared at the bachelor's degree level, and (2) technical nurses, who would complete an associate degree program. These were proposed as entry-level categories; nurses already licensed were covered by a grandfather clause that would allow them to retain their licenses to practice as RNs. A grandfather clause would not, however, confer a bachelor's degree.

In order for the ANA proposal to be implemented, each state legislature would need to amend its statutes governing RN licensure. To date, eight states have a BSN requirement plan that includes a target date; another eight have expressed no support for the ANA position. The remainder have taken positions ranging from support of the ANA position without a mandated BSN requirement to an accepted BSN requirement plan without a target implementation date.[10]

Many nursing organizations issued statements addressing the entry into practice issue. AACN supported the bachelor's degree in nursing as the minimal academic credential for entry into professional practice.[11] AACN also supported grandfathering of all currently licensed RNs who do not hold a bachelor's degree in nursing. Recognizing that a majority of its members fall into the latter category, AACN was unique among the organizations in pledging to pursue solutions to obstacles that hinder registered nurses from achieving bachelor's degrees in their field. The association established an educational advancement scholarship program as part of this pledge.

Certification

Nurses may choose to augment their professional credentials by obtaining specialty certification or graduate academic degrees. Certification is defined as

> the process by which a nongovernmental agency or association grants recognition to an individual who has met certain predetermined qualifications specified by that agency or association. Such qualifications may include: (a) graduation from an accredited or approved program; (b) acceptable performance on a qualifying examination or series of examinations; and/or (c) completion of a given amount of work experience.[12]

Specialty certification may be mandatory (as it is for nurse anesthetists) or voluntary (as it is for critical care nurses).

Certification denotes that a nurse has achieved and has maintained minimal competency in a field of specialization. Certification differs, however, from licensure, which verifies that a nurse has the minimal knowledge needed to practice general nursing. The main objective of certification is to protect the consumer by assuring quality nursing care within a particular specialty. Certification also encourages specialization and advanced practice, provides credentials for possible reimbursement by third party payers, and expands opportunities for mobility and advancement. Certification may also motivate nurses to increase their participation in continuing education activities and may increase their prestige and recognition by peers in clinical practice. Critical care nurses are certified as CCRNs by the AACN Certification Corporation, a wholly-owned subsidiary of the American Association of Critical Care Nurses. The CCRN certification process is described in Appendix 5–B.

Graduate Study

After receiving a bachelor's degree, nurses may continue their academic studies for the master's or the doctoral degree. The bachelor's degree curriculum focuses on generalized nursing practice (whether the degree is completed at the entry into practice level or after a nurse is licensed as an RN); a master's degree program allows a nurse to strengthen clinical expertise in a particular area of specialty practice. The program also develops the nurse's skills in conducting research and in establishing a leadership role in professional practice or education.

Should the nurse wish to continue for a doctoral degree, the master's program provides a foundation for the doctoral course of studies. The degree designation awarded upon completion of a master's level nursing curriculum varies according to the institution granting the degree. The most commonly awarded degrees are the

MSN (Master of Science in Nursing), the MS (Master of Science), the MN (Master of Nursing), the MA (Master of Arts), the MEd (Master of Education), and the MPH (Master of Public Health).

Doctoral study in nursing focuses primarily on developing and testing nursing theory and on in-depth research of nursing and the problems nurses deal with in clinical practice. Doctoral programs are designed to prepare nurses for academic, clinical, and administrative positions, including major roles in health policy planning. As in the case of master's degrees, doctoral degree designations vary according to the program's focus and the institution granting the degree. PhD programs strongly emphasize research, whereas professional doctorates (DNS, DNSc, DSN) emphasize the application of research findings and existing knowledge to nursing in clinical practice, education, or administration. The trend for nurses to seek doctorates in their own discipline continues to increase, but many nurses still seek doctorates in related fields like the basic sciences, behavioral sciences, and education.

THE NURSE'S ROLE IN DRUG THERAPY

In general, nurses function dependently, interdependently, or independently, according to the requirements of a particular situation. In *dependent* functions the nurse has no direct control over the treatment outcome, and depends on another professional (usually a physician) for assessment and decision making. *Interdependent* functions are shared. Nursing aspects of patient care are controlled by the nurse, who also participates in assessment and decision making. The nurse entirely controls assessment and is fully accountable and responsible for the outcome when functioning *independently*.

Drug administration is one of nursing's most important responsibilities. It also carries probably the greatest risk of legal liability. The nurse's role in drug therapy usually is described as a dependent one because a written order from a physician or dentist is required and a pharmacist must dispense the preparation before the nurse is permitted to administer it. The actions surrounding the actual administration of a drug are actually a series of independent functions carried out within the context of the nursing process.

In the first phase of this process, the nurse assesses the patient before administration of the prescribed drug. This comprehensive assessment includes a review of pertinent past history and an evaluation of current physical and emotional status. When it is appropriate, the nurse also assesses how much the patient knows about the drug. Assuming all assessment data are in line, the nurse's plan is to administer the drug. If PRN medications are involved, the nurse uses data from this assessment in deciding whether to administer the drug and, when more than one drug may be used, in selecting the most appropriate one. Assessment data also could lead the nurse to withhold the drug and to seek consultation with the physician. The importance of nursing judgment when administering drugs to critically ill patients cannot be underestimated.

The actual administration of a drug is a medically delegated action. Drug administration is guided by the so-called *five rights*: right drug, right time, right dose, right route, right patient. Sometimes a sixth is added: right technique. The evaluation phase begins immediately after a drug is administered. During this phase the nurse observes and assesses the patient to determine drug efficacy and drug-induced adverse effects.[13] The intensity and the extent of observation during the evaluation phase depend on the drug administered and the patient's overall condition. In critical care, the complexity of drug regimens and the acuity of a patient's condition mean that evaluation after the administration of one drug overlaps frequently with the assessment that precedes administration of another.

Patient and family teaching are integrated throughout the process. This teaching includes information about the use and the expected effects of the drug, along with possible adverse or side effects. It will also include special instructions concerning drug administration and precautions that may be required after administration. Some years ago patient and family teaching was thought to take place only during uninterrupted time set aside expressly for teaching purposes. Increased familiarity with adult learning theory and research has shown that learning takes place in a multitude of ways, often depending on a person's own learning style. For this reason, nurses now integrate patient and family teaching throughout the patient care process.

The appropriateness of drug information teaching is carefully considered when working with critically ill patients and their families. Not only may a patient's condition preclude learning, but even when the patient's condition itself is not a barrier, the complexity of the regimen may be overwhelming. Nevertheless, drug information teaching is not automatically excluded when a patient is critically ill.

In some situations the patient is alert, oriented, and wants to follow the plan of care. In coronary care units, for example, patients begin to receive drugs, such as antiarrhythmics and antianginals, that they will be expected to take on a long-term basis. Clearly, every opportunity for drug information teaching in these situations should be taken.

LEARNING ABOUT DRUGS

Basic Curricular Approach

Nurses first learn about drugs and their use in patient care as part of their basic educational program. Many programs integrate the information throughout the curriculum. Drugs used to treat particular problems are discussed in relation to the problems themselves. This integrated presentation considers drugs as only one of several therapeutic solutions to a health problem—solutions that must not be isolated from one another. The integrated presentation supports a holistic approach to patient care.

Other nursing programs present pharmacology as a separate content area. Students in those programs take a pharmacology course that focuses on basic principles and detailed information about drug categories. The information is usually presented from the perspective of the drugs themselves, not the types of problems for which they may be used.

Either presentation has pros and cons. The integrated presentation has become widely accepted because it presents drug information as one of various components of a comprehensive patient treatment plan. The thoroughness with which the information is presented depends, however, on the instructor's expertise and preference. The same situation occurs in the case of other integrated content areas, such as nutrition.

Although the second approach seems to offer the nurse a stronger base in pharmacology, it may be lopsided because most of the information is learned from a drug-related perspective. One solution could be to integrate pharmacology content throughout the course of studies while offering a brief introductory course in basic pharmacologic principles. The latter could be required or optional, depending on the needs of the program's students.

Regardless of the curricular approach used in their basic educational program, nurses become familiar with the many sources of drug information available to them. Basic pharmacology texts are supplemented by quick-reference handbooks that focus on information essential for administering drugs and evaluating their effectiveness. Nursing journals and periodicals overflow with drug information. Presented in many ways, this information includes case presentations, articles on new drugs or new uses for existing drugs, and self-assessment tests. Self-assessment tests often include continuing education credit options. The credits may be used by nurses applying for relicensure in states where mandatory continuing education regulations are in effect and by nurses applying for specialty recertification in critical care.

Noncurricular Sources

Nurses learn about other drug information sources during their clinical experience as students. A variety of drug formularies and the *Physicians' Desk Reference* (PDR) are standard issue in most patient-care facilities; there nurses also become aware of drug inserts and other descriptive literature prepared by manufacturers. Furthermore, the differences between drug information prepared by manufacturers and that prepared by unbiased experts in the field are emphasized when nursing students learn about drugs.

In recent years nurses have begun to recognize the pharmacist as a major source of current and accurate drug information. The pharmacist's wide range of specialized expertise in the field has been a well-kept secret for many reasons. Whether in hospital pharmacies or in retail establishments, pharmacists have most often been dispensers of drugs, not of drug information. The information they did dispense was usually the repetition of the directions for administration given by the physician.

As pharmacists have assumed a very active clinical role, their prominence as significant members of the health care team has dramatically increased. Nurses who have had student experiences in facilities with well-developed clinical pharmacy services are especially acquainted with the role. They know that, at the very least, the pharmacist is a phone call away, readily available with current drug information or the sources in which it can quickly be obtained. Increasingly often, those nurses see the pharmacist in patient care areas, participating in interdisciplinary patient care conferences and informational update sessions.

Nurses without these experiences also have become familiar with pharmacists and their role. While clinical pharmacy services have become more prominent, pharmacists have gained the attention of thousands more nurses through very active speaking and publishing schedules. Drug-related presentations at continuing education programs for nurses are often given by a pharmacist or by nurse-pharmacist teams. Such joint ventures also have led to coauthored textbooks. Two of the general nursing publications with the highest circulation have made drug information a featured part of each issue.

Nursing 84 features regular columns on new drugs, case histories of medication errors, and self-assessment tests. Each of these columns is presented from a nursing perspective. The publisher also markets various drug handbooks for nurses and employs a pharmacist with a doctoral degree as full-time drug information manager. Each issue of the *American Journal of Nursing* includes the most recent edition of *Nurses' Drug Alert*, an eight-page newsletter prepared by a panel of pharmacists and nurses for an independent publisher. Drug information also features prominently in many of the journal's clinical articles.

Staying Current after Graduation

After graduation, nurses in practice maintain current knowledge about drugs and their use in patient care by using many of the resources already described. Although initial familiarity with available resources depends heavily on classroom and clinical exposure during their basic educational program, nurses in practice quickly expand their horizons about clinical drug use in response to the demands of clinical practice.

In critical care, this expansion may come about through formal courses to prepare for work in a critical care unit. The AACN *Core Curriculum for Critical*

Care Nursing is often used by clinical educators as the framework for critical care orientation courses and for advanced courses as well. The core curriculum presents information according to body systems and fully integrates information and references on the use of drug therapy in treating critically ill adults.

Unfortunately, a nurse who is familiar with the widest possible range of drug information sources may become frustrated by their lack of availability and by time constraints. Most critical care units have several basic printed reference sources available. However, these may not be the most up-to-date sources. More current information may be unavailable or difficult to locate on short notice. Seeking recourse in the hospital's library, a nurse may be further frustrated because these often are "medical" libraries that lack the kind of clinical practice information nurses need.

Time constraints are another obstacle to nurses seeking current drug information. The nurse usually needs this information on short notice in order to administer appropriately an unfamiliar medication that has been newly ordered for a patient. Often, little or no time is available to go to the library. However, should that time be available, the nurse often finds closed doors because critical care units are open around-the-clock; hospital libraries are not. Sadly, drug information services established by pharmacy departments frequently use the same scheduling as that used by libraries. Their usual 40-hour work week covers less than a quarter of the 168 hours per week that nurses are working in critical care units. Fortunately, the increase in computerized hospital information systems offers a welcome remedy to the problem, but it is a remedy that will be applied only as quickly as immediate and up-to-date drug information available around-the-clock is acknowledged to be a major hospital priority.

FREQUENTLY ASKED DRUG QUESTIONS

Under the best circumstances, achieving effective drug therapy may pose a challenge to the skilled professional. Achieving effective drug therapy becomes an olympian feat when treating the complex, often multisystem problems that plague most critically ill persons. Faced with the responsibility of administering and evaluating drug therapy on a 24-hour basis, the critical care nurse often turns to the clinical pharmacist for information that can make drug therapy more effective and less prone to unnecessary complications.

In our experience, the questions most often asked by critical care nurses can be grouped into five major categories:

1. compatibilities and admixtures
2. dosage alteration
3. special administration techniques

4. clinical effects
5. interpretation of serum drug levels

These categories are not all-inclusive, nor are they mutually exclusive.

Compatibilities and Admixtures

Except for the operating suite, no clinical area relies on intravenous drug administration as heavily as does the critical care unit. Altered levels of consciousness, impaired oral intake, and the need for rapid action make it impossible to consider other routes. The critical care nurse is faced with the administration of drugs by routes not usually used for those drugs, and with the dilemma of simultaneously administering multiple drugs through a limited number of intravenous access sites. Frequently asked questions include the following:

- If several drugs must be administered in sequence, which order is preferred and why?
- Which, if any, of several drugs are compatible for simultaneous administration?
- Can particular drugs be administered through a line in which blood or blood products are simultaneously infusing?
- Which, if any, of several titratable drugs may be administered simultaneously through the same line (e.g., vasopressors, antiarrhythmics, anticoagulants)?

Dosage Alteration

Drug dosages must be adjusted frequently when treating critically ill persons. A person taking oral medications to treat a preexisting condition (often the case with elderly persons or those who are chronically ill) usually requires dosage adjustment when the route of administration is changed, or may require dosage adjustment because of acute changes in his or her condition. A variation of the problem occurs when enteral administration is effective for treating a specific condition, but parenteral administration is not as effective. For example, a patient's hypertension may be controlled with an oral preparation; yet, the same control may not be achieved by intravenous administration of the same drug, and intramuscular administration may be contraindicated. Physicians and nurses alike may be uncertain about the extent to which a drug's dosage should be changed.

Although the *PDR* and various formularies offer reliable guidelines for dosage alteration, these guidelines deal in general terms and do not address the multitude of other treatments—including drugs—that may be prescribed for a specific person at a specific time. This uncertainty occurs especially among newly graduated nurses and physicians—whether house officers or attendings—who lack training and experience in critical care. The pharmacist is often approached in these situations for validation of a decision—a validation based on the pharmacist's knowledge of the patient's entire drug treatment regimen.

The pharmacist should be aware that even when validation is given to a physician, a nurse also may require the same type of verification because of liability for any harm caused by failure to adhere to acceptable standards of care in drug administration. Indeed, nurses have the legal right to refuse to administer a drug when they think it will harm a patient. The nurse may exercise this right in situations when, for example, an inappropriate dosage is ordered or when the drug appears contraindicated because of the patient's condition or the possible interaction with other drugs the patient has received.

Special Administration Techniques

Critical care nurses seek information about special techniques required to administer a particular drug. These techniques may include the need to dilute the drug in a specific type of solution, to administer it through specific types of vascular access catheters or infusion devices, or to take special precautions in the event of extravasation. Nurses are familiar with the usual techniques required to administer a particular drug, but they are not likely to have the same access as pharmacists to the most recent pharmacologic research data. For example, the finding that sodium nitroprusside (Nipride) remains stable in solution for longer than four hours was first reported in the pharmacy literature and communicated to critical care nurses at our institution by clinical pharmacists.

When titratable drugs like sodium nitroprusside are used, nurses also are concerned about how long the solution will remain sterile after it is prepared and connected to an infusion system. The same question applies to flush solutions for hemodynamic monitoring. Clinical pharmacists and infection control nurses may conduct joint research to seek answers to this question in varied clinical situations. In unit-dose systems, the information is consistently relayed on container labels. In hospitals in which solutions are prepared by the nurses in the critical care unit, it is essential that the pharmacist consistently relay this type of information to the unit.

Critical care nurses must be informed of the most recent findings and directives about handling potentially dangerous drugs, such as cytotoxic preparations. The American Society of Hospital Pharmacists took the lead in issuing recommendations about handling, preparing, administering, and disposing of these drugs.[14] Pharmacists, who would be the first to become aware of the recommendations, should consider it their responsibility to share the information with others who may be affected.

Clinical Effects

"How soon can I expect to see the effects of this drug?" This question is probably the most frequently asked question about the clinical manifestations of a drug's action. The nurse usually asks the question when, after administration of a drug, new or different signs and symptoms are identified. The nurse's observations are further complicated by the knowledge that the assortment of drugs being administered to the typical critically ill person may also have potentiating, synergistic, or antagonistic effects among one another. Finally, the nurse is already familiar with the drug's expected action and may be faced with a clinical response that is faster, slower, stronger, or weaker than expected. The nurse may seek consultation from the pharmacist at times like this.

Interpretation of Serum Drug Levels

Serum drug levels are measured to evaluate the effectiveness of many of the drugs used to treat critically ill persons. The critical care nurse is responsible for obtaining the necessary blood specimens directly or through a technician. Here are some of the most frequently asked questions about serum drug levels:

- When should specimens be obtained?
- What is the difference between peak and trough levels?
- Why do some drugs require peak levels and others trough levels?
- Does it make a difference whether an arterial or a venous blood sample is obtained?
- How about mixed arteriovenous samples, such as those from arteriovenous fistulas?
- How are drug level results interpreted?
- What are therapeutic levels for particular drugs?
- What can cause values above or below acceptable therapeutic levels?
- Given the drug level results for a particular patient, are drug dosage and frequency of administration being correctly adjusted to meet that person's therapeutic needs?

CRITICAL CARE NURSE-PHARMACIST COLLABORATION

Critical care nurses and pharmacists have fertile ground for collaboration in three major areas: (1) education, (2) clinical research, and (3) interdisciplinary activities. Because of the shared nature of activities in each of these areas, either discipline may appropriately take the initiative in their initial development.

Education

Pharmacists may participate in every phase of a nurse's education. Nursing students may use a pharmacology text coauthored by a nurse and a pharmacist. Subsequently, the students may be exposed to an active clinical pharmacy service during their clinical experiences that leaves an indelible mark of the pharmacist as a useful and accessible drug information resource. This exposure is strengthened when pharmacists actively participate in education and orientation programs for critical care.

A pharmacist probably is most active in ongoing educational activities and informally may help the nurse in finding answers to the kinds of questions presented in the preceding section. The pharmacist may supplement or even may anticipate the need for information by regularly providing it in scheduled inservice presentations or by establishing a current awareness program of journal articles on drug-related topics. A current awareness program can be easily established with help from the hospital librarian. In its simplest form, pharmacists, nurses, and the librarian identify the journals and newsletters that publish drug information most useful to nurses. (This plan may require that the library subscribe to some new publications.) Every month the librarian sends a copy of the contents page of each publication to the pharmacists or nurses, who select articles of particular interest. In keeping with the limitations of copyright laws, the librarian makes available copies of the selected items. In institutions with closed circuit broadcast capability, the pharmacist may provide this information to many more participants by taping a presentation for rebroadcast at times that are convenient for the nurses.

Another timely, efficient, and cost-effective approach is available where a computerized hospital information system is in place. Ideally, a major national formulary, the hospital's own formulary, and information updates would be available on-line. Minimally, the updates alone could be available. Where on-line computer capability is unavailable but pharmacists and nurses have access to a microcomputer, the same information can be put on disk.

Even where there is no computer capability, many hospital pharmacy departments publish a printed newsletter to keep practitioners informed. Curiously, those newsletters often are distributed only to physicians. This oversight can easily be rectified by including the hospital's critical care nurses on the distribution list. Rather than sending copies in bulk to the critical care unit, attach a copy of the newsletter to each critical care nurse's paycheck—a more effective and personal approach.

Pharmacists are welcome participants in formal nursing continuing education programs offered within and outside the hospital. National AACN and its local chapters frequently sponsor these programs, which often include content experts from other disciplines. Program planning committees will usually consider proposals from potential speakers, especially when the proposed presentations address a topic in ways that are interesting and useful for practicing critical care nurses. Of course, there also are numerous potential publishing opportunities in which pharmacists or nurse-pharmacist author teams can reach nursing audiences. (Some examples were described earlier.) Finally, pharmacists can collaborate with nurses in helping patients, where possible, and their families learn about the ways in which drugs are used as part of their comprehensive treatment plan.

Clinical Research

Comprehensive Structure Standard XI for nursing care of the critically ill requires that clinical research be conducted and used as part of critical care nursing practice, and that this should be done "independently and/or in collaboration with others."[8(pp 47-50)] Clinical research is a logical arena for nurse-pharmacist collaboration. The nurse brings expertise in assessing patients before, during, and after drug administration, and expertise in drug administration itself—all within a holistic patient care framework. The pharmacist brings in-depth knowledge of drugs and their expected actions when used singly and in combination.

What directions should this research take? Each of the frequently asked questions that were discussed earlier could form the basis of a collaborative clinical research design. Studies also can be designed to investigate ethical issues in drug research and the use of drugs in clinical practice, including the allocation of scarce and costly drug preparations. Related issues that would benefit from collaborative research are the consumer's right to information about drugs and the use of experimental drugs after brain death is established.

The complexities of patient compliance with drug regimens are yet another direction for collaborative research. Critical care nurses usually are not involved in many of the nursing activities that influence compliance, but they frequently work with patients who have been admitted because of poor adherence to a drug regimen. In short, the possibilities for collaborative nurse-pharmacist clinical research are endless.

Interdisciplinary Activities

"Collaboration has been identified as a pivotal component in the delivery of quality health care . . . [and] the impetus for true collaboration must originate with health care professionals themselves."[15] The activities presented here focus on interdisciplinary collaboration between critical care nurses and pharmacists, although many of the activities can and should expand to include other disciplines such as medicine, nutrition support, and social service.

Interdisciplinary patient care conferences can become the focal point of interdisciplinary collaboration if they are held on a frequent and regular basis. These conferences zero in on the individual needs of specific patients and how each discipline can best contribute to meeting those needs.

Clinical pharmacists who actively participate in the care of critically ill patients can be major participants in these conferences. Active participation should include a careful daily review of each patient's drug profile that is followed by bedside rounds in which the pharmacist monitors the effectiveness of the overall drug therapy regimen. Ideally, these rounds should be joint rounds with nurses and physicians, but conflicting schedules may require that joint discussions be held during the conference itself instead of at the bedside.

During an interdisciplinary patient care conference, drug therapy is discussed as one component—albeit a major one—of a patient's comprehensive plan of care. The informed clinical pharmacist should be able to discuss the effectiveness of the overall regimen and to make recommendations about continuing or discontinuing drugs, perhaps suggesting other drugs or drug combinations that can offer effective treatment. Recommendations should always be based on the most current clinical and research data available and, equally important, should consider the cost of the recommendations.

Furthermore, pharmacists may promote collaborative practice by serving on interdisciplinary committees. Numerous hospital-wide committees invite representation from various disciplines. Pharmacists can be especially important members of infection control, quality assurance, and cardiopulmonary resuscitation committees. When a committee does not have a primary critical care focus, the clinical pharmacist with experience in critical care can be a strong advocate for the unique needs of that specialty. Conversely, when a hospital's pharmacy committee does not have nursing representation, the pharmacist's awareness of the nurse's important role in drug therapy can facilitate adding a nurse to the committee.

Pharmacists can also consider participating in the design of new and renovated critical care units, new designs and modifications for drug administration equipment, and numerous other possibilities limited only by their willingness and ingenuity.

In summary, effective nurse-pharmacist collaboration strengthens the patient care in critical care units. It enhances the thoroughness with which critical care nurses participate in drug therapy regimens (which are a key part of successful care for critically ill persons), and truly makes the clinical pharmacist an active participant in patient care.

REFERENCES

1. Nightingale F: *Notes on Nursing: What It Is and What It Is Not*, facsimile of 1859 ed. Philadelphia: WB Saunders, 1946, p 79.

2. Henderson V: *The Nature of Nursing*. New York, Macmillan, 1966, p 15.

3. Blake M: The Peplau developmental model for nursing practice, in Riehl JP, Roy SC (eds): *Conceptual Models for Nursing Practice,* ed 2. New York, Appleton-Century-Crofts, 1980, p 53.

4. Johnson DE: The behavioral system model for nursing, in Riehl JP, Roy SC (eds): *Conceptual Models for Nursing Practice,* ed 2. New York, Appleton-Century-Crofts, 1980, p 207.

5. Rogers ME: Nursing: A science of unitary man, in Riehl JP, Roy SC (eds). *Conceptual Models for Nursing Practice,* ed 2. New York, Appleton-Century-Crofts, 1980, pp 329–330.

6. American Nurses' Association: *Nursing: A Social Policy Statement.* Kansas City, Mo, The Association, 1980, p 9.

7. American Association of Critical Care Nurses: *Monthly Report to Chapters.* Newport Beach, Calif, The Association, March 1984.

8. American Association of Critical Care Nurses: *Standards for Nursing Care of the Critically Ill.* Reston, Va, Reston, 1981, pp 5–6, 47–50.

9. Kelly LY: *Dimensions of Professional Nursing.* ed 4. New York, Macmillan, 1981, p 425.

10. Nurse's Reference Library: *Practices.* Springhouse, Pa, Springhouse Corp., 1984, pp 317–323.

11. American Association of Critical Care Nurses: AACN's position statement on entry into practice. *Focus on AACN* 1981; 8(6):5–8.

12. Kelly LY: *Dimensions of Professional Nursing.* ed 4. New York, Macmillan, 1981, p 412.

13. Johnson GE, Hannah KJ: *Pharmacology and the Nursing Process.* Philadelphia, WB Saunders, 1983, p 18.

14. Hospitals told to take precautions in handling cytotoxic drugs. *Hosp Week* 1983 8(July):3.

15. Adler D, Ayres S, Disch J, Greenbaum D, et al: The organization of human resources in critical care units. *Focus Crit Care* 1983; 10(1):43–44.

BIBLIOGRAPHY OF AACN PUBLICATIONS

Adler DC, Shoemaker N: *Organization and Management of Critical Care Facilities.* St Louis, CV Mosby, 1979.

American Association of Critical Care Nurses: *Core Curriculum for Critical Care Nursing.* ed 2. Philadelphia, WB Saunders, 1981. (ed 3 and companion review book in press)

American Association of Critical Care Nurses: *Standards for Nursing Care of the Critically Ill.* Reston, Va, Reston, 1981.

Guzzetta CE, Dossey BM: *Cardiovascular Nursing: Bodymind Tapestry.* St. Louis, CV Mosby, 1984.

Hazinski MF: *Nursing Care of the Critically Ill Child.* St. Louis: CV Mosby, 1984.

Kinney MR, et al: *AACN's Clinical Reference for Critical Care Nursing.* New York, McGraw-Hill, 1980. (ed 2 in press)

Mann JK, Oakes AR: *Critical Care Nursing of the Multi-injured Patient.* Philadelphia, WB Saunders, 1980.

Millar S, Sampson L, Soukup SM, Weinberg SL: *Methods in Critical Care: The AACN Manual.* Philadelphia, WB Saunders, 1980. (ed 2 in press; retitled *AACN's Procedure Manual for Critical Care*)

Oakes AR: *Critical Care Nursing of Children and Adolescents.* Philadelphia, WB Saunders, 1980.

Vestal KW, MacKenzie CAM: *High Risk Perinatal Nursing.* Philadelphia, WB Saunders, 1983.

Appendix 5-A

What Is AACN?

The AACN is the largest specialty nursing organization in the world. AACN's almost 50,000 members include critical care nurses from the United States and associate members from other nations. Fourteen thousand of the members also belong to 1 of more than 200 local AACN chapters in the United States and its overseas military bases. AACN was established in 1969 to promote the health and welfare of mankind by advancing the science and art of critical care nursing. This is fulfilled through the following organizational goals stated in the bylaws:

- to promote standards for care of the critically ill
- to promote educational standards in critical care nursing
- to provide educational opportunities for nurses caring for the critically ill
- to promote professionalism and accountability of nurses caring for the critically ill
- to facilitate effective communication among critical care nurses
- to encourage scientific investigation in critical care
- to maintain effective communication between critical care nursing and its public

AACN is the parent of the AACN Certification Corporation, which was established to develop, to maintain, and to promote high standards of critical care nursing practice. The AACN Certification Corporation administers the CCRN Certification Program, which is described in Appendix 5-B.

AACN's wide range of activities are designed to carry out the association's goals. *Standards for Nursing Care of the Critically Ill* were published in 1980, funded in part by a grant from the US Health Resources Administration—Division of Nursing. The standards are based on AACN's philosophy and represent statements of quality that can be used as a model for nursing care of critically ill patients. The AACN *Standards* are endorsed by the Society of Critical Care Medicine. To complement these clinical practice standards, AACN has commissioned a task force to develop academic and clinical education standards for critical care nursing.

The association is noted for its wide-ranging educational programs. The annual National Teaching Institute™ (NTI) is considered by many to be the most important annual learning event in critical care nursing. In addition to the NTI, the national association presents a variety of educational programs on topics that are current and relevant to the practicing critical care nurse. Programs are offered in numerous locations in the United States to increase accessibility to members. AACN chapters offer equally varied educational programming at the local level. In 1982, AACN sponsored its first international intensive care nursing conference in London as an effort in promoting international communication and collaboration in critical care nursing. International conferences are scheduled at regular intervals with the next one to be held in The Hague in 1986.

Publications are among AACN's most visible enterprises. *Heart & Lung, The Journal of Critical Care* is a bimonthly scientific journal with a circulation of more than 62,000 nurse, physician, and other health professional subscribers. Reflecting the important role of interdisciplinary collaboration in AACN's activities, *Heart & Lung* is the only publication of its kind to have a nurse and a physician as co-editors. *Focus on Critical Care*, AACN's bimonthly magazine, evolved in 1982 from *Focus on AACN*, an in-house newsmagazine for members. *Focus* features articles on clinical practice and other topics of interest to critical care nurses. Both periodicals are published under contract with The C.V. Mosby Company.

AACN is also an active publisher of books. The association has published ten books to date, and new editions of several of them are in preparation. A list of AACN books is included in the bibliography. Through an author recognition program, the association recognizes members for their many published contributions to critical care nursing by sending each author a letter of commendation and printing the citation of their publication in *Heart & Lung* on a space-available basis.

AACN produces nonprint media as well. *Condition Critical: The Nurse Makes a Difference* is a 30-minute videotape depicting vignettes of critical care nursing practice situations. The videotape was produced for use in a variety of settings, especially those directed towards consumers. Other nonprint media productions include videotape presentations of advanced clinical topics and a project to develop audiovisual programs that will augment the critical care nursing core curriculum. To recognize accurate, realistic, and meaningful media portrayals of critical care nursing, AACN presents annual multimedia awards in broadcast and print categories. Nominations are submitted by association members.

Awards and scholarships extend beyond the multimedia awards. AACN offers educational advancement scholarships to member RNs who return to school for the bachelor's degree in nursing. Authors of award winning manuscripts on designated topics receive scholarships to attend the NTI. The scholarships are awarded in collaboration with a corporate sponsor. Annual awards also are made for creativity in critical care nursing and for critical care nurses who exemplify the art and the science of critical care nursing. Recognizing the importance of scientific investigation in the development of critical care nursing, AACN collaborates with corporate sponsors to present special awards for outstanding research. The award winners are among the presenters of research abstracts during the Scientific Sessions at each year's NTI.

To provide direction for research that would most benefit critical care nursing, AACN conducted a Delphi study that identified research priorities.[1] The association has since issued a compilation of research abstracts based on these priorities and established a grant program for research conducted by beginning nurse investigators. Grant applicants are encouraged to submit proposals for research that examines priorities from the Delphi study. Future research-oriented projects include developing a research design for study of a selected clinical topic by a nationwide group and establishing postdoctoral fellowships in critical care nursing. In recognition of the paramount importance of ethical standards in critical care research, a special task force has been commissioned to develop a position paper that will reflect the association's views on the subject.

Legislative and political issues exert an ever-increasing influence on the activities of all health care professionals. AACN's public affairs activities include careful monitoring of legislative and political issues with significant information reported to members through various publications and inhouse newsletters. An updated nursing resource list is available for local chapter members to link with other nursing groups in addressing issues of local or regional importance. AACN is a founding member of the National Federation for Specialty Nursing Organizations (NFSNO). The federation is a group of 28 nursing organizations that meet on a regular basis to "work toward coordination and cooperation among participating nursing organizations in matters that relate to nursing practice, education, and other matters of mutual concern." (NFSNO Minutes, June 28, 1981)

REFERENCE

1. Lewandowski LA, Kositsky AM: Research priorities for critical care nursing. *Heart Lung* 1983; 12:35–44.

Appendix 5–B

What Is a CCRN?

AACN established the CCRN Certification Program in 1975 in order to recognize professional competence in critical care nursing. Almost 18,000 critical care nurses hold current certification.[1] The certification program is administered by the association's subsidiary AACN Certification Corporation. The program is designed to promote professional competence in the nursing care of critically ill persons and their families by promoting high standards of care. Its specific objectives are—

- to establish the body of knowledge necessary for CCRN certification;
- to test through written examination the common body of knowledge needed to function effectively within the critical care setting;
- to recognize professional competence by granting CCRN status to successful certification candidates;
- to assist and to promote continual professional development of critical care nurses.[2]

Critical care nurses who currently are licensed as registered nurses in the United States and who submit documentation of at least one year's clinical experience caring for critically ill patients are eligible for candidacy. "Caring for critically ill patients" is defined according to the AACN scope of critical care nursing practice described earlier.

Candidates need not be members of any association or organization in order to apply for certification, nor are they required to join any association or organization upon certification. They take an examination that tests their ability to use data, to formulate problems, and to plan nursing care for critically ill patients and their families. This ability is tested in the context of critical illness in the following body systems: cardiovascular, pulmonary, renal, neurologic, endocrine, psychosocial, gastrointestinal, and hematologic. The examination stresses decision making and assesses knowledge of anatomy, physiology, and psychosocial aspects beyond that expected of a beginning graduate nurse.

CCRNs must recertify every three years in order to maintain the credential. Those who meet the recertification requirements, which include validation of current clinical practice in direct care of critically ill patients, can recertify either by accruing continuing education recognition points in designated categories—the option chosen by most recertifying CCRNs—or by retaking the certification examination.

In 1983, the Certification Corporation began a comprehensive role delineation and CCRN validation study. The study was designed to document the actual knowledge and skills required for the competent practice of critical care nursing. This information will provide the certification program with a sophisticated data base from which the certification examination can be further refined.[3]

REFERENCES

1. Sanford S: The challenge of adolescence. *Heart Lung* 1984; 13(4):26A.

2. AACN Certification Corporation: *CCRN Certification Program for Critical Care Nurses*. Irvine, Calif, The Corporation, 1982.

3. CCRN certification program study in progress. *Focus Crit Care* 1984; 11(2):70.

Chapter 6
Critical Care Nursing Education in a Neurotrauma Center—A Learning Contract

Jane E. Aumick and Susan T. Roberts

The impact of the critical care nurse on medicine today is significant because, as a professional, the nurse takes the initiative in answering the question, Why? The focus is on teaching, planning, implementation, assessment, and understanding; so with these skills, the critical care nurse is able to formulate nursing diagnoses and to deliver optimum patient care.

CRITICAL CARE NURSING EDUCATION

The components of critical care nursing skills include highly technical skills, a broad knowledge base, and an in-depth problem solving capability. The nurse then integrates these skills with a humanistic approach. Basic nursing experience must be obtained and educational requirements must be met before the nurse enters a critical care setting. Ideally, such a candidate would have previous experience in an intensive care unit.

One of the most important attributes of a critical care nurse is the ability to make a nursing assessment. A detailed physical assessment is completed, and—with additional clinical data—the interpretation of that assessment is followed by a nursing diagnosis. This nursing diagnosis then becomes the basis of the care the critically ill patient receives. The previous chapter discusses general aspects of critical care nurse training. In this chapter, we present specific examples of the total training program in neurotrauma, including drug use.

The nursing diagnosis begins by addressing the most immediate needs of the patient. To do this, the diagnosis is formulated in order of priority. Clearly, the critical care nurse must be an astute observer, determining the needs of the patient on the basis of time spent at the bedside and being the major care provider. The critical care nurse knows how, when, and what to report to the physician.

At the Maryland Institute for Emergency Medical Services Systems (MIEMSS) Neurotrauma Center (NTC), an orientation program has been started for the graduate nurse so that the nurse can gain intensive care experience while being aided in the transition from graduate nurse to critical care nurse (Exhibit 6–1). This process involves learning the skills needed to care for the unit's subacute population under a formalized learning contract. The learning contract uses the format and the concepts of adult learning and is designed to be completed independently. Although this contract is specifically related to this nursing unit, it could be adapted to any critical care area. The contract includes unit activities, protocols, primary nursing, and a total systems approach to the critically ill patient. Appendixes 6–A through 6–F provide copies of material used at the MIEMSS—NTC.

The graduate nurse is assigned a preceptor who evaluates the nurse's progress. A resource person to answer questions and to clarify any problems that might arise, the preceptor functions as a facilitator throughout the experience. At the NTC, the staff has found that the knowledge and the experience gained helps the graduate nurse in setting priorities that are essential in the care of critically ill patients.

The established registered nurse who enters the neurotrauma unit with several years experience receives a six-week orientation program that incorporates the use of a "Buddy Book" and a unit teacher (UT) as a mentor. The unit teacher assigns patients who will most benefit the nurse's learning experience to insure the nurse's

Exhibit 6–1 NTC Graduate Nurse Orientation Guidelines

Orientation is achieved in three phases:

Phase 1 *Special Care Unit Orientation*
- 1–2 wk of technical observation with the same clinical components
- 6–8 wk of clinical orientation with a unit teacher/preceptor
- Functions independently as a staff member in the special care area *only* for a period of 12 wk, after successful completion of Phase 1

Phase 2 *Independent Clinical Practice Special Care Area*
- Clinical learning contract provided by unit teacher
- Utilize unit teachers/primary nurses to assist in completing contract, and as clinical resources
- Independent learning focused on the Neurotrauma Center

Phase 3 *Intensive Care/Critical Care Unit Orientation*
- Begins after successfully demonstrating ability to care for the special care patients during 12-wk period completing learning contract
- 8 wk of clinical orientation with a unit teacher in the intensive care/critical area of NTC

adequate integration into the system. Inasmuch as education is an ongoing process, in-service programs, seminars, workshops, and staff days are provided also for the current staff. In addition, the staff nurse may request educational time whenever staffing allows. This system allows the staff nurse to pursue any area of special interest.

CRITICAL CARE NURSING AND PHARMACOLOGY

In any critical care area, questions about medications always arise. Several of these questions are common to all areas, and the nurse learns the answers to the commonly asked questions, along with suggestions about the procedure for finding answers to other questions. Commonly asked questions include the following:

- Will this drug be effective?
- Does this combination of drugs have any potential for incompatibility?
- How long will the effects of this drug be seen?
- Why is drug A being used, rather than drug B?
- What other medications may be infused through this same intravenous line?
- Can any crystalloid solution be used to infuse this drug?
- Does the line need to be flushed before and after this drug is infused?
- What side effects can be expected?
- How much time must elapse before this drug is totally eliminated?
- Will this drug continue to accumulate in the body?

Critical care nursing requires a solid working knowledge of medications—their indications, their common side effects, and the unique side effects of specific agents. Calculations such as drip rates, compatibilities and incompatibilities, and recommended dosages must be part of that working knowledge. Before any medication is administered, the dose, the route of administration, and the dosage must be specifically delineated. Although the physician makes these decisions, the nurse is held accountable for all actions and must accept responsibility for those actions. The nurse's responsibility begins with knowing the proper dosage, the effect to be expected when the medication is begun, and the side effects that may be expected that are unique to that specific agent. Knowing whether a drug is compatible with the solution through which it is infused and whether other medications can be simultaneously infused through the same line are also important factors in assessing drug therapy. Many times the nurse must anticipate the route and dose that the physician may desire. Throughout the educational process, information is given to the graduate nurse about how questions can be adequately answered.

Learning about medications and general pharmacology begins in the nursing school, and each institution develops its own plan for initiating the student nurse into the field of pharmacology. With the pharmacology book, the learning process is started. Drug cards also become a way of life, but after a graduate nurse has joined the ranks of professional nursing, many ask where a nurse can go from there to continue the educational process concerning drugs. The real understanding of drugs becomes apparent when the nurse is able to relate the knowledge of drugs to actual experience.

Each unit or floor in any given institution has a *Physician's Desk Reference* (PDR) and the hospital drug formulary, and so these reference books have become the backbone of drug information. At the MIEMSS neurotrauma unit, there is also an IV flowrate book that gives all of the vasoactive and cardiotonic agents in a variety of concentrations and also the flowrate in µg/kg/min and mL/h, depending upon the pump system used. Drugs found in this book include dopamine, dobutamine, sodium nitroprusside, epinephrine, norepinephrine, and lidocaine.

Another book developed at the MIEMSS center is a drug reference book that lists drugs by categories—narcotics, analgesics, corticosteroids, pressors, antibiotics, and others. This book lists the basic action of the drug; the effects and side effects common to that particular group of drugs, as well as recommended dosage

Exhibit 6–2 Most Widely Used Drugs in NTC

Neuro	*CVS*	*Drugs Common to Neuro and CVS*
methylprednisolone	KCl	naloxone
droperidol-fentanyl citrate	sodium nitroprusside	lidocaine
phenobarbital	nitroglycerin	furosemide
pentobarbital	αmethyldopa	pitressin
phenytoin	diazoxide	
mannitol	diphenhydramine	*Infection*
pancuronium bromide	Aquamephyton	ticarcillin disodium
d-tubocurare	dopamine	amikacin
diazepam	dobutamine	gentamicin
morphine sulfate	isoproterenol	tobramycin
meperidine hydrochloride	norepinephrine bitartrate	clindamycin
fentanyl citrate	calcium chloride	chloramphenicol
pitressin	atropine	nafcillin
furosemide	digoxin	
lidocaine	propranolol	*Respiratory*
naloxone	cimetidine	succinylcholine chloride
dexamethasone	$D_{50}W$	isoetharine
thiopental	insulin	
chlorpromazine	regular	*GI*
baclofen	NPH	Maalox
		Amphojel

ranges; the routes of administration; and the compatibilities for specific drugs. In an institution that uses nursing care plans, a drug teaching-tool may be included in the care plan for the patient receiving that drug. The drugs phenytoin and vasopressin are included at the MIEMSS center. Exhibit 6-2 provides a list of the drugs used most widely at the NTC.

A newer method used for learning about medications and formulating dosage and drip rates is the use of the bedside computer. Ideally, each two to three beds is a workable situation. The computer program—a joint effort on the part of the pharmacy, the nursing staff, and the physician—helps to eliminate or, at least, to decrease the chance of dosing error.

Drug surveillance programs have been instituted by the MIEMSS pharmacy to alert the physician and the nurse of potential interactions. Furthermore, the pharmacist, who has a more extensive library and up-to-date information, is available at all times to help solve problems concerning medications. The clinical pharmacist makes rounds daily, reviewing charts, making recommendations, and changing orders when necessary.

With the educational process and the learning contract completed, an examination is given to the graduate nurse. Upon passing the examination the nurse begins work in the neurotrauma unit in the critical care area.

Appendix 6-A
Learning Contract

Source: MIEMSS Neurotrauma Center.

Critical Care Nursing Education 107

Learning Objectives	Learning Strategy	Evidence of Accomplishment
Neurological		
Perform an accurate comprehensive assessment of head & spinal cord patients (acute & stable).	Read guidelines on neuro assessment. Read supplied articles. Seek out physical therapist; go over muscles on cord-injured patient. With assistance of bedside (if available) nurses in acute area, assess spinal cord or head patient and their assessment. Read ICP protocols; set up times to observe UT or PN while balancing Richmond screw or IVC.	Can assess cord- and head-injured patient accurately. Can repeat procedure.
Be able to care for patient on Stryker frame.	Read hints for turning patient on Stryker frame. Observe patient being cared for on Stryker frame (preferably UT). UT will give explanation of parts. UT will demonstrate procedure for safely pulling patient down on frame, TBurg and reverse TBurg X3.	Can repeat procedure to UT.
Be familiar with frequently used neuro drugs list.	Make drug cards for drugs related to neuro list enclosed.	Can complete drug questionnaire.

108   PRACTICE OF CRITICAL CARE PHARMACY

Learning Objectives	Learning Strategy	Evidence of Accomplishment
Be able to care for patient in halo tx or cervical tx (Gardner-Wells, halo vest).	Read emergency removal of halo vest article; see resource files and resource book. Outline procedure for pin care, CPT, skin care. UT will demonstrate safety checks.	Can repeat procedure for UT.
Be able to care for head-injured patient.	Read principles of hyperventilation. Describe signs and symptoms of herniation. Identify concussion, contusion, basilar skull, brain-stem injuries. List patient behaviors/symptoms acutely produced by injury. Review and read article on Glasgow coma scale.	Can repeat to UT what adequate range PCO_2 should be. Can give at least 3 S & S of herniation. Can score 3 patients with Glasgow coma scale.
Be able to care for spinal cord patient (acute & stable).	Refer to master care plan. Read articles provided for intermittent cath, bowel regimen, halo vest, spinal shock, autonomic dysreflexia, muscle testing and sensation levels, psychosocial and sexual problems. Initial spinal cord workbook.	Can show UT an accurate assessment and can list potential problems the cord patient may have.

Critical Care Nursing Education 109

Be familiar with diagnostic tests on the neuro-trauma patient.	Define CT scan, myelogram, lumbar puncture, arteriogram, ice water calorics, evoked potentials, tomograms. Check traveling schedule for day and assist patient and bedside nurse to area (preferably PN or UT).	Can tell UT procedure to travel with patient.

Respiratory

Perform an accurate assessment of respiratory system.	Read provided articles, listen to various patients' lungs, and check with resource person for verification of accurate assessment.	Show UT drawing of lungs; can describe different lung sounds; can demonstrate use of AMBU.
Identify anatomical landmarks of lungs and lung sounds.	Draw diagram—anterior and posterior view of all lobes.	
Be aware and know functions of equipment in intubation tray.	Read procedure book on intubation and extubation; read respiratory protocols; take short quiz after reading protocols.	Passing grade.
Identify ETT and trachs, face masks.	List sizes and types of respiratory airways and the differences between them.	
Be familiar with normal values for ABGs.	Read articles provided; describe technique for drawing ABGs; punch up various ABGs on computer, and see if you can recognize any abnormalities.	Discuss with UT whether answers are correct.

Learning Objectives	Learning Strategy	Evidence of Accomplishment
Acquaint yourself with Bear® ventilator.	Seek out respiratory therapist to get inservice on Bear® vent.	Date when received.
Be aware and know function of chest tubes and drainage chambers.	Read procedure for insertion of chest tube; read provided drainage chamber insert; using opened chamber in quiet area, familiarize self with different chambers; fill different chambers.	
Be able to state technique for stripping chest tube.	After reading protocol, practice stripping chest tube on open drainage chamber in quiet area.	Check with UT or PN; date and initial.
Be aware of a patient in acute respiratory distress.	Read provided articles; state S & S of respiratory distress.	State to UT the necessary nursing intervention for patient in distress.
Be able to perform chest physiotherapy (CPT) on acute head and spinal cord patient.	Set up time with physical therapist to receive inservice on CPT.	Perform CPT on patient with PT, UT, or PN present.
Cardiovascular (CVS)		
Be able to perform an accurate assessment of CVS.	Read articles.	Do assessment with UT.
Become familiar with monitoring system.	Call biomedical engineer and get inservice on monitor.	Take EKG, A-line, ICP strip.
Be able to identify PQRST wave forms in cardiac cycle.	Read provided article.	Take EKG strip measure QRS.

Critical Care Nursing Education   111

Be able to perform 12-lead EKG.	Initial demonstration by UT on placement of leads, marking strip, and trouble shooting machine.	
Be able to identify NSR, sinus brady, PVCs, ventricular tachycardia, and ventricular fibrillation and asystole.	Read provided article; measure PR, QRS intervals; determine rate and rhythm.	Have UT or PN check sheets.
Be familiar with normal values for CBC, electrolytes.	Collect data off computer of several patients; identify abnormals; read provided article.	Check with UT or PN for accuracy.
Be able to identify accurate wave forms for A-line, PA line, PCWP, CVP.	Read provided articles on invasive monitoring; observe monitors that have those lines on patient; draw wave forms for each; and take readings.	Show drawing to UT; state measurements, and explain what they mean.
Be aware of signs of shock (septic, hypovolemic) and treatment of each.	Read provided articles, make drug cards for drugs that may be used, do case study exercises.	Have drug cards and exercise checked by UT.
Be familiar with blood products, RBCs, FFP, plasma, platelets, volume expanders, albumin, and dextran.	Read provided article; read procedure for type and crossmatch and fill mock slip with Typenex®; if possible, observe patient getting plasma or fluid challenge.	State to UT the procedure for blood reaction.

Gastrointestinal (GI)

Be able to do accurate assessment of GI systems.	Read article; pick 2 patients in unit who are receiving tube feedings or had a minilap or some other abdominal incision or drain, and do assessment.	Check with UT whether assessment was correct.

112 PRACTICE OF CRITICAL CARE PHARMACY

Learning Objectives	Learning Strategy	Evidence of Accomplishment
Familiarize yourself with different types of gastric and intestinal tubes (Levine®, Salem®, Keofeed®, Dobhoff®); gastrostomy, jejunostomy.	Read provided information; pick 2 patients—each with different tubes—check placement and residuals, if being tube fed.	Answer 3 questions T or F: 1. Can you aspirate from a Dobhoff®? 2. A patient will receive Osmolite via a jejunostomy? 3. If residuals are > 200, will hold T.F.?
Be able to set up gastric wall, and Gomco® suction.	Use NTC attendance as resource to demonstrate how to set up; then, repeat procedure.	Demonstrate to UT or PN how to set up suction.
Be able to care for patient with elimination problems and need for bowel training.	Read articles provided.	Discuss why impaction is serious in head and spinal cord patients, and state to UT.
Be familiar with common GI drugs used in NTC.	Make drug cards for antacid, cimetidine, Peri-Colace, metoclopramide, and bisacodyl.	Be able to state to UT bowel regimen protocol.
Genitourinary (GU)		
Be able to do an accurate assessment of GU system.	Read bladder training program; test urine SP, *pH*, S/A, heme.	Describe bladder credé; demonstrate technique for intermittent cath sterilization.
Be able to understand and to execute actions pertaining to bladder training—with rationale.	Read procedure for insertion of Foley and intermittent cath (I.C.); locate cord patient on I.C.—read I & O fluid restriction and cath residuals.	Discuss purpose of fluid restriction; state why I & O is important.

Ortho/Skin

Be able to perform an accurate assessment of the musculoskeletal systems.	
Be aware of the traumatized patient's ability to breakdown skin.	Read procedure for care of Hoffman, Steinmann pins and for care of patient in cast. Demonstrate for UT (date and initial).
	List nursing responsibilities in restraining patient; have physical therapist demonstrate range of motion; read procedure book on application of Aqua K pad; find out 3 different ways to care for decubitus ulcer.

Infection Control

Be familiar with clean and sterile technique for dressing changes, opening trays, bottle and line changes.	Read Infection Control Manual; perform at least one complex and one simple sterile dressing under supervision of UT. Consistently follows standards by changing bottle, lines, and dressings as needed.
Be familiar with antibiotics used in NTC.	Make drug cards: amikacin, tobramycin, ticarcillin, nafcillin, cefoxitin. Be able to state to UT common side effects.
Be familiar with different types of isolation.	Use infection control officer as resource. Briefly describe the following blood and needle wounds: silk and strict.
Be familiar with fever pack.	Read protocol and procedure for patient with fever; if possible, observe patient getting one done. Return demonstration.

Critical Care Nursing Education 113

Learning Objectives	Learning Strategy	Evidence of Accomplishment
Primary Nursing		
Be familiar with and support primary nursing system.	The primary nurse on your team and UT will provide education to new clinical nurses in collaborative effort. Review the PN booklet: • How to fill out forms • Role of clinical nurse in primary nursing • Purpose of team system Do in-basket exercise (see Appendix 6-D).	Will cover for PN at least 2–3 times while on buddy system. Consistently utilizes PCP; show PN 2 data base forms complete; show PN 2 initial interviews complete; have PN check in-basket exercise for feedback.
Be able to admit patient and get necessary information for PCP.	Observe UT or PN admit patient; sit in on family interview, and read through various forms after filled out. Will attend at least 1 family conference.	Can repeat to UT or PN what needs to be done when patient is admitted.
Approximately 2 wk before completing orientation, you will have clear understanding of PN in NTC.	Meet with PN preferably on your team: review form/roles; answer questions; develop working relationship.	Can repeat to PN—to her satisfaction—what, how, and when forms and interaction with family take place.

| To be aware of the responsibilities of the charge nurse in NTC. | Read the Charge Nurse Handbook. Spend time with charge nurse, and observe her in action (sick call, report, status sheet). | Able to state to PN or UT charge nurse's responsibilities on each shift. |
| | Read disaster manual and role of NTC Charge Nurse. | Procedure for disaster. |

Appendix 6-B

Learning Contract Questions

1. What is a fever pack?
2. When is a fever pack done?
3. What does a fever pack consist of?
4. When does a doctor's verbal order need to be signed by the doctor?
5. How routinely are IV-line dressings changed?
6. How often do you change a hyperalimentation IV dressing?
7. What materials are needed to change an IV-line dressing?
8. What is considered cubicle "emergency equipment"?
9. What are the contents of the intubation tray?
10. What is a Thora-Drain III?
11. How often are narcotics counted in 24 hours?
    In the NTC, who is responsible for doing the narcotic count?
12. What is an IVC?
13. What is a Richmond screw?
14. Who can draw arterial blood gases?
15. What is the protocol for drawing arterial blood gases?
16. What is the procedure to follow in the case of an arrest in the NTC?
17. Who responds to the arrest call in the NTC?
18. How often is the distilled water at the bedside changed?
19. What is the major difference between the Bear® respirator and the Engstrom® respirator?
20. When you are doing patient care in the NTC, where will (could) your signature appear?
21. If a patient has blood on hold and you need three units available to you quickly, where can it be stored?
22. Who must check a unit of blood before it is hung?
23. What is the procedure for checking blood?

Critical Care Nursing Education   117

24. What is the nurse's responsibility before hanging the blood on the patient (assuming all the numbers check out)?
25. What equipment is needed to insert a chest tube? Where are the items located?
26. What equipment is needed to insert a pulmonary artery catheter? Where are items found?
27. What equipment is needed to insert a radial arterial line? Where are items located?
28. List the equipment needed to insert a femoral arterial line. Where is it located?
29. Who does 24-hour patient assessments?
30. Who copies over the treatment sheet?
31. What is a mini-lap? When is it usually done? Where?
32. What is a combo tray?
33. Who can remove sutures from a mini-lap incision?
34. What is the aortogram cart? When is it used?
35. When is a complete systems assessment done on a patient?
36. How often do tube feeding setups get changed?
37. How often do irrigation setups get changed?
38. Who updates the diet Kardex?
39. What are the nurse's responsibilities in administering insulin?
40. What are the nurse's responsibilities in administering digoxin?
41. What is Cidex? Where is it?
42. Volume expanders—what are they? What is available in the NTC? Where are they located?
43. What is the stock refrigerator? Where is it located? What medications are in the refrigerator?
44. IV stock solutions—what is available in NTC?
45. Emergency drug box—what are the contents?
46. Name three instances when you would stat page physicians.
47. Where is the oxygen turn-off valve?
48. Where is the extension cord for arrests in subacute?
49. What are the red plug outlets for?
50. What do you do if you have an arrest in subacute area? Where can you get a Doppler machine? Where are the x-ray machine outlets?

Appendix 6-C

Respiratory Therapy Quiz

1. Who is responsible for ventilating the patient during an arrest?
2. Who is responsible for intubating a patient?
3. Who will make order changes on ventilator?
4. What is the nurse's responsibility when a patient is extubated?
5. When will the respiratory therapist accompany the patient being transported?
6. What is the name of the test performed to test collateral circulation in the hand before getting radial blood gas?
7. What are the nurse's responsibilities when RT is doing cardiac output on a patient?
8. List some adverse problems that may be encountered 15 seconds after an endotracheal suctioning.
9. How often should a ventilated patient be suctioned? What may he be lavaged with?
10. How often are the ventilator circuits changed?

Appendix 6-D

Case Study Exercises

Situation 1

A 17-yr-old white girl has been admitted to NTC with a gunshot wound to the left temporal area. At present, she remains in coma (GCS of 4); she is being hyperventilated and has a Richmond screw. You are covering for the PN. You were updated by her about the situation at home. You find out that the circumstances surrounding the shooting are unclear; Mom and Dad are not convinced that the GSW was self-inflicted. There was no evidence of drugs or alcohol on board. The pregnancy test was negative.

Mom and Dad are extremely anxious; how can you help?
Several phone calls are coming in from the girls' school; to whom should you direct them?
Police want information on the case; who can give it to them?
An impromptu family conference has been arranged; where would you document this?

Situation 2

The patient was admitted to AA with C5C6 subluxation after a diving accident; he is 16 yr old, president of his class, and an A student. John needed to go to OR for reduction upon admission at 7 P.M. He arrived in the NTC at 2400 hours. His parents have been waiting in the waiting room since admission and have received little information.

As the admitting nurse, you have gotten the patient admitted and situated. What would you do next?
What forms do you need to fill out?
How would you go about setting up a calling schedule and visitation?

Situation 3

Mr. Hanes is a 30-yr-old white man admitted to NTC after a traffic accident. He has a closed head injury. His condition is deteriorating. His wife is the family spokesperson. You are covering for his primary nurse. Numerous phone calls are coming into the unit about him. You find out he is an aide to the Governor.

What information can be given out?
Who should handle the numerous phone calls coming in?
What are your responsibilities as a relief nurse?

Appendix 6-E

Unit Questions

1. What is the procedure for using the reference books in the Quiet Area?
2. What is the Communication Book? Where can you find it?
3. Where are the resource files, and who may use them?
4. What is the in-service book, and where is it located?
5. What is "green time"? Who may get it? How can you get it?
6. What is an anecdotal? Who writes them? How are they used?
7. How many personal leave days are you allotted? How are they used?
8. What is a sick letter?
9. What times does shift report begin?
10. How do you find out when staff meetings occur?
11. How much vacation time can you take in the summer months?
12. Who is the Associate Nurse Supervisor?
13. Who is the clinical specialist in NTC?
14. Where are two places in which you would find telephone numbers of the staff?
15. Where is the personnel office located?

Appendix 6-F

Drug Questionnaire

1. What is the lethal side effect of pentobarbital?
2. In which tube is a pentobarbital serum level sent? Which slip, and how is it marked? Which laboratory is it sent to?
3. Can tube feedings be given to a patient in pentobarbital coma?
4. How fast can phenytoin be given IV?
5. Through what solution must phenytoin be given? Why?
6. What side effect must the nurse be aware of when giving phenytoin IV?
7. Do patients on pancuronium bromide need pain medication? Why?
8. What two simultaneous side effects of pancuronium bromide must the nurse be aware of (related to CVS)?
9. Can you put a patient who is on pancuronium bromide on continuous positive airway pressure?
10. What is dopamine used for?
11. What changes would you see in a patient's urine and serum osmolarity after giving pitressin?
12. For what must a nurse check mannitol before injection?
13. Where should an IM injection be given to a spinal cord patient? Why?
14. Why is lidocaine used for a head patient?
15. What two drugs should be checked with another nurse before administration?
16. What are two drugs you must flush with NSS before and after administration? What happens if you don't?
17. What is the difference between mannitol and Osmitrol?
18. Why do you wrap the IV tubing and bag in foil when administering sodium nitroprusside?
19. What drug is given to reverse the effects of narcotics?
20. What is succinylcholine chloride, and where is it kept?
21. In what aspect could thiopental sodium be used in NTC?

Critical Care Nursing Education 123

22. What is fentanyl citrate, and how is it used?
23. What are the side effects of giving potassium IV?
24. State a reason for giving methylprednisolone to head and spinal cord patients.
25. List two things you need to be aware of in the use of methylprednisolone.
26. What is baclofen? Why is it used? What are the major side effects?
27. What is another name for cimetidine? What is it used for? What is a side effect of its use?
28. State the antagonist used for heparin and warfarin?
29. When using IV solutions or meddrips made up by the pharmacy, what is your responsibility?

Part II
Present and Future Roles

Chapter 7

The Pharmacist in Surgical Intensive Care and Anesthesiology

Deborah K. Armstrong, Joseph F. Dasta, Michael Schobelock, and Philip J. Schneider

The three objectives in developing pharmacy services in critical care areas are meeting the needs of the patient, the medical and nursing personnel, and the Pharmacy Department. To meet these needs, the current medication distribution system should be evaluated for three to six months. This review reveals problems with the current system and ways to develop medical and nursing personnel trust and confidence. Such a preliminary period can also be used to develop clinical pharmacy services and to establish the pharmacist as an important member of the critical care team.

With the implementation of prospective payment programs in hospitals, approval of new services would be contingent then on the ability to reduce overall costs rather than on the generation of revenues. An evaluation of the pharmaceutical needs of the surgical intensive care unit (SICU) and operating room (OR) must consider several areas. Justification of the pharmacy services can be accomplished through cost containment measures, improved drug distribution systems, development of clinical pharmacy services, education, and research. Areas of cost containment include improved drug control, accurate charging methods, decreased drug inventories, and promotion of rational drug therapy. Pharmacy services are traditionally poorly accessible to critical care areas and the OR. This is true because of the large volume of drug use and the need for immediate availability of medications. A properly designed satellite pharmacy can alleviate many of the problems of a more traditional drug distribution system and can improve the rapport between nursing and pharmacy by providing drugs in a timely manner.

The positive impact that pharmacy services have had on the anesthesiology department, the OR, and the critical care areas has been reported.[1-7] These reports have described pharmacy satellites in OR or ICU areas that improve the drug distribution system and enable rapid response to the immediate needs of these perioperative areas. In addition to the reduction in floor stock, inventory, and lost charges, the pharmacist developed rapport with and generated support from nurses and anesthesiologists.[2,3,5,7,8] In one study, efficient drug distribution systems and accurate patient billing have been reported to save up to $12,000 annually upon the implementation of an anesthesiology-OR satellite pharmacy.[9] Improved drug control in the OR has also been reported as a result of the establishment of anesthesiology medication exchange trays.[3,7,9]

Promoting rational drug therapy through clinical pharmacy services can potentially result in decreased drug costs and improved patient care. By providing direct consultative services, conducting inservice lectures and developing drug therapy protocols, the clinical pharmacist can influence prescribing patterns. Along with these basic pharmacy services, education of pharmacy students and research designed to answer therapeutic questions are also responsibilities of the critical care pharmacist—particularly in a teaching hospital.

DESCRIPTION OF THE SICU AREA

The fourth floor of the Ohio State University (OSU) hospitals contains 21 ORs, a 12-bed recovery room, a pre-op holding area, and the SICU. The SICU is divided into three areas: general surgery intensive care (10 beds), thoracic surgery intensive care (11 beds), and neurosurgery intensive care (6 beds). The typical patient population in the general surgery section includes those who have had major abdominal surgery, gun shot wounds, multiple trauma, and vascular surgical procedures. It also includes any patient admitted to the general surgery department who requires intensive monitoring and support. The cardiac surgery patient is admitted postoperatively to the thoracic ICU.

In 1982, the number of patients admitted to the general and thoracic surgery units was 1,210. The average length of patient stay was three days. The neurosurgery unit, which opened in July 1982, admitted 280 patients during the first five months. Patients admitted to this unit have undergone major neurosurgical procedures or have suffered major head trauma requiring close monitoring. The average daily census figures for the three units are shown in Table 7–1.

Each patient cubicle is equipped with bedside patient monitors capable of displaying, recording, and trending systolic, diastolic, and mean arterial blood pressure, heart rate, EKG, central venous or pulmonary artery pressures, and intracranial pressure. Because most patients require ventilatory support, several different types of ventilators are used, including an investigational high-frequency jet ventilator.[10] Three respiratory therapists are assigned to the area each shift and are responsible for the maintenance and operation of the ventilators. They also generate a list of respiratory parameters on each ventilated patient and perform blood gas determinations.

Table 7-1 SICU Admission and Discharge Data

	Sun.	Mon.	Tues.	Wed.	Thur.	Fri.	Sat.
Total average daily census	15.6	14.4	18.2	20.3	19.5	20.1	15.7
Average daily admissions—thoracic surgery	0.3	3.3	3.1	1.4	3.0	3.2	0.4
Average daily admissions—general surgery	1.2	3.2	2.6	1.7	1.6	3.2	1.0
Average daily admissions—neurosurgery	0.5	1.5	1.1	1.0	1.0	1.5	0.4
Total average daily admissions	2.0	8.0	6.8	4.1	5.6	7.9	1.8
Total average daily discharges	3.6	5.1	5.2	5.2	5.9	7.5	4.7

Source: Ohio State University Hospitals.

Each patient is assigned to one nurse. Nurses administer all medications with the exception of certain intravenous (IV) push drugs. Pertinent patient information is transcribed onto a nursing flowsheet (Exhibit 7-1). This form has sections for recording vital signs, input and output, pulmonary information, and blood or urine chemistry data. A new sheet is generated every day. Nursing assessment notes are written on the back of the form. The information on these flowsheets is widely used by physicians, pharmacists, students, and the nursing staff because it provides a current record of patient status. Dosing charts for dopamine, dobutamine, nitroglycerin, nitroprusside and epinephrine are located at the bedside. Dosages of these drugs are often ordered in micrograms per kilogram per minute and the pharmacist works closely with the nurse in calculating proper flow rates of drugs.

ADMINISTRATIVE CONSIDERATIONS—DRUG DISTRIBUTION CONTROL

Control of drug distribution is a challenge throughout the hospital but poses a particular problem in the perioperative area. This area annually consumes about twice the dollar value of drugs in comparison to traditional patient care areas. The critical nature of drugs extends throughout the perioperative units, with problems attendant to each division. Controlled substance discrepancies, due to either poor record keeping or drug diversion, are a continuing problem. Excessive or inaccurate drug ordering causes inefficiencies of labor and potential patient harm. The OR is often supplied by systems that do not meet the recommendations of the Joint Commission on Accreditation of Hospitals (JCAH). A review of the OR is likely

130 PRACTICE OF CRITICAL CARE PHARMACY

Exhibit 7–1 Nursing Flowsheet

Surgical Intensive Care and Anesthesiology 131

Exhibit 7-1 continued

Exhibit 7–1 continued

Exhibit 7-1 continued

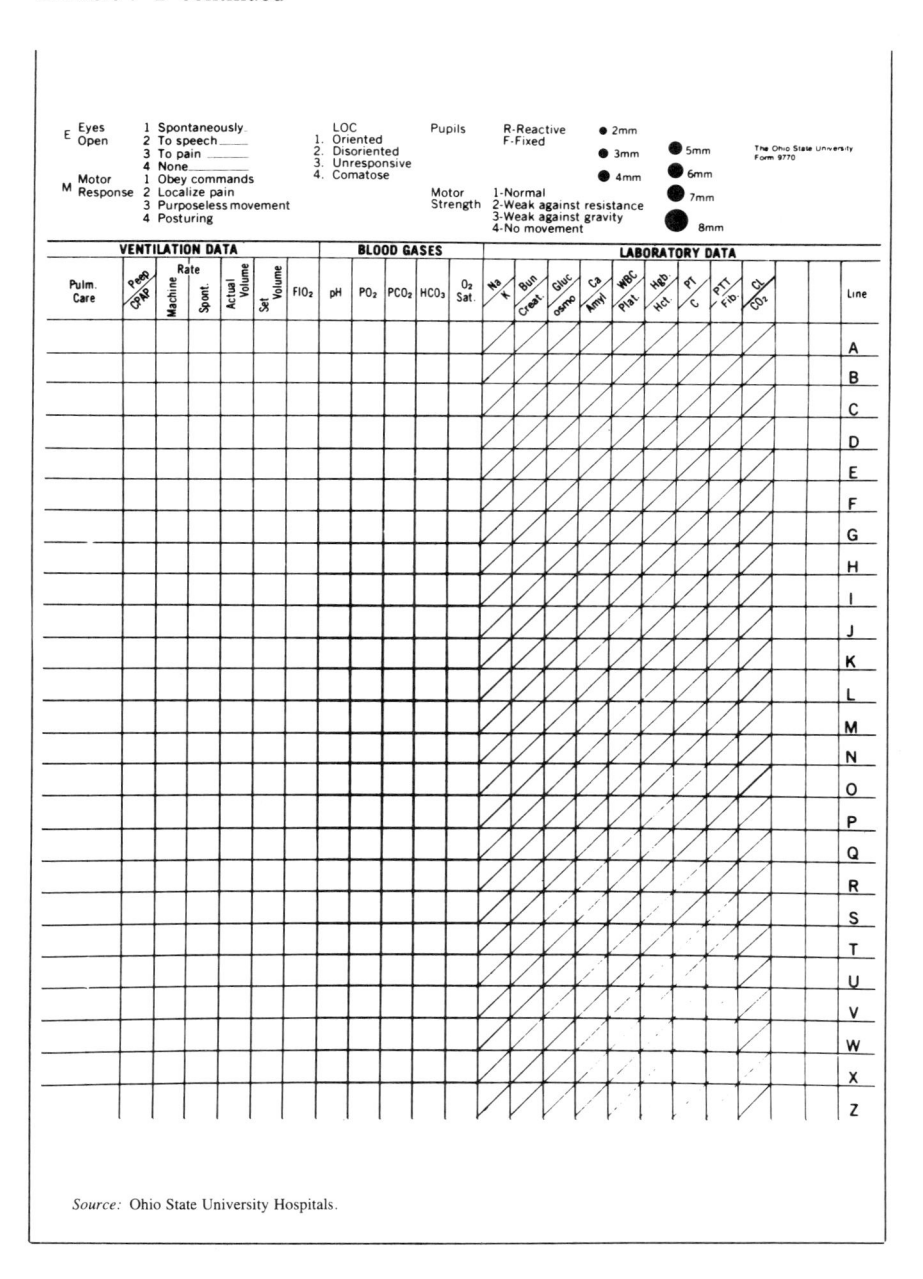

E Eyes Open	1 Spontaneously 2 To speech 3 To pain 4 None	LOC 1. Oriented 2. Disoriented 3. Unresponsive 4. Comatose
M Motor Response	1 Obey commands 2 Localize pain 3 Purposeless movement 4 Posturing	

Pupils R-Reactive F-Fixed
● 2mm
● 3mm
● 4mm
● 5mm
● 6mm
● 7mm
● 8mm

The Ohio State University
Form 9770

Motor Strength
1-Normal
2-Weak against resistance
3-Weak against gravity
4-No movement

VENTILATION DATA	BLOOD GASES	LABORATORY DATA	Line
Pulm. Care	Peep/CPAP	Rate Machine	Spont.	Actual Volume	Set Volume	FIO₂	pH	PO₂	PCO₂	HCO₃	O₂ Sat.	Na/K	Bun/Creat	Gluc/osmo	Ca/Amyl	WBC/Plat	Hgb/Hct	PT/C	PTT/Fib	Cl/CO₂	

Lines A through Z

Source: Ohio State University Hospitals.

to reveal drug control problems, including the presence of expired drugs and lack of security precautions for controlled substances such as prefilled sodium thiopental syringes left on a tray in an unsupervised supply room.

A method of supply common to all service areas is usually the floor-stock system. The JCAH discourages use of this system for several reasons:

- There is no routine monitoring for expired drugs.
- There is poor continuity in removing recalled drugs from inventory.

A decentralized pharmacy in the perioperative area addresses these problems by eliminating the need to maintain most floor stocks of medications, ensuring the proper charging of medications, preventing the supply of expired or recalled medications to patient care areas, and involving the pharmacist in the distribution and control of drug products.

The appropriate assignment of charges for medications and inventory control is also a problem in the perioperative system. The critical nature of patient care makes charge assignment a relatively low priority activity for nursing and associated personnel. The high volume of drug use in the area further complicates the problem.

Drug products used in the area are usually supplied through an anesthesia storeroom. To resolve this problem, a "blanket" drug charge is usually assessed regardless of the drugs used. This system does not allow the accurate assignment of the cost of drugs used for each patient. Identification of individual patient care expenses is a fundamental premise of any drug reimbursement program and makes patient charges easier to understand and to justify. Further, maintenance of drug stockrooms requires that drugs be charged twice through the hospital accounting system: once to transfer from the pharmacy to the OR and once from the OR to the patient.

Intensive care areas are usually supplied medications from the pharmacy in multiday patient supplies. Medications left over when orders are changed or patients discharged are frequently retained on the unit and sent to the pharmacy when time allows. Delay in processing these credits reduces the pharmacy's ability to credit the patient's account for drugs not used.

When floor-stock systems are used, problems occur if vouchers are not returned and patients are not charged. When new supplies are needed for the unit and vouchers have not been sent, the nursing unit is charged, increasing the unit's costs of operation. The hospital can substantially reduce these lost charges if a 24-hour unit-dose system is implemented to reduce or eliminate the need for floor-stock supplies of medications. Charging for drugs can occur at the point of distribution. Credits can be more efficiently processed there because of the proximity of the patient care area and increased pharmacy awareness of order changes and patient transfers.

Also needing improvement are the availability of medications and pharmacist interaction in the areas. A decentralized approach allows the provision of more types of drugs commonly used in the area within a few steps of the patient's bedside. When medications that are not stocked in the perioperative areas are needed, it is usually necessary to obtain them from the main pharmacy. Considerable time and inconvenience can be saved when these orders are supplied in the patient care area through a satellite pharmacy. Access to a satellite eliminates the supplier's need to manipulate protective attire in order to obtain medications. Proximity to the units also allows pharmacy personnel to become familiar with and to observe closely the routine of the areas. Their familiarity as well as the increased communications that the satellite concept fosters helps to decrease medication supply and patient charging problems.

The JCAH Standards for Pharmaceutical Services specify pharmacist involvement in patient care as an integral feature of the accredited hospital. It is recommended that the pharmacist review all medication orders before dispensing medication. According to the JCAH, the pharmacist should also review a direct copy of the physician's orders and maintain a profile of the patient's medication orders, neither of which is possible under a floor-stock system.

Another responsibility of the pharmacist under the standards is to compound IV admixtures under optimal conditions. When the department of pharmacy cannot actually compound admixtures, it is charged with the duty of supervising admixture techniques. Nurses and anesthesiologists usually compound a variety of admixtures that should be prepared by pharmacy personnel to ensure optimal conditions and proper labeling and technique. Nonpharmacy personnel may continue to compound some admixtures, but the pharmacist can be available to assure proper technique, stability, and compatibility.

Thus, the pharmaceutical needs of the perioperative area are amply justified. It is usually easy to obtain support from the surgery, anesthesia, and nursing departments once they recognize the adverse impact of these problems on the quality of patient care, their own time to practice, and the legal posture of their areas of practice. This support is invaluable in gaining administrative approval for a proposal to develop a decentralized pharmacy program in the perioperative areas.

PROGRAM DESCRIPTION

Preliminary Activities

Clinical pharmacy activities began when a faculty member of the College of Pharmacy became interested in developing a practice in the SICU. With the approval of the co-directors of the SICU and after discussions with the Department of Pharmacy, he began attending teaching rounds in January 1981. It quickly became evident that there was a great need for clinical pharmacy involvement and a substantial potential for practice, teaching, and research. Because of the Department of Pharmacy's clinical program in other areas of the hospital the physicians were familiar with the pharmacist's contributions. The SICU nurses' main contact with a pharmacist, however, was by telephone for medications needed for their patient and drug information questions. To gain exposure and to develop rapport, a series of nursing inservice lectures was presented on topics such as basic pharmacokinetics, antibiotics, catecholamines, and vasoactive drugs. Also, an all day seminar on drug therapeutics was developed and was attended by over 100 nurses from Ohio and neighboring states. The pharmacist was available for questions by nurses and an active effort was made to inform the nurses of pertinent information about the drugs they were administering to their patients.

The first substantial clinical involvement was to formulate a protocol for ordering and drawing blood for drug level analysis. Before this protocol, random blood samples for drug analysis had been drawn, and the results of tests were often uninterpretable. Basic principles of pharmacology and therapeutics were discussed during teaching rounds, and recommendations of changes in drug therapy were made. Although the faculty members' time allocated to clinical practice in the SICU was limited primarily to the morning, the role of the clinical pharmacist as a provider of drug therapy information was established.

During the second year of the SICU program, the College and Department of Pharmacy jointly developed a cardiovascular and critical care residency. Two post-Pharm.D. residents were recruited; each spent three months in the SICU. The physicians and nurses were becoming accustomed to continual clinical pharmacy coverage.

Several audits of the area were conducted at this time by the Department of Pharmacy. The results revealed certain violations of JCAH guidelines and a significant number of lost charges. In an effort to improve drug distribution, to establish appropriate drug control measures, and to develop a continuity of clinical services, a satellite pharmacy was proposed and approved. Two pharmacists with Pharm.D. degrees and residencies were hired in August 1982. These two persons and a faculty member share in the provision of the unit's clinical services and educational activities 16 hours per day with a rotating on-call system for weekends.

Clinical Services

Because surgeons spend much time in the OR, an SICU co-management team was formed. The team cares for the acute needs of the patient and provides an interface between the patient and the physicians performing the surgery. The SICU team consists of the SICU co-directors (an anesthesiologist and a surgeon), an anesthesiology and surgical resident, two to three medical students, the nurse caring for the patient, and the clinical pharmacist.

Monitor Patient Medication

The clinical pharmacist is an active member of the multidisciplinary team and attends daily patient care rounds to offer expertise in the selection of appropriate drug therapy. Many of the critically ill patients have multiple system organ failure and often receive 10 to 20 medications.[11,12] The pharmacist provides expertise in patient medication monitoring to ensure that the appropriate dosage, route of administration, and duration of drug therapy are optimized. Many surgical patients require close hemodynamic monitoring to ensure maximum cardiac output and tissue oxygenation.[13] The pharmacist's guidance in the selection of appropriate cardioactive medications is essential to ensure maximum cardiac function. A hemodynamic profile flowsheet is used for selected patients (Exhibit 7–2). A hand-held calculator has been programmed to calculate many of these parameters. Based upon the data generated, the response to drug therapy can be quickly assessed and necessary changes can be implemented. The use of pulmonary artery catheters is common in these patients. Because drugs are frequently infused through these devices, the pharmacist is careful to evaluate potential drug incompatibilities and to assess the time required for drug-containing fluids to be delivered to the patient. A recent study reported that the time required for fluids to traverse from the outer connection hub to the proximal injectate port of the pulmonary artery catheter ranged from 28 seconds at a flow rate of 99 drops/min to 335 seconds at a flow rate of 10 drops/min.[14] This delay in drug delivery must be considered when evaluating the patient's response to drugs.

Monitor Patient Nutrition

Many critically ill surgical patients require nutrition support; here the pharmacist's ability to monitor the patient is beneficial. At OSU hospitals, a pharmacist is a full-time member of the nutrition support team. All problems and major changes with the solutions are coordinated with the SICU pharmacist in order to assure accurate interpretation of orders and to decrease wasted solutions.

Pharmacokinetic Consultation

Another key area in which the pharmacist's expertise is used is pharmacokinetics. With complex medical problems, the SICU patient requires close monitoring of drugs with narrow therapeutic indices (i.e., theophylline, lidocaine, procainamide, phenytoin, and the aminoglycosides).[15] The aminoglycoside antibiotics are an important component of the antibiotic therapy for intraabdominal sepsis, a common problem in the SICU. Triple antibiotic coverage (tobramycin,

Exhibit 7–2 Hemodynamic Profile Flowsheet

Patient Name and Number				
Diagnosis				
Surgery/Date				

Hemodynamic Monitoring Flowsheet

Date/Time				
Drugs/Fluids	DOP __ ug/kg/min DOB __ ug/kg/min Epi __ ug/min Norepi __ ug/min NTG __ ug/min NTP __ ug/kg/min ISO __ ug/min	DOP __ ug/kg/min DOB __ ug/kg/min Epi __ ug/min Norepi __ ug/min NTG __ ug/min NTP __ ug/kg/min ISO __ ug/min	DOP __ ug/kg/min DOB __ ug/kg/min Epi __ ug/min Norepi __ ug/min NTG __ ug/min NTP __ ug/kg/min ISO __ ug/min	DOP __ ug/kg/min DOB __ ug/kg/min Epi __ ug/min Norepi __ ug/min NTG __ ug/min NTP __ ug/kg/min ISO __ ug/min
PRESS A*				
CO (4-6.5) 1				
Sys Press 1				
Dias Press 2				
MAP (80-95) 3				
HR (80-95) 4				
MPA (10-25) 5				
PAO (2-12) 6				
CVP (2-12) 7				
(BSA) 8				
PRESS B*				
SV (45-60)				
CI (3-4)				
SI (30-35)				
RVSW (10-15)				
RVSWI (4-8)				
LVSW (60-80)				
LVSWI (44-68)				
SVR (1200)				
PVR (200)				
MVO$_2$C				
PEEP/FIO$_2$				
IMV/V$_t$				
Hgb (11-13) 0				
FIO$_2$ 1				
PaCO$_2$ (35-45) 2				
PaO$_2$ 3				
Art Sat 4				
P$_v$O$_2$ 5				
Ven Sat (65-80) 6				
PRESS C*				
C$_c$ (18-20)				
C$_v$ (11-14)				
Ca (16-19)				
A-VO$_2$ (4-5)				
O$_2$Del (1000)				
O$_2$ Cons (250)				
O$_2$ Util (25%)				
Qs/Q$_t$ (2-6%)				
Qs/Qt Flow				
Pul Cap Flow				

Source: Ohio State University Hospitals.

ampicillin, and clindamycin) is used to treat the likely abdominal source of pathogens such as Gram-negative rods, enterococci, and anaerobic microorganisms.[16] Surgical patients may require larger volumes of intravenously administered fluids and blood products during surgery that can affect the disposition of the aminoglycosides. An example of a tobramycin pharmacokinetic consultation often seen in SICU is shown in Appendix 7–A.

Surgical patients spend three to four days in the SICU during which time their hemodynamic status can change markedly. These changes often require adjustments of their aminoglycoside dosage. A pharmacokinetic flowsheet has been developed (Exhibit 7–3) to improve follow up on their dosage adjustments. The pharmacokinetic flowsheets are also used as data collection forms for various research projects.

Aggressive therapy and monitoring of the aminoglycosides are necessary to assure maximal drug concentrations. In a recent study, 59% of peak serum tobramycin concentrations were less than 5 µg/mL when critically ill patients received the standard 2 mg/kg loading dose.[17] Pharmacokinetic parameters of the aminoglycosides are frequently generated after the first dose. After the subsequent dosage regimen is implemented, peak and trough serum concentrations are frequently obtained (daily in some patients). Problems such as liver and renal failure, "third spacing" of fluid, and hemodynamic instability affect the disposition of these and other drugs. The pharmacist's pharmacokinetic expertise is an important contribution to the critical care team, because a pharmacist's primary role is to maximize the therapeutic effects of drugs.

Inasmuch as infections are a common problem in surgical patients,[18] the clinical pharmacists have also established a bacteriologic data collection sheet that contains the culture reports of the patients. The need for monitoring the culture and sensitivity data was determined after an audit demonstrated up to a five day delay before the final report entered the patient's chart. The pharmacist (or student) obtains data from the bacteriology laboratory daily, records the information on the data collection sheet, and helps to interpret minimum inhibitory concentrations of the drugs for the organism and the site of infection in order to determine the most appropriate antibiotic regimen. This information is discussed with the physician, and antibiotic therapy is instituted or changed when the need arises.

IV Phenytoin Preparation

Another area of clinical involvement was the preparation of guidelines for IV infusion of phenytoin. All patients were previously receiving phenytoin by IV push (50 mg/min), which required administration by a physician. Problems encountered with this system included erratic timing of doses due to physician surgery schedules, too rapid administration of phenytoin resulting in hypotension, and administration of phenytoin through IV lines containing incompatible fluids or drugs.

After the literature on the stability of phenytoin in IV solutions had been reviewed,[19-24] guidelines for IV infusions of phenytoin were prepared (Exhibit 7–4). The goals of the program were to implement a system whereby

Exhibit 7-3 Pharmacokinetic Flowsheet

DRUG	Tobramycin	DATE STARTED	1/2/83	PATIENT NAME

DIAGNOSIS	MODIFYING FACTORS	MEDICATION PROFILE	C&S MIC
Colon CA; *Pseudomonas* pneumonia; 1/7/83, colon resection (exp.lap.)	☐ Liver disease ☐ Smoker ☐ Obesity ☐ CHF ☒ Renal compromise ☐ Other	Ticarcillin, 3 g IV q 6 Flagyl, 500 mg IV q 6	1/2—*Pseudomonas* Sputum MIC tobramycin ≤ 1 ticarcillin 4 1/7—Sputum 3⁺ *Pseudomonas aeruginosa* blood ⊖, urine ⊖ 1/8—Sputum 3⁺ *Pseudomonas* tobra ≤ 1, ticar 4 Blood—*E.coli* tobra ≤ 1, ticar 8 Urine—*E.coli* tobra ≤ 1, ticar 8

Sex __F__ Ht (in) __66__ LBW(kg) __59.3__ pre-op(kg) __72__   Consult date __1/7/83__   Billed __X__

Date*	Wt(kg)	WBC*	Tmax	BUN/Cr*	CrCl (mL/min)	I/O	Dosage*	Time Dose*	Levels mg/L*	Time of Levels*	Kel (h⁻¹)*	t1/2 (h)	Vd (L/kg)*	Cl (mL/min)	Comments
1/7	72 preop	19⁴	101ᴿ	30/3.0	19.5 est	4280 1800	80 mg IV q 12 h	— 11P.M.							Received 18 L crystalloid during surgery
1/8	82	16⁵	101⁸ᴿ	27/2.7		2500 2700	80 mg q 12 h	11A.M. 11P.M.	2.2 mg/L 4.3 mg/L 2.5 mg/L	11A.M. 12:30A.M. 10P.M.	.057	12	31.9 L (0.39 L/kg)	30.3	Cpo = 4.6 mg/L; change to 180 mg IV q 24 h
1/9	78	14⁰	100ᴿ	23/2.5	24-h CrCl pending	2700 2580	180 mg	8A.M.							
1/10	76	10²	99ᴷ	20/2.5	28	2450 4690	180 mg	8A.M. 8A.M.	14 mg/L 7.2 mg/L	8A.M. 9:30A.M.	.071	9.7	31.0 L (0.41 L/kg)		Transferred to floor

Note: * = Items are mandatory.
Source: Ohio State University Hospitals, Department of Pharmacy.

Exhibit 7–4 Guidelines for IV Infusion of Phenytoin

1. Phenytoin is compatible only with 0.9% and 0.45% NaCl.
2. A standard concentration of 3 mg/mL is to be used to decrease the incidence of microcrystallization.
3. The intravenous line must be flushed with 20 mL of 0.9% NaCl before *and* after infusing phenytoin to prevent crystallization of drug in the tubing.
4. The infusion rate is not to exceed 25 mg/min.
5. All infusions must be filtered with 0.45 micron, in-line filter.
6. All infusions must be prepared in glass bottles to allow visual inspection for crystals.
7. The infusion should be administered within four hours of preparation.
8. In the event of hypotension or arrhythmias, the infusion should be stopped and the physician should be notifed.

Source: Ohio State University Hospitals, Department of Pharmacy.

nurses could administer the drug safely and provide consistent delivery of the medication to the patient. After the guidelines were approved by the medical director of the unit and nursing administration, an inservice lecture was given to the nursing staff on IV infusions of phenytoin.

Since the start of this program, 94 patients have received IV infusions of phenytoin during the first nine months—a total of 394 doses. No cases of visible precipitation of phenytoin have occurred. Because of the implementation of this program, delivery of the medication to the patient has been improved. This improvement has been accomplished by allowing consistent timing of daily doses, decreasing the incidence of hypotensive episodes, and increasing staff awareness of the incompatibilities of phenytoin. The physicians and nurses have been pleased with this project. A similar system has since been reported in the literature.[25]

Emergency Drug Dosing

Finally, cardiac arrest situations are coordinated by the SICU personnel. An emergency drug box is located on the unit. An emergency drug dosing chart has been prepared and is kept in each drug box. The chart is reproduced in Table 7–2.

Drug Distribution Services

The original drug distribution system in the SICU consisted of a three-day supply of medications prepared by the central pharmacy. Oral medications were delivered to the unit in unit-dose packages, whereas IV drugs were sent unreconstituted or in syringes prepared by the manufacturer. The expansion of the therapeutic role of the pharmacist has served as a strong foundation for the development of the SICU pharmacy satellite at OSU hospitals. The challenge was

Table 7-2 Emergency Drug Dosing Chart

Drug	Usual Dose	Maximum Dose	Administration	Adverse Effects
Atropine	0.5 mg q 5 min[3]	2.0 mg[3]	IV: 30 sec[2]	< 0.5 mg—paradoxical bradycardia
Bretylium	5–10 mg/kg[2,3]	30 mg/kg[2,3]	IV: 1 min (v fib)[4] IVPB: 8–10 min (v tach)[3] Infusion: 1–4 mg/min[6]	Increasing arrhythmias, hypotension
Calcium Chloride	500 mg q10 min[3]	N/A	IV: 4–5 min[2]	Hypotension, bradycardia, vein irritation
Dobutamine	2.5 μg/kg/min[3]	20 μg/kg/min[3]	IV Infusion	Tachycardia, arrhythmias
Dopamine	2.5 μg/kg/min[6] (2–5 μg/kg/min)[1]	30 μg/kg/min[6]	IV Infusion	Tachycardia, vasoconstriction
Epinephrine	0.5–1 mg q5 min[3]	N/A	IV: slow push Infusion: 1–8 μg/min[6] (1–5μg/min)[2]	Vasoconstriction, rapid push: arrhythmias, increased blood pressure
Isoproterenol	1–4 μg/min[6] (0.5–5 μg/min)[4]	N/A	IV Infusion	> 120 beats/min causes ventricular arrhythmias
Lidocaine	Loading dose[3]: 1 mg/kg	N/A	IV: 50 mg/min[2] Infusion: 1–4 mg/min[2,3]	CNS disorders, ventricular arrhythmias
Norepinephrine	8–16 μg/min[1,6] (8–12 μg/min)[4]	N/A	IV Infusion	Reflex bradycardia, hypertension, arrhythmias, vasoconstriction
Phenylephrine	0.1–0.5 mg[4]	1 mg[3] (single dose)	IV: rapid push	Hypertension, bradycardia

Procainamide	Loading dose: 14–17 mg/kg[7]	1 gm[1,3] (single dose)	IV: 50 mg/min[1,2] Infusion: 1–4 mg/min[3]	Hypotension, ventricular tachycardia
Propranolol	1 mg q5 min[3]	N/A	IV: 1 mg/min[4]	Bradycardia, intensifies AV block
Sodium Bicarbonate	1 mEq/kg[3]	N/A	IV: push	Metabolic alkalosis, hypokalemia, hypernatremia
Verapamil	0.075–0.15 mg/kg[2,4]	N/A	IV: 2–3 min[4] Infusion: 0.125–0.375 mg/min[5]	AV block, rapid IV push causes hypotension

Notes:

1. *Physicians' Desk Reference*, ed 38. Oradell, NJ, Medical Economics, 1984.
2. Katcher BS, Young LY, Koda-Kimball MA (eds): *Applied Therapeutics: The Clinical Use of Drugs*, ed 3. San Francisco, Applied Therapeutics, 1983.
3. Advanced cardiac life support. *JAMA* 1980;244:484–487.
4. McEvoy GM (ed): *American Hospital Formulary Service: Drug Information*. Washington, DC, American Society of Hospital Pharmacists, 1984.
5. Reiter MJ, Shand DG, Pritclett ELC: Comparison of intravenous and oral verapamil dosing. *Clin Pharmacol Ther* 1982;32:711–720.
6. Standard clinical practice at the Ohio State University Hospitals.
7. Taylor WJ, Finn AL (eds): *Individualizing Drug Therapy: Practical Applications of Drug Monitoring*. New York, Gross, Townsend, Frank, 1981, vol 3.

Source: OSU Hospitals, Department of Pharmacy; prepared by Deborah K. Armstrong and Lori J. Kratz.

to provide consistent pharmacy services to all critical care areas on the fourth floor with the resources allocated: 2.0 full-time equivalent (FTE) pharmacists and 2.8 FTE technicians.

Evaluation

It was first necessary to evaluate the current system and to propose alternatives for existing problems. The areas considered were these:

- improving the existing drug control system to decrease lost charges and drug costs and to meet JCAH accreditation standards
- improving the accessibility of pharmacy services to the perioperative area
- decreasing the waste of drugs associated with the multiday supply
- improving the quality of drugs prepared for parenteral administration
- improving the control of narcotics used in OR
- decreasing drug inventory (i.e., floor stock).

Several projects were implemented to evaluate these areas, including:

- inventory of medications located in the OR and floor stock in each unit
- evaluation of lost charges with subsequent list posted for nurses on high cost items (e.g., albumin) charged to unit
- data collection of medication orders to evaluate efficiency of current pharmacy services
- observation of techniques used by nonpharmacy personnel in preparation of medications for parenteral use or naso-gastric tube administration (e.g., crushing tablets)
- review of narcotic discrepancies.

Some of these projects were completed by the SICU pharmacists; remaining projects were finished by a pharmacy technician. All projects will be reevaluated after the institution of the satellite pharmacy in order to assess its impact on these problem areas.

Other projects were completed to evaluate the workload and timing of functions for the proposed services of the satellite. Data were collected to evaluate the number of orders written per day (categorized into the hours as well as the number of doses of medication to be distributed per day). This information was used along with the number of admissions in order to determine optimal staffing patterns.

A major project was to tabulate the information available on the stability of drugs (Appendix 7–B)—especially antibiotics prepared in syringes. The nurses in the unit administer most IV medications and all IV fluids through a volume control system in order to document fluid intake accurately. After much debate, it was decided to prepack most medications in syringes (unless this option was limited by lack of stability). The reasons for this approach include the lower cost of syringes versus the minibag, less fluid added to patient's intake, and the variable rate of administration and drug delivery with conventional minibag and administration sets.[26] A drug compatibility chart was prepared for drugs commonly used in our unit (Table 7-3). An emergency drug dosing chart also was prepared, including recommended doses, rates of administration, and common adverse effects (see Table 7-2). These charts are kept on each crash cart.

Implementation

The implementation of the satellite pharmacy is occurring in several steps. The presatellite phase has involved the integration of the pharmacists into the SICU team. During this period, the projects previously described were completed (i.e., evaluating the needs of the area, the patients, and the staff).

Phase I, currently being implemented, will provide a 24-hour unit-dose medication supply system. The hours of service will be 7:00 A.M. to 11:00 P.M. Monday through Friday; Saturday and Sunday, 8:30 A.M. to 5:00 P.M.; but because of a delay in space renovation, the pharmacy services will operate from the central pharmacy. Another service that will be initiated in Phase I is the restructuring of the narcotic supply system in the OR. Currently, the anesthesiologists sign out narcotics (in the pre-op holding area) needed for the day. In anticipation of the amount of drugs needed to cover all cases, excessive quantities are often signed out. Poor record keeping leads to large discrepancies in annual audits of narcotic usage. In an attempt to improve narcotic accountability, a narcotic medication box exchange system will be implemented. The anesthesiology resident or certified registered nurse anesthetist will sign out a narcotic box each morning. A plastic lock will be broken, and the contents will be verified (4 fentanyl 50 µg/mL, 20 mL ampules; 2 morphine sulfate 15 mg/mL syringes; 2 meperidine 100 mg/mL syringes; 2 diazepam 5 mg/ml syringes). The anesthesiologist will keep a balance sheet of the amount of medication used per case. At the end of the day the anesthesiologist will waste opened ampules and syringes. This procedure will be witnessed and verified on the balance sheet. The box will be relocked with the second plastic lock (in the box); then it will be placed back in the locked cabinet. During the evening shift, the pharmacy technician will collect all boxes used during the day and will replace all narcotics used. The next day, any discrepancies are discussed with the anesthesiologist who had signed out the box. This system provides stricter record keeping as well as a mechanism to charge each patient for the medication given. In our previous system, it was difficult to trace discrepancies. A smaller amount of narcotics for use in emergencies is provided in the pre-op holding area. The last goal of Phase I will be to decrease available floor stock after the initiation of the 24-hour medication supply system.

Table 7-3 Drug Compatibility Chart

Drug (pH)	Aminophylline	Atropine	Bretylium	Calcium Chloride	Digoxin	Dobutamine	Dopamine	Epinephrine	Isoproterenol	Lidocaine	Nitroglycerin	Norepinephrine	Phenylephrine	Potassium Chloride	Procainamide	Sodium Bicarbonate	Verapamil
Aminophylline (8.6–9)	N/A	N/A		X	C		C	X	X	C	C	X	C	C	C	C	C
Atropine (3.5–6.5)	N/A		N/A	C	C	C	C	X		C	C	X				X	C
Bretylium (5–7)		N/A		C					C	C				C		C	
Calcium Chloride (6–7.5)	X	C		N/A	N/A	#	C	X	C	C		C				X	C
Digoxin (6.6–7.4)	C					N/A								#			
Dobutamine (2.5–5.5)	C	C		C			C	X		C				C		X	
Dopamine (3–4.5)	C	C		C		N/A		X		X				C		X	
Epinephrine (2.5–5)	X	X		X					N/A	X		X		X		X	
Isoproterenol (3.5–4.5)	X			C				N/A		N/A				C		C	
Lidocaine (6–7)	C		C	C	C			X	X		C	X	C	C		C	C
Nitroglycerin (3–6.5)	C						C	X	X	C		X	C	C			C
Norepinephrine (3–4.5)	X	X	C	C		C	C	X	C	X	N/A		N/A	C		X	
Phenylephrine (3–6.5)	C									C	N/A	C		C		C	
Potassium Chloride (4–8)	C		C	C		C	C	X	C	C		C	C				C
Procainamide (4–6)	C									C						N/A	
Sodium Bicarbonate (7–8)	C	X	C	X		X	X	X	X	C		X	C		N/A		N/A
Verapamil (4.1–6)	C	C			C									N/A	C	N/A	

Notes: X = Incompatible; C = Compatible; # = Compatible up to 4 hours; blank space = Insufficient information; N/A = Not applicable.

1. King JC: *Guide to Parenteral Admixtures*. St. Louis, Cutter Laboratories, 1984.
2. Trissel LA: *Handbook of Injectable Drugs*. Washington, DC, American Society of Hospital Pharmacists, 1983.
3. Personal communications from manufacturers.

Source: OSU Hospitals, Department of Pharmacy; Prepared by Deborah K. Armstrong and Lori J. Kratz.

Phase II will be implemented after Phase I is fully operational. This next step will involve the preparation of all IV admixtures and solutions and the prepackaging of standard concentrations of dopamine, dobutamine, and nitroglycerin, as well as maintenance solutions containing KCl. Although Phase II may be instituted without renovation of satellite space, it will not be able to provide "stat" medications and will require the nurses to compound some medications, such as IV methylprednisolone.

Phase III will be completed as the pharmacy satellite opens and expands pharmacy services to provide for "stat" medications to the SICU, the OR, and the recovery room. Implementation of this last phase will allow for a further reduction in floor-stock medications for all perioperative areas. The satellite pharmacy will continue to provide service during the hours of 7 A.M. to 11 P.M., Monday through Friday; coverage for Saturday and Sunday will be provided by a technician supervised from the central pharmacy area. Although it would be ideal, 24-hour service cannot be provided without additional personnel.

The satellite pharmacy will be 235 sq. ft. It will contain a laminar flow-hood, computer terminal for patient profiles, billing, and IV labels, and a refrigerator-freezer, and storage space for medications needed to fill the unit-dose cart and to prepare parenteral medications for the OR, the recovery room, and the SICU. The stocking of the satellite will be done daily by the technician.

Educational Programs

The SICU is a required one-month rotation during the second year of the Pharm.D. program (Exhibit 7–5). The student is responsible for monitoring three to five patients in the general surgery section and participating in patient care rounds. The Pharm.D. preceptors meet with the students daily to discuss assigned patients. In addition, the following topics are discussed during the month: use of ventilators, hemodynamic monitoring, acid-base balance, fluid therapy, use of vasoactive and inotropic drugs, antibiotic therapy, stress ulcer prevention, and pharmacokinetics in the critically ill patient. These discussions center around principles of patient monitoring and drug therapeutics while the student is being challenged about therapeutic alternatives. Students complete written pharmacokinetic consultations that are reviewed by the preceptor before they are placed in the patient chart. The students present one formal patient case and several informal inservice lectures to nurses and medical students.

This area is also a required three-month rotation for students in the advanced residency in critical care pharmacy. Enrollment in this program requires an advanced degree and a desire to specialize in critical care pharmacy practice. During the year, residents also rotate through medical and coronary intensive care, emergency medicine, nutrition support, and other internal medicine areas. Residents are responsible for monitoring all patients in the SICU; however,

Exhibit 7–5 SICU Pharm.D. Clerkship Syllabus

A. Introduction and Goals

The SICU clerkship is a one-month required experience for Pharm.D. II students. The student is required to complete a minimum of 200 clock hours during this rotation. The goals of the SICU clerkship include the following:

1. To provide the student with the opportunity to develop his/her knowledge of pharmacotherapeutics through the application of drug knowledge in the setting of acute patient care
2. To enhance the quality of patient care via the student's acceptance of responsibility in providing clinical pharmacy service
3. To develop the student's confidence in his/her abilities to practice in an interdisciplinary setting
4. To guarantee that the student attains a set of competencies in the practice of clinical pharmacy and attains a minimum knowledge base in the specialty area of critical care

B. Objectives

In order to successfully pass the clerkship, the Pharm.D. student must demonstrate by written examination, oral challenge, and daily performance, his/her ability to do the following:

1. To communicate drug information to other members of the health care team either verbally or in writing
2. To detect any drug-induced problems that may be contributing to the patient's current illness, including adverse drug effects, drug-drug interactions, and interference with laboratory tests
3. To recommend an appropriate approach to the management of drug-induced problems
4. To assess the risk to benefit ratio of various therapeutic alternatives and develop a therapeutic plan and expected therapeutic endpoints
5. To develop individualized dosage regimens based on a knowledge and application of pharmacokinetics
6. To communicate the plan of therapy to the SICU team both verbally and in writing
7. To select appropriate subjective and objective parameters to assess the patient's response to therapy
8. To actively follow the patient's course and progress in an organized fashion to assess the response to therapy
9. To recommend rational alternative treatment when the initial plan fails to achieve therapeutic endpoints or results in adverse effects
10. To retrieve, evaluate, and communicate information obtained from the medical literature regarding pharmacotherapeutics
11. To establish an effective and cooperative working relationship with other members of the SICU team
12. To develop educational skills by providing inservice lectures to nurses and physicians

Exhibit 7–5 continued

C. Specific Activities

1. Conduct one nursing inservice lecture.
2. Attend daily workrounds (7:00 A.M.) and teaching rounds (9:00 A.M.).
3. Attend selected lectures in the medical student orientation series and Department of Anesthesiology resident lecture series.
4. Attend weekly SICU grand rounds.
5. Present one formal case presentation per week.
6. Monitor therapy of patients.
7. Be responsible for pharmacokinetic consultations.
8. Present selected articles at journal club.

Source: Pharm.D. Program, OSU College of Pharmacy, Division of Pharmacy Practice.

emphasis is placed on general surgery and on patients in thoracic and neurosurgery with special pharmacological needs. Residents are given more responsibility than Pharm.D. students for patient care activities, such as attendance at work rounds and follow-up on problems. They also provide several informal case presentations, nursing inservice lectures, and one formal seminar.

This one-year residency was begun in 1981 and was one of the first to be offered. Since that time, several critical care residencies have been developed. For example, in the 1983 to 1984 Residency and Fellowship Programs listing by members of the American College of Clinical Pharmacy, there are five critical care pharmacy residencies or fellowships, including the program at OSU. It is clear that critical care is becoming an important area of specialization, and the SICU plays an important role in its development.

Finally, second-year students in the combined M.S. and residency program in hospital pharmacy can elect this area for a one-month rotation. They are exposed to clinical pharmacy practitioners and are responsible for monitoring the drug therapy of assigned patients.

Research Activities

The loss of nitroglycerin to pulmonary artery catheters is an example of research projects that have been completed to date.[27] This study was begun because of the increased use of the drug and the lack of information available on the sorption characteristics of nitroglycerin to patients with pulmonary artery (Swan-Ganz®) catheters.

Another study was designed to determine the proper sampling time for obtaining peak tobramycin levels in abdominal surgery patients. The results suggested that the initial distribution period of tobramycin among our patients was variable.[28] Patients with infected ascitic fluid are often treated with tobramycin. The penetration characteristics of tobramycin into this fluid are incompletely understood. A study was designed to characterize the disposition of tobramycin into ascitic fluid in two patients with abdominal catheters placed to drain fluid. Simultaneous serum and ascitic fluid samples were obtained for tobramycin. Adequate concentrations in ascitic fluid were found with peak concentrations occurring three to six hours after the infusion of the drug.[29]

Infected patients with renal failure who received amikacin were also studied, because the hemodialyzability of amikacin is poorly documented. The hemodialysis clearance of amikacin was evaluated in eight patients. Minimal drug is lost during the three to four hour dialysis period, suggesting that routine supplemental doses of the drug are not always needed in this setting and should be guided by a two hour post dialysis serum level.[30]

Other projects that are in progress include the use of a continuous verapamil infusion in supraventricular arrhythmias, evaluation of the potential interaction between dopamine and haloperidol, tobramycin pharmacokinetics in trauma patients, evaluation of the effect of dopamine on tobramycin clearance, and cost containment methods in the ICU.

These research efforts have one common theme: the attempt to answer questions encountered in clinical practice with the ultimate goal of improved patient care. The critical care environment provides a constant stimulus for clinical investigation, and the pharmacist can play a vital role in the development and implementation of research projects.

REFERENCES

1. Moritani D, Stein ZLG: Operating room pharmacy: A new subspecialty. *US Pharm* 1981;6:H2–H6.

2. McAllister JC, Murray WJ, Skolaut MW, et al: A new look at pharmacy services in the operating suite and recovery room. *Contemp Pharm Pract* 1980;3:6–10.

3. Evans, DM, Guenther AM, Keith TD, et al: Pharmacy practice in an operating room complex. *Am J Hosp Pharm* 1979;36:1342–1347.

4. Rose BF: Planning and operation of a surgical suite pharmacy. *Hospitals* 1976;50:107–109.

5. Caldwell RD, Tuck BA: Justification and operation of a critical-care satellite pharmacy. *Am J Hosp Pharm* 1983;40:2141–2145.

6. Holt MR: The ICU pharmacy, in Chernow B, Lake CR (eds): *The Pharmacologic Approach to the Critically Ill Patient.* Baltimore, Williams & Wilkins, 1983, pp 133–139.

7. Powell PJ, Maland L, Bair JN, et al: Implementing an operating room pharmacy satellite. *Am J Hosp Pharm* 1983;40:1192–1198.

8. Edmondson G: Impact of a satellite pharmacy IV service upon ICU nurses' attitudes. Abstracts, 18th Annual Midyear Clinical Meeting, American Society of Hospital Pharmacists. Atlanta, 1983, p 125.

9. Hague B, Maland L, Powell PJ, et al: The anesthesiology/operating room pharmacy. *Anesthesiology* 1983;59:A478.

10. O'Rourke PP, Crone RK: High-frequency ventilation. A new approach to respiratory support. *JAMA* 1983;250:2845–2847.

11. Borzotta AP, Polk HC: Multiple system organ failure. *Surg Clin North Am* 1983;63:315–336.

12. Campos RA, Herraez FX, Marcos RJ, et al: Drug use in an intensive care unit and its relation to survival. *Intensive Care Med* 1980;6:163–168.

13. Sibbald WJ, Calvin JE, Holliday RL, et al: Concepts in the pharmacologic and nonpharmacologic support of cardiovascular function in critically ill surgical patients. *Surg Clin North Am* 1983;63:455–482.

14. Kahn JK, Kirsh MM: The infusion delivery time of the flow-directed pulmonary artery catheter: Clinical implications. *Heart Lung* 1983;12:630–632.

15. Dasta JF: Pharmacokinetics of drugs in critically ill patients. *Syva Monitor* 1982;11:1–10.

16. Snyder SK, Hahn HH: Diagnosis and treatment of intra-abdominal abscess in critically ill patients. *Surg Clin North Am* 1982;62:229–239.

17. Summer WR, Michael JR, Lipsky JJ: Initial aminoglycoside levels in the critically ill. *Crit Care Med* 1983;11:948–950.

18. Meakins JL, Wicklund B, Forse RA, et al: The surgical intensive care unit: Current concepts in infection. *Surg Clin North Am* 1980;60:117–132.

19. Baumann JL, Siepler JK, Fitzloff AH: Phenytoin crystallization in intravenous fluids. *Drug Intell Clin Pharm* 1977;11:646–649.

20. Cloyd JC, Besch DE, Sawchuk RJ: Concentration-time profile of phenytoin after admixture with small volumes of intravenous fluids. *Am J Hosp Pharm* 1978;35:45–48.

21. Salem RB, Yost RL, Torosian G, et al: Investigation of the crystallization of phenytoin in normal saline. *Drug Intell Clin Pharm* 1980;14:605–608.

22. Pfeifle CE, Adler DS, Ganaway WL: Phenytoin sodium stability in three intravenous solutions. *Am J Hosp Pharm* 1981;38:358–362.

23. Giacona N, Bauman JL, Siepler JK: Crystallization of three phenytoin preparations in intravenous solutions. *Am J Hosp Pharm* 1982;39:630–634.

24. Carmichael RP, Mahoney CD, Jeffrey LP: Solubility and stability of phenytoin sodium when mixed with intravenous solutions. *Am J Hosp Pharm* 1980;37:95–98.

25. Ganaway WL, Wilding DC, Siepler JK, et al: Clinical use of intravenous phenytoin sodium infusions. *Clin Pharm* 1983;2:135–138.

26. Armistead JA, Nahata MC: Effect of variables associated with intermittent gentamicin infusions on pharmacokinetic predictions. *Clin Pharm* 1983;2:153–156.

27. Jacobi J, Dasta JF, Reilley TE, et al: Loss of nitroglycerin to pulmonary artery delivery systems. *Am J Hosp Pharm* 1983;40:1980–1982.

28. Dasta J, Jacobi J, Armstrong D, et al: Importance of sampling time on determining tobramycin pharmacokinetics in abdominal surgery patients. Abstract, American Society of Hospital Pharmacists, Atlanta, 1983.

29. Hodgman T, Dasta JF, Armstrong DK, et al: Tobramycin disposition into ascitic fluid. *Clin Pharm* 1984;3:203–205.

30. Armstrong D, Hodgman T, Visconti J, et al: Hemodialysis of amikacin in critically ill patients. *Drug Intell Clin Pharm* 1983;17:437.

Appendix 7–A

Pharmacokinetic Dosing Service Consult Protocol

1. Provide a patient care summary, including patient's age, weight, recent antibiotic therapy (recent serum drug levels), recent bacteriologic culture data, and OR procedure and volume of fluid received in OR.
2. Pertinent laboratory data should be listed for last 24 to 36 hours, including temp. profile, WBC (differential if available), BUN/SCr, urine output trends, and 24-hour Crcl—if available.
3. Provide a summary of previous aminoglycoside dosing regimen, including LD (if given), date, time, and MD regimen.
4. Provide a summary of aminoglycoside serum levels (date, time).

Assess the above data, and recommend appropriate dosing regimen to achieve therapeutic serum concentrations; include calculated volume of distribution (Vd, L/kg), elimination half life (t½), and total clearance.

Case Example

A 71-year-old white woman admitted 1/1/83 with a history of colon CA and *Pseudomonas* pneumonia has been treated with ticarcillin and tobramycin (MIC *Pseudomonas* 1/2/83 to tobramycin, ≤ 1 mg/L). Patient admitted to SICU 1/7/83 post colon resection and exp. lap. Patient received 18 L crystalloid during surgery. Post op wt, 82 kg (ideal body weight, 57 kg; pre op wt, 72 kg). Patient is currently receiving ticarcillin, 3 gm, IV q 6 hr; tobramycin, 80 mg, IV q 12 hr; and flagyl, 500 mg, IV q 6 hr. No tobramycin serum levels are available.

Source: OSU Hospitals, Department of Pharmacy.

	Date	I/O	BUN/SCr	WBC	Seg/band	Tmax
Other laboratory data	1/1/83	...	45/4.3	26[4]	72/18	103°
	1/7/83	4280/1800	30/3.0	19[4]	...	101[R]
	1/8/83	...	27/2.7	16[5]	...	101[8R]

Tobramycin 100 mg LD given 1/2/83, followed by 80 mg IV q 12 hr; last dose of tobramycin given at 11 P.M. upon admission to SICU after surgery. Recommend obtaining tobramycin serum levels on next dose (11:00 A.M.) as follows: predose level, 60 min post dose level after 30 min infusion, and a level 10 hours after this dose. Latest cultures from 1/7/83 of sputum: 3+ pseudomonas aeruginosa (Gram stain 4+ WBC, 3+ Gram-neg rod). Blood and urine cultures negative. Intraoperative cultures pending. Because of the large amount of fluid this patient required, patient may have large aminoglycoside volume of distribution which necessitates increasing the dose until patient diureses the extra fluid. Patient's renal function appears to be improving, but a 24-hour urine for creatinine will help our assessment.

Will follow with you.   Thank you.

                                     _____
                                     Name

                                     _____
                                     Beeper No.

Follow-up Note:

Tobramycin: Serum levels obtained on 80-mg IV dose on 1/8

Date	Serum Levels	Time
1/8	2.2 mg/L	(predose) 11 A.M.
	4.3 mg/L	(60 min postdose) 12:30 P.M.
	2.5 mg/L	(10.5 h postdose) 10:00 P.M.

Other Data:

Date	BUN/SCr	I/O	WBC	Tmax	Wt	Crcl
1/8	27/2.7	2500/2700	16[5]	101[8R]	82 kg	...
1/9	23/2.5	...	14[0]	100[R]	78 kg	Pending

Recent Cultures:

1/8	Leukens	—3⁺ *Pseudomonas*	MIC tobramycin ≤ 1 mg/L, ticar 4 mg/L
1/8	Blood	*E. coli*	MIC tobramycin ≤ 1 mg/L, ticar 8 mg/L
	Urine	*E. coli*	MIC tobramycin ≤ 1 mg/L, ticar 4 mg/L

From the above information and the tobramycin serum concentration/time curve this patient's calculated volume of distribution is 31.9 L (.39 L/kg) and elimination half life is 12 hours. To achieve therapeutic serum concentrations in the patient with *Pseudomonas* pneumonia and *E. coli* bacteremia, a dosing regimen of 180 mg IV q 24 hours should provide peak serum concentration of 6.5 to 7.0 mg/L and a predose serum concentration 1.5 to 2.0 mg/L.

Recommend predose level and 60 min postdose level on 2nd dose of 180 mg tobramycin. Dosing regimen will need to be aggressively followed as patient begins diuresing.

Thank you. Will follow patient with you.

Appendix 7–B

Stability Data on Concentrated Intravenous Drugs

Solution	Concentration	Temperature	Stability	Reference
AMPICILLIN				
Sterile water for injection	Up to 30 mg/mL	Room	8 h	1
Sterile water for injection	30 mg/mL	Refrigerate	48 h	1
Sterile water for injection	Up to 20 mg/mL	Refrigerate	72 h	1
Sterile water for injection	In vial	27°C	1 h	2
Sterile water for injection	In vial	5°C	4 h	2
Sterile water for injection	In vial	−20°C	48 h	2
CEFAMANDOLE				
Sterile water for injection	Not given	Room	24 h	3
Sterile water for injection	Not given	Refrigerate	96 h	3
Sterile water for injection	1 g/3 mL	−20°C	52 wk[a]	4 (p 81)
Sterile water for injection	1 g/3.5 mL	−20°C	9 mo[b]	4 (p 81)

Source: OSU Hospitals, Department of Pharmacy.

Solution	Concentration	Temperature	Stability	Reference
CEFAZOLIN				
Sterile water for injection	In vial	Room	24 h	5
Sterile water for injection	250 mg/mL	25°C	4 d	4 (p 85)
Sterile water for injection	In vial	5°C	96 h	5
Sterile water for injection	In vial	−20°C	12 wk[a]	5
Sterile water for injection	1 g/2.5 mL	−20°C	26 wk	4 (p 85)
Sterile water for injection	10 g/45 mL	−20°C	26 wk	4 (p 85)
Sterile water for injection	1 g/3 mL	−20°C	9 mo[b]	4 (p 85)
CEFOTAXIME[d]				
Sterile water for injection	50–180 mg/mL	Room	24 h	6
Sterile water for injection	50–180 mg/mL	Room	24 h[c]	6
Sterile water for injection	50–180 mg/mL	Refrigerate	10 d	6
Sterile water for injection	50–180 mg/mL	Refrigerate	5 d[c]	6
Sterile water for injection	50–180 mg/mL	Frozen	13 wk	6
Sterile water for injection	50–180 mg/mL	Frozen	13 wk[c]	6
CEFOXITIN				
Sterile water for injection	1 g/10 mL	Room	24 h	7
Bacteriostatic water	1 g/2 mL	25°C	48 h	4 (p 88)
Sterile water for injection	1 g/10 mL	Refrigerate	1 wk	7
Bacteriostatic water (benzyl alcohol)	1 g/2 mL	5°C	1 mo	4 (p 88)

Surgical Intensive Care and Anesthesiology

Solution	Concentration	Temperature	Stability	Reference
CEFOXITIN continued				
Sterile water for injection	1 g/10 mL	Refrigerate	48 h[e]	7
Sterile water for injection	1 g/10 mL	Room	24 h[e]	7
Sterile water for injection	1 g/10 mL	Frozen	48 h	7
Bacteriostatic water (benzyl alcohol)	1 g/10 mL	−20°C	30 wk[f]	4 (p 88)
CEPHALOTHIN, NEUTRAL				
Sterile water for injection	Not given	Room	12 h	8
Sterile water for injection	Not given	Refrigerate	96 h	8
Sterile water for injection	Not given	−20°C	12 wk[g]	8
Sterile water for injection	100–230 mg/mL	−20°C	6 wk	4 (p 92)
Sterile water for injection	1 g/5 mL	−20°C	9 mo[b]	4 (p 92)
CEPHAPIRIN[h]				
Sterile water for injection	20–400 mg/mL	Room	12 h	9
Bacteriostatic water	20–400 mg/mL	Room	48 h	9
Sterile water for injection	20–400 mg/mL	Refrigerate	10 d	9
Bacteriostatic water	20–400 mg/mL	Refrigerate	10 d	9
Sterile water for injection	20–400 mg/mL	−15°C	60 d	9
Bacteriostatic water	20–400 mg/mL	−15°C	60 d	9
CHLORAMPHENICOL				
Sterile water for injection	1 g/10 mL	Room	30 d	4 (p 105)
Sterile water for injection	1 g/10 mL	Frozen	6 mo	4 (p 105)

Solution	Concentration	Temperature	Stability	Reference
DOBUTAMINE HYDROCHLORIDE				
D_5/LR	1 mg/mL	25°C	48 h[i]	10
D_5/0.9	1 mg/mL	25°C	48 h[i]	10
0.45 NaCl	1 mg/mL	25°C	48 h[i]	10
GENTAMICIN				
	. . .	. . .	30 d[j]	4 (p 202)
ISOPROTERENOL				
D_5W	4 mg/L	Room	30 m[k]	4 (p 253)
MEZLOCILLIN				
Sterile water for injection	10–100 mg/mL	Room	48 h	11
Sterile water for injection	Up to 250 mg/mL	Room	24 h	4 (p 304)
Sterile water for injection	10–100 mg/mL	Refrigerate	7 d	11
Sterile water for injection	10–100 mg/mL	−12°C	28 d	11
MOXALACTAM				
Sterile water for injection	1 g/3 mL	25°C	96 h	2
Sterile water for injection	1 g/3 mL	5°C	96 h	2
NAFCILLIN				
Sterile water for injection	Up to 250 mg/mL	Room	3 d	4 (p 317)
Sterile water for injection	Up to 250 mg/mL	Refrigerate	7 d	4 (p 317)
Sterile water for injection	250 mg/mL	−20°C	9 mo[b]	4 (p 317)
NITROPRUSSIDE				
D_5W	5 mg/100 mL	Room	24 h	12

Solution	Concentration	Temperature	Stability	Reference
PENICILLIN G K				
Sterile water for injection	Not given	Refrigerate	1 wk	13
Sterile water for injection	Not given	Refrigerate	3 d[l]	13
Sterile water for injection	1,000,000 U/mL	−18°C	12 wk	4 (p 350)
Sterile water for injection	500,000 U/mL	−18°C -	35 d	4 (p 350)
PENICILLIN G SODIUM				
Sterile water for injection	Not given	Room	24 h	14
Sterile water for injection	Not given	Refrigerate	1 wk	14
Sterile water for injection	100,000 U/mL	Refrigerate	1 wk	4 (p 360)
PIPERACILLIN				
Sterile water for injection	1 g/5 mL	Room	24 h	15
Sterile water for injection	1 g/5 mL	Refrigerate	1 wk	15
Sterile water for injection	1 g/5 mL	Frozen	1 mo	15
Sterile water for injection	2 g/5 mL	Frozen	32 d[e,j]	4 (p 387)
PROCHLORPERAZINE				
In ampule	5 mg/mL	Room	3 m[m]	4 (p 408)
TICARCILLIN[n]				
Sterile water for injection	200 mg/mL	Room	24 h	16
Sterile water for injection	10–100 mg/mL	Room	72 h	16
Sterile water for injection	200 mg/mL	Refrigerate	72 h	16
Sterile water for injection	10–100 mg/mL	Refrigerate	14 d	16
Sterile water for injection	10–100 mg/mL	Frozen	30 d	16

Solution	Concentration	Temperature	Stability	Reference
TOBRAMYCIN				
In ampule	40 mg/mL	25°C	2 mo[e]	17
In ampule	40 mg/mL	4°C	2 mo[e]	17
TRIMETHOBENZAMIDE				
In ampule	100 mg/mL	Room	3 mo[o]	4 (p 477)
VANCOMYCIN				
Sterile water for injection	Not given	Room	14 d	18
Sterile water for injection	Not given	Refrigerate	96 h	4 (p 482)

Notes: Stability is the time limit in which the drug may be further diluted.
a. In original container
b. In glass hypod
c. In viaflex, glass, or plastic syringe
d. Thawing—do not heat; stable as if stored frozen; do not refreeze
e. In plastic syringe
f. Thawed stability—24 h at 25°C and 7 d at 5°C
g. Thawing—can be heated UNTIL thawed; do not refreeze
h. Thawing—at room temperature; stable for 12 h at room temperature or 10 d refrigerated
i. In glass container
j. In glass syringe
k. Some substances leached from the PVC bag during the study
l. Lilly brand
m. In tubex cartridge
n. Stability of thawed solutions are identical to the unfrozen solution
o. In one 2-mL tubex cartridge

REFERENCES

1. *Omnipen*. Wyeth Laboratories, package insert, February 15, 1978.
2. King, JC: *Guide to Parenteral Admixtures*. St. Louis, Cutter Laboratories, 1984.
3. *Mandol*. Eli Lilly & Co., package insert, May 21, 1982.
4. Trissel, LA: *Handbook on Injectable Drugs*, ed 3. Bethesda, Md, ASHP, 1983, pp 81, 85, 88, 92, 105, 202, 253, 304, 317, 350, 360, 387, 408, 477, 482.
5. *Kefzol*. Eli Lilly & Co., package insert, May 26, 1982.
6. *Claforan*. Hoechst-Roussel Pharmaceuticals, package insert, July 1982.
7. *Mefoxin*. Merck, Sharp & Dohme, package insert, February 1982.
8. *Keflin*. Eli Lilly & Co., package insert, May 26, 1982.
9. *Cefadyl*. Bristol Laboratories, package insert, November 1981.

10. Kirschenbaum HL: Compatibility and stability of dobutamine hydrochloride with large-volume parenterals and selected additives. *Am J Hosp Pharm* 1983;40:1690.

11. *Mezlin*. Miles Pharmaceuticals, package insert, July 1981.

12. *Sodium Nitroprusside*. Elkins-Sinn, package insert, September 1982.

13. *Penicillin G Potassium*. Eli Lilly & Co., package insert, September 12, 1980.

14. *Penicillin G Sodium*. ER Squibb & Sons, package insert, December 1980.

15. *Piperacil*. Lederle Laboratories, package insert, April 1982.

16. *Ticar*. Beecham Laboratories, package insert, September 1981.

17. Seitz DJ, Archambault JR, Kressel JJ, et al: Stability of tobramycin in plastic syringes, *Am J Hosp Pharm* 1980;37:1614.

18. *Vancocin*. Eli Lilly & Co., package insert, January 6, 1982.

Chapter 8

The Pharmacist in Neurosurgery Intensive Care

Christine M. Quandt

Over the past decade an acceleration in the understanding of acute central nervous system (CNS) physiology and pathology, the development of advanced neurologic monitoring techniques and treatment modalities have occurred.[1,2,3] Inasmuch as patients with acute neurologic disorders have problems that are different from those of patients in other intensive care units (ICUs), the treatment of patients with systemic disorders frequently needs modification in the management of concomitant CNS injury. Management of these patients frequently involves complex pharmacologic therapy with drugs that have a narrow therapeutic index. Careful monitoring of these drugs is necessary to maximize therapeutic effects and to minimize adverse reactions. Because of the specialized needs of these patients, the neurosurgery intensive care unit (NICU) has emerged as an important entity in many hospitals, and the provision of pharmacy services to this area is an important component of patient care.

An important factor in establishing an NICU is the availability of specialized neuroradiology diagnostic equipment and CNS-monitoring devices. Another critical element is the presence of staff with both neurologic and intensive care training and skills. Physicians, nurses, and clinical pharmacists are all important members of this multidisciplinary approach to treatment. The clinical pharmacist actively participates in the management of the neurotraumatized patient and has responsibilities for organizing, coordinating, and monitoring drug therapy in addition to education and research activities.

NEUROSURGERY INTENSIVE CARE ENVIRONMENT

The neurotraumatized patient may be managed in a surgical or general ICU, but often such a patient is treated in an NICU. Generally, these neurologic units are found in tertiary care hospitals, that is, referral centers or university hospitals, in which a high degree of specialization exists. The NICU may be organized according to clinical syndrome, such as stroke or head injury, but more often these units accommodate patients with a variety of neurologic disorders.

The location of this unit within the hospital may be dictated by the predominant patient population. For example, a unit with many neuro-trauma patients is best located near the emergency department or room; with an abundant surgical population, this unit may be near the operating room. In many institutions, the NICU is in an area integrated with other specialized ICUs that also contains a laboratory, a pharmacy, and other support facilities. In general, this unit is often close to the neurosurgery care floor or unit in order to maintain a smooth flow of staff and patients. There are usually six to ten beds per nursing station, arranged so that each bed is visible from the nurse's desk. The nurse-patient ratio is 1:1 to 1:2, 24 hours a day, depending on the complexity of care, patient load, and nurse availability. At least one isolation room for serious infections is essential. Also common to many NICU areas is a single enclosed room with full monitoring capabilities for patients with subarachnoid hemorrhage. It is important that patients with this condition be in an ICU, but they must be in a quiet room away from noxious stimuli in order to decrease the chances of rerupture of the aneurysm.

ADMISSION-DISCHARGE GUIDELINES

Patients are usually admitted to the NICU because of an altered state of consciousness, fluctuating neurologic signs, or inappropriate ventilatory capacity or a loss of airway protective reflexes. The most common admitting diagnoses are brain tumor, head injury, ruptured aneurysm or other cerebrovascular accidents (CVAs), and posthypoxic encephalopathy. Patients may also be admitted for immediate postoperative observation and stabilization after a craniotomy. Less commonly, patients are admitted for spinal cord trauma, status epilepticus, and various infectious, metabolic, and hypertensive encephalopathies.[4,5] The recovery period for a neurologic disorder is frequently longer than that of other disease states. The average stay of the patient in the NICU is eight to ten days, but the stay may extend to several months.[4] For example, head-injured patients may be in a coma for several weeks, requiring intensive care. Patients with spinal cord injuries and quadriplegia may require intensive care for several months because of ventilator dependency.

NEUROLOGIC ASSESSMENT

Assessment of neurologic status is an important function of the NICU staff. Frequent determinations of neurologic status, chiefly involving changes in level of consciousness, gross motor response, and brain-stem reflexes, are essential for determining the effects of therapy or the course of the intracranial disease.[6,7] Continual assessment and recording of the neurologic function in critically ill patients is probably best accomplished by use of a neurologic assessment sheet (Exhibit 8–1). These flow charts vary among institutions but they generally include the Glasgow Coma Scale or one of its modifications. The Glasgow Coma Scale is a simple scoring system in which responsiveness and neurologic status are measured in terms of motor responsiveness, verbal performance, and eye opening.[8] This scale, however, does not provide a complete guide to the patient's overall neurologic and medical status. The NICU flowsheet (Exhibit 8–2), therefore, also contains the patient's vital signs, blood gases, intake and output, pupillary size and reactivity, and intracranial pressure (ICP).

Pupillary size and reactivity, the respiratory pattern, the oculovestibular reaction, and the pattern of motor reactions to painful stimuli are important for assessing the neurologic status of the comatose patient.[9] In a patient with loss of consciousness, these brain-stem reflexes may serve to localize the lesion and to assess progression of the intracranial disease process.[5,9]

When the clinician assesses any of the neurologic functions and evaluates the disease process, drugs that can cause neurologic changes must be considered. Many antihypertensives (such as reserpine, methyldopa, propranolol, and nitroprusside) can cause mental confusion and drowsiness.[10] A number of drugs have effects that may confuse the interpretation of pupillary changes in coma. Atropine and scopolamine ingested in large amounts produce dilated and fixed pupils, often accompanied by delirium and stupor. Reports have indicated that transdermal scopolamine, which has been recently introduced for motion sickness, may cause a unilateral fixed dilated pupil for up to 48 hours.[11,12] Anticholinergics, such as atropine, are frequently given during resuscitation after cardiac arrest and may produce mydriatic pupils that respond poorly or not at all to light.[13] Glutethimide poisoning causes midposition or moderately dilated pupils that are unequal and frequently fixed to light.[10] Opiates, particularly heroin and morphine, produce pinpoint pupils.[14] Dopamine in doses greater than 30 µg/kg/min may cause fixed and dilated pupils by stimulating alpha-receptors in the radial muscle of the iris.[15] Barbiturates, neuromuscular blockers, phenytoin and ototoxic drugs can block oculovestibular responses.[16–19]

SPECIALIZED CNS MONITORING

Monitoring of the NICU patient requires a four-channel monitor with electrocardiographic, intraarterial pressure, pulmonary artery catheter, and ICP measurement capabilities. A pulmonary artery catheter is important for managing the fluid status of these patients.[20] The neurosurgical patient does not tolerate excessive fluid administration well because of his greater tendency to develop water

Exhibit 8–1 Example of Neurologic Assessment Sheet

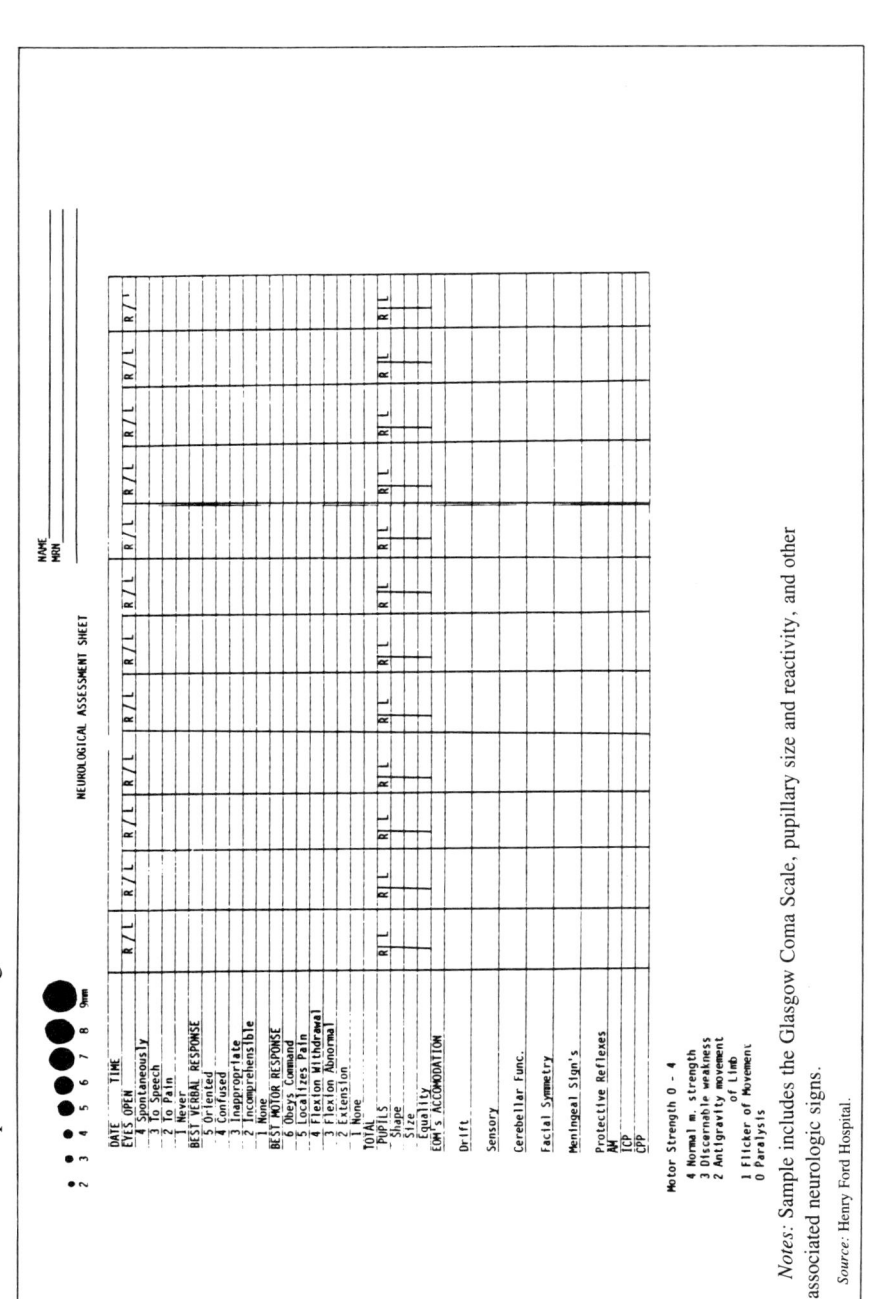

Notes: Sample includes the Glasgow Coma Scale, pupillary size and reactivity, and other associated neurologic signs.

Source: Henry Ford Hospital.

Exhibit 8-2 Example of NICU Flowsheet

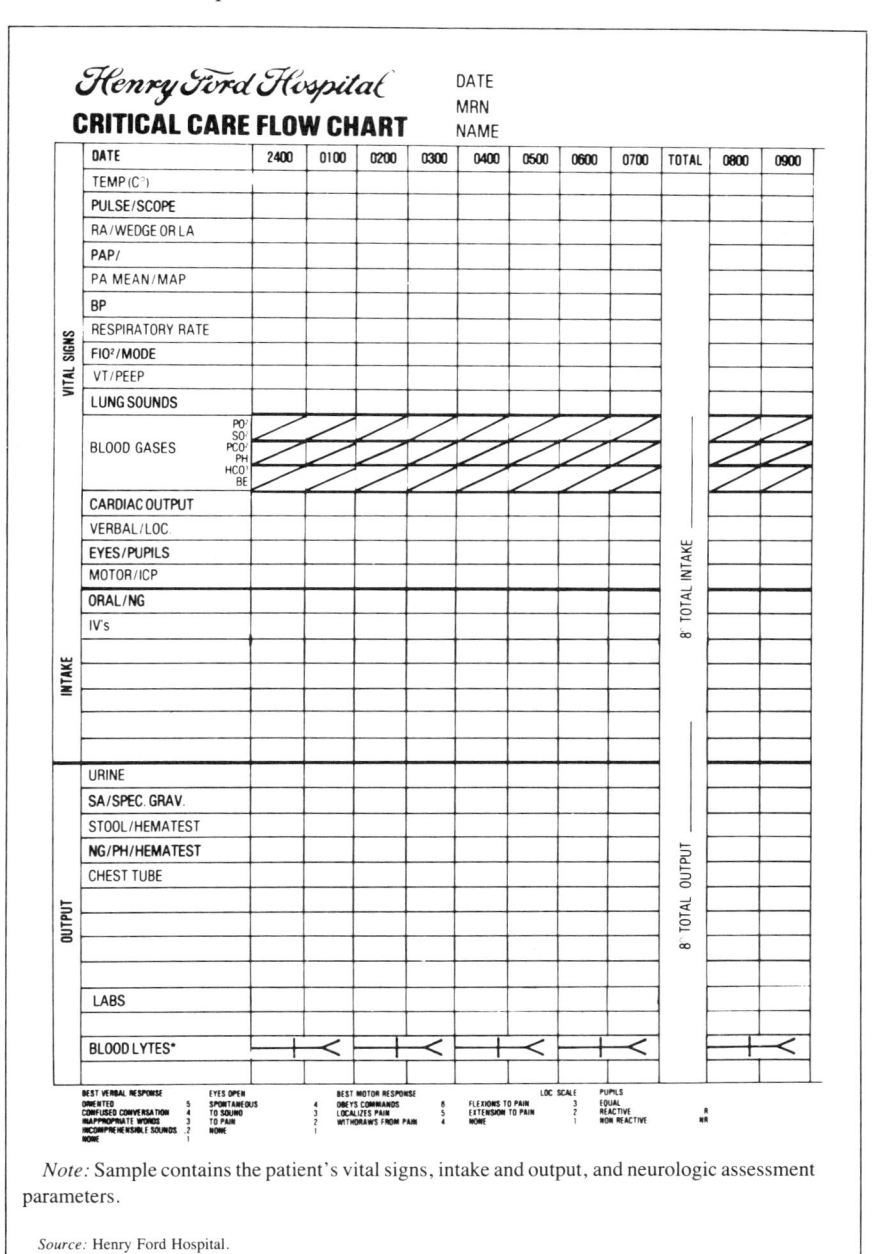

Henry Ford Hospital
CRITICAL CARE FLOW CHART

DATE
MRN
NAME

	DATE	2400	0100	0200	0300	0400	0500	0600	0700	TOTAL	0800	0900
VITAL SIGNS	TEMP (C°)											
	PULSE/SCOPE											
	RA/WEDGE OR LA											
	PAP/											
	PA MEAN/MAP											
	BP											
	RESPIRATORY RATE											
	FIO₂/MODE											
	VT/PEEP											
	LUNG SOUNDS											
	BLOOD GASES (PO/SO/PCO/PH/HCO/BE)											
	CARDIAC OUTPUT											
	VERBAL/LOC.											
	EYES/PUPILS											
	MOTOR/ICP											
INTAKE	ORAL/NG									8° TOTAL INTAKE		
	IV's											
OUTPUT	URINE											
	SA/SPEC. GRAV.											
	STOOL/HEMATEST											
	NG/PH/HEMATEST									8° TOTAL OUTPUT		
	CHEST TUBE											
	LABS											
	BLOOD LYTES*											

BEST VERBAL RESPONSE		EYES OPEN		BEST MOTOR RESPONSE		LOC SCALE	PUPILS	
ORIENTED	5	SPONTANEOUS	4	OBEYS COMMANDS	6	FLEXIONS TO PAIN 3	EQUAL	
CONFUSED CONVERSATION	4	TO SOUND	3	LOCALIZES PAIN	5	EXTENSION TO PAIN 2	REACTIVE	R
INAPPROPRIATE WORDS	3	TO PAIN	2	WITHDRAWS FROM PAIN	4	NONE 1	NON REACTIVE	NR
INCOMPREHENSIBLE SOUNDS	2	NONE	1					
NONE	1							

Note: Sample contains the patient's vital signs, intake and output, and neurologic assessment parameters.

Source: Henry Ford Hospital.

intoxication, increased ICP, and brain swelling.[5] Cardiac output readings from the pulmonary artery catheter are important for patients who are managed with high-dose barbiturates for increased ICP and for patients who are undergoing intravascular volume expansion and vasopressor therapy for cerebral vasospasm.[21,22] The ICP, measured by either an intraventricular catheter or a subarachnoid bolt (Figure 8–1), is essential for managing patients with intracranial hypertension.[23,24] The ICP measurement may also serve as a prognostic tool for neurotraumatized patients. Systemic mean arterial pressure (MAP) and ICP measurements permit continuous computation of overall cerebral perfusion pressure (CPP, i.e., CPP = MAP − ICP) and may forewarn of impending cerebral ischemia.[25]

Figure 8–1 ICP Measurement

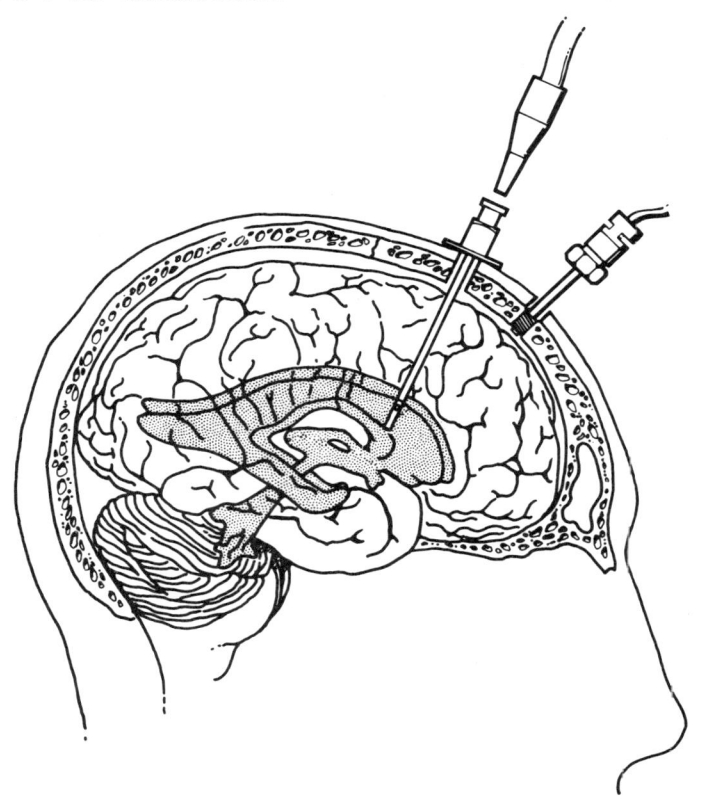

Note: Artistic depiction of the intraventricular catheter (*left*) and subarachnoid bolt (*right*), either of which may be used for measuring ICP.

Direct total and regional cerebral blood flow (CBF) measurements may also be performed in NICU patients. Measurements of CBF are usually performed by tracing the clearance of an inhaled gamma-emitting radioactive isotope—usually ^{133}Xe—with external scintillation counters. Computer analysis of the clearance curves is then performed.[26] Measurement of CBF may provide prognostic indices in the management of head-injured patients as well as a guide to therapy. However, because of the cost and complexity of CBF measurements, their application at present is limited to specialized treatment centers.

Continuous electroencephalography (EEG) provides a valuable noninvasive measurement of cerebral function in the NICU patient.[1] The EEG can localize the pathologic process and may be used to monitor high-dose barbiturate therapy.[27] Sensory evoked potentials, the technique of analyzing the EEG responses to specific stimuli (visual, auditory, somatosensory, etc.), although still in its infancy, may also be useful for identifying and localizing the CNS injury.[28,29]

Appropriate management of the airway and ventilation is important in the treatment of patients with intracranial abnormalities; therefore, the NICU must be equipped with ventilators. Frequently, endotracheal intubation is necessary because of the prolonged state of impaired consciousness, particularly when the patient has poor function of the lower cranial nerves.[5] The abnormality can result in a depressed cough reflex, proneness to aspiration, or relaxed pharyngeal musculature that might lead to obstruction. Mechanical ventilation is, therefore, often necessary for severe head and spinal cord injuries.[21,30] In the case of patients with intracranial hypertension, controlled hyperventilation to a PCO_2 level of 25 to 30 torr is a therapeutic tool to decrease cerebral blood volume and to decrease ICP.[31]

PHARMACIST'S ROLE

Drug Distribution

The dispensing of medication to the NICU at Henry Ford Hospital (HFH) is facilitated by the critical care pharmacy. This satellite pharmacy serves not only the NICU, but also three other ICUs in the immediate area, serving a total of 48 patients. The patients are serviced 24 hours a day, seven days a week, from this pharmacy.

The critical care pharmacy utilizes a 24-hour dispensing procedure. Copies three and four of the Medication Order Form (MOF) are received in the pharmacy from the nursing units by the pneumatic tube or on a routine delivery. The dispensing pharmacist reviews the order for completeness, accuracy, and appropriateness. If this pharmacist discovers a problem with the MOF, he notifies the clinical pharmacist who clarifies the order.

The order is processed according to its nature (intravenous admixture or non-admixture). Orders for intravenous admixtures (IV) are entered into a computerized patient profile. One copy of the order is attached to a workcard for preparation of the IV; the other copy is placed into the patient's Medication Profile Book. Depending on the urgency of the medication, the initial dose may be sent immediately through the pneumatic tube or may be placed on a standard administration time and delivered later.

Non-IV medications are dispensed as a 24-hour unit-dose supply. When an order is received, the medication is initially dispensed in the appropriate quantity to supply the patient until the next medication cart exchange. One copy of the order is placed in the Medication Profile Book. The technician then transcribes the order on a 24-Hour Dispensing Profile, which is maintained in front of each patient's complete medication profile. The transcribing is later verified and initialed by the pharmacist. This dispensing profile is used by the technicians to determine the appropriate medications and the number of doses needed for each patient when they are filling the unit-dose cassettes. After the technician has completed filling the cassettes for all critical care patients, the cassettes are checked by the dispensing pharmacist and delivered to the nursing units each afternoon.

Clinical Pharmacy Services

The clinical pharmacist is an integral part of the NICU team. The position of neuro-intensive care pharmacist at HFH was developed as a progression of clinical pharmacy services within the hospital. The pharmacist's first direct contact with the neurosurgery patient and staff was as a clinical pharmacist on the neurosurgical inpatient floor. The role of the pharmacist was to monitor drug therapy by medication profile review. The goal of the clinical pharmacy program was to identify drug-related problems and to make recommendations to the physician and nurse of possible solutions. The pharmacist provided information concerning the proper dosing of drugs for patients with hepatic and renal disease. He also provided information about adverse effects and drug interactions. The pharmacist monitored not only the neurosurgical and neurology patients, but also was responsible for drug therapy review of at least one other nursing unit as well. This service was initially provided eight hours a day, five days a week. The total patient load for the clinical pharmacist was approximately 80 to 100 patients, of whom 10% represented the NICU patients.

As a result of the increased demand and the patient load of the clinical pharmacist, only a limited amount of time could be spent monitoring the NICU patients. Clearly evident was the need for a full-time critical care pharmacist to provide intensive drug monitoring and to work closely with the NICU staff on the acute management of the neurosurgical patients. The neurosurgeons, as well as other ICU staff, recognized the need for a full-time pharmacist in this area. Their verbal and written support to the hospital administration was instrumental in creating this position. The critical care pharmacist provides coverage eight hours a day, five days a week, to an average patient load of 12 to 15 patients. On weekends, these patients are monitored by the staff clinical pharmacist covering several nursing units.

The pharmacist's salary can be generated solely from the Pharmacy Department budget, from the Department of Neurosurgery, or from a combination of both. Funding from the Neurosurgery Department can be obtained from research grants or patient generated revenue. At HFH, the pharmacist's salary was provided by the Pharmacy Department; however, a proposal to combine funds from departments (neurosurgery and pharmacy) was discussed.

Organization

Before the creation of the full-time position, the clinical pharmacist worked in the NICU on a consultative basis. These consultations were mainly to monitor patients with severe head injury and intracranial hypertension. The use of complex regimens of potent pharmacologic agents was well-adapted to pharmacist input in treating these patients.[32] There was a need to identify specific drug protocols and to educate the NICU staff in the proper dosing and administration of these drugs and in the possibility of adverse patient reactions. As a result, one of the first responsibilities of the NICU pharmacist was to develop a protocol for the pharmacologic management of severe head injury (Exhibit 8–3). This protocol included developing a dosing regimen for the continuous infusion of thiopental and pentobarbital which was based on pharmacokinetic parameters. A sequence of drug therapy based on the extent of ICP was established. Guidelines for proper dosing and other monitoring criteria were also established.

Another initial responsibility of the pharmacist was to create a stock list of drugs that showed appropriate concentrations and quantities for the pharmacy servicing the NICU (Table 8–1). This list included 25% mannitol. Because the usual dosage of mannitol for treating cerebral edema is 1 g/kg initially, followed by 0.25 g/kg/ q 4 h, several 50-mL ampules must be stocked in the pharmacy. A warming chamber must be provided for the storage of mannitol to maintain the solution in a crystal-free condition.[33] Other important drugs for the NICU patient include several grams of pentobarbital or thiopental for treating intracranial hypertension; intravenous glycerol and dexamethasone for treating cerebral edema; and aminocaproic acid for treating subarachnoid hemorrhage. Adequate quantities of phenytoin must be included for treating head injury-related seizures.

If the Pharmacy is not in close proximity to the NICU and rapid delivery to the NICU cannot be assured, a small stock of emergency drugs for treating neurologic injuries should be stored on the unit. This stock may include mannitol, dex-

Exhibit 8-3 Protocol for Management of Acute Head Injury

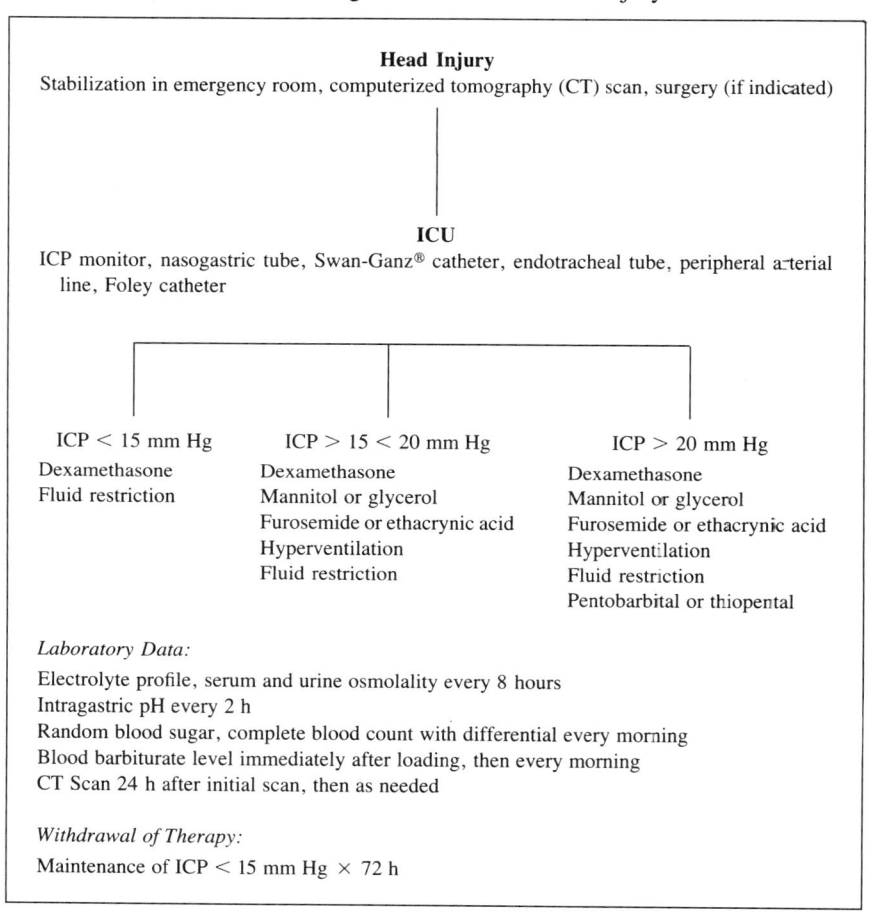

Head Injury
Stabilization in emergency room, computerized tomography (CT) scan, surgery (if indicated)

ICU
ICP monitor, nasogastric tube, Swan-Ganz® catheter, endotracheal tube, peripheral arterial line, Foley catheter

ICP < 15 mm Hg	ICP > 15 < 20 mm Hg	ICP > 20 mm Hg
Dexamethasone	Dexamethasone	Dexamethasone
Fluid restriction	Mannitol or glycerol	Mannitol or glycerol
	Furosemide or ethacrynic acid	Furosemide or ethacrynic acid
	Hyperventilation	Hyperventilation
	Fluid restriction	Fluid restriction
		Pentobarbital or thiopental

Laboratory Data:
Electrolyte profile, serum and urine osmolality every 8 hours
Intragastric pH every 2 h
Random blood sugar, complete blood count with differential every morning
Blood barbiturate level immediately after loading, then every morning
CT Scan 24 h after initial scan, then as needed

Withdrawal of Therapy:
Maintenance of ICP < 15 mm Hg × 72 h

---

amethasone, phenytoin, and pentobarbital. The storage and the quantities of these drugs should be coordinated by the clinical pharmacist.

Coordination

The clinical pharmacist coordinates the pharmacologic management of the NICU patients by recommending appropriate therapy according to the established protocol or current literature. The pharmacist assures rapid availability of drugs and advises proper drug administration by the nursing staff. As part of the intensive care team, the pharmacist attends daily rounds and reviews each patient's pharmacologic management. The pharmacist also suggests proper ther-

Table 8–1 Stock List of Drugs for NICU Patients

Drug and Concentration	Quantity
Aminocaproic acid injection, 250 mg/mL (20-mL vial)	40
Amobarbital injection, 50 mg/ampule	4
Dexamethasone injection, 10 mg/mL (10-mL vial)	24
Dexamethasone injection, 4 mg/mL (1-mL vial)	250
Dexamethasone injection, 4 mg/syringe	150
Glycerol injection, 10% (500-mL bottle)	5
Mannitol injection, 25% (50-mL vials)	200
Mannitol injection, 20% (500-mL bottles)	12
Pentobarbital Na injection, 50 mg/mL (2-mL tubex)	10
Pentobarbital Na injection, 50 mg/mL (50-mL vial)	10
Phenytoin injection, 100-mg/mL syringe	300
Thiopental Na injection, 2.5% (5-g vial)	2

apy or adjusts current drugs according to the patient's clinical status. Drug information and education, especially regarding new drugs, is also provided to the intensive care staff.

Upon initiation of an established drug protocol for a patient, the physician first contacts the clinical pharmacist. The pharmacist reviews the patient's chart and assesses the patient's current status, along with the patient's age, height, weight, previous medications, and medical history as it relates to precautions or contraindications to therapy. For example, if a patient is to be started on mannitol for cerebral edema and has a history of congestive heart failure, the pharmacist will recommend pretreatment with furosemide approximately 15 minutes before mannitol infusion to prevent circulatory overload.[21]

The pharmacist also assists in the institution of drug therapy according to protocol by calculating initial doses and recommending the proper concentration and diluent for these drugs. In patients with intracranial hypertension, the use of 5% dextrose in water should be avoided, because the solution may lower the osmolarity of the blood and increase cerebral edema.[21] The pharmacist, therefore, recommends that all intravenous piggyback medication be put in 0.9% NaCl. These patients must also be fluid restricted to 65% to 75% of normal to prevent fluid overload and increased ICP.[24] The pharmacist, therefore, minimizes the fluid volumes of all IV medications.

The presence of the clinical pharmacist on the nursing unit facilitates the dispensing and the delivery of these medications to the patient and insures the earliest possible institution of therapy. Often, the physician or nurse contacts the clinical pharmacist when certain medications are indicated. The pharmacist contacts the critical care pharmacy to communicate the urgency of the drug and to give any special dispensing instructions required. The transfer of the order from the chart to the pharmacy is then expedited by the clinical pharmacist. In addition, the pharmacist coordinates the accurate administration of drugs by the nursing staff, by calculating infusion rates and assuring that the drug is infused with the proper administration set and in the proper infusion site. For example, thiopental and pentobarbital must be infused through a central, rather than a peripheral, IV line to prevent thrombophlebitis; mannitol infusions must be given through an administration set with a filter[33]; and phenytoin should be administered at a rate no greater than 25 mg/min in the presence of dopamine infusions because of their potential for causing hypotension and bradycardia.[34]

Monitoring

The high dosage of drugs often required in treating NICU patients has a great potential for producing adverse effects. The clinical pharmacist continually monitors these drugs and recommends dosage changes to avoid adverse reactions. The pharmacist is often the first person on the NICU staff to recognize potential problems and to alert the physician when a change in therapy is needed. For example, high-dose steroids used for cerebral edema may increase blood sugar and cause gastrointestinal bleeding, requiring daily monitoring of glucose, hemoglobin, hematocrit or a heme-positive nasogastric aspirate.[35,36] If signs of gastrointestinal bleeding are noted, the steroid may have to be withdrawn or tapered, antacid coverage may be increased, or, in some cases, blood transfusions may be needed. When osmotic diuretic therapy is instituted, the pharmacist monitors serum and urine osmolarity along with serum electrolytes to prevent severe dehydration or electrolyte imbalance.[21]

Dosing of barbiturates for intracranial hypertension must be titrated to specific guidelines (Exhibit 8–4) requiring constant monitoring and frequent dosage adjustments.[21] Barbiturates can cause myocardial depression and reduce cardiac output, both of which effects can alter the pharmacokinetics of certain drugs and necessitate dosage changes.[21,37] The serum concentrations of barbiturates are

---

Exhibit 8–4 Guidelines for Monitoring Barbiturates

Serum concentration:	25–40 μg/mL
Intracranial pressure (ICP):	< 15 mm Hg
Cerebral perfusion pressure (CPP):	> 50 mm Hg
Mean arterial pressure (MAP):	90–120 mm Hg
Controlled ventilation PO_2:	90–100 mm Hg
PCO_2:	25–30 mm Hg

recorded daily by the pharmacist and correlated with the measured ICP. If the ICP remains high or increases during the course of therapy or if any adverse effects are detected, the pharmacist recommends a dosage adjustment.

Pharmacologic therapy for the management of seizures requires close monitoring by the clinical pharmacist. For example, status epilepticus must be treated rapidly; if the usual drugs, diazepam and phenytoin, are not effective, the pharmacist recommends alternative therapy, such as barbiturates or paraldehyde.[38] Because pharmacokinetic dosing of phenytoin is important in these patients, dosages are based on frequent monitoring of serum concentrations.

Other important areas for clinical pharmacist involvement include the treatment of patients with meningitis or encephalitis and the nutritional management of the NICU patient. The clinical pharmacist can aid in the selection of appropriate antibiotics and antifungal agents based upon the drug's ability to cross the blood-brain barrier.[39] When the intrathecal or intraventricular route is used for the administration of drugs, it is imperative that the vehicle for delivery of the medication be preservative free and as close to CSF characteristics as possible.[40] The pharmacist may, therefore, need to compound the drug in the proper vehicle to assure its safe administration. Patients with CNS infections require close monitoring, inasmuch as antibiotics are often used in higher doses than usual, causing an increased risk of toxicity.

Nutrition support is very important in managing the NICU patient, especially those who may be unconscious or unable to feed normally for extended periods of time. Although enteral feeding is preferred, this route is sometimes impractical in such a patient because of an unprotected airway, a fluctuating level of consciousness, or the impairment of gastric absorption. Parenteral therapy is often necessary, then, to prevent muscle wasting, to provide immunologic competence, and to promote healing.[41,42] Adequate nutrition has also been shown to improve survival in these patients.[43] Because both enteral and parenteral therapy require close monitoring to prevent complications, the pharmacist plays an important role in managing the nutrition support of the neurosurgical patient.

Education

Another important responsibility of the NICU pharmacist is to provide inservice education to nurses, physicians, and pharmacists. Lectures on drug therapy for neurologic injuries are periodically given at physician and pharmacy conferences. The pharmacist is also involved in teaching formal neurologic intensive care classes to nurses. The nurses are also instructed on drug protocols, because their collection of blood samples for drug analysis and recording of monitoring parameters are vital for proper dosage adjustments.

Problem Solving

The pharmacist can expect to encounter many opportunities for involvement while working in the NICU. These opportunities revolve around clinical as well as drug distribution activities. Examples of input with drug distribution include assuring the proper storage and handling of barbiturates, compounding of special solutions for treating neurologic disorders, and assuring rapid availability of all required medications.

A problem of storing and handling barbiturates arose when high doses of these drugs were recognized as a treatment for refractory intracranial hypertension. This treatment regimen required storage of many vials of pentobarbital and thiopental. Controlled substances, such as barbiturates, were routinely stocked on the nursing unit, and the nurse was responsible for preparing and administering these medications. Barbiturate infusions, however, require careful preparation, because these drugs have limited solubility, and calculation of the precise infusion rate is important for pharmacokinetic dosing of these drugs.[44] The storage and preparation of barbiturates for the treatment of intracranial hypertension were, therefore, transferred to the Pharmacy Department.

The limited stability of barbiturate infusions also required pharmacist input. Pentobarbital initially had been recommended for administration by the IV push route because it was felt that the drug would precipitate if it was diluted as an IV infusion.[44,45] Pentobarbital often had to be administered at hourly intervals to maintain a normal ICP—a procedure that placed large demands on nursing time.[45] Also, IV push administration of high doses of barbiturates has been associated with vascular thrombosis.[46] Therefore, the concentration of pentobarbital for intravenous infusion was developed on the basis of stability data and the physical characteristics of the drug.

The management of many neurologic disease states requires the administration of drugs by unconventional routes—intrathecal and epidural drug administration. Therapy sometimes involves drugs that are not commercially available by this route, and so the pharmacist must compound the medication to ensure its stability and sterility. For example, morphine sulfate has recently been used for intractable pain by the intrathecal and epidural routes.[47] Because morphine sulfate injection was available only with preservatives, a sterile, preservative-free solution had to be prepared by the pharmacy. Another compounding challenge for the pharmacist involved intravenous glycerol. This drug was not commercially available as an IV solution; it was available only as an oral solution. Because the injectable form is preferred for treating cerebral edema—especially in the comatose patient—an intravenous solution was formulated by the pharmacist.[21,48] Ideally, these solutions should be prepared in bulk form in the Sterile Products Department within the Pharmacy. The amount of medication should depend on the projected needs of the ICU and on the shelf life of the drug. If this department is not available, the pharmacist can prepare these solutions using sterile technique under a laminar flow hood for short-term use. The solutions can be autoclaved, if necessary, in the laboratory and in other designated areas of the hospital.

These special solutions and other medications must be readily available in the pharmacy for rapid delivery to the patient. To ensure the service, the pharmacy personnel must be made aware of the application and the importance of the drugs. Stock levels and a method for the replacement of these items should be determined. These activities should be coordinated with the Purchasing and Sterile Products Department and the stockroom personnel. Occasionally, there may be a need to stock certain drugs on the NICU. The clinical pharmacist should coordinate the proper storage of these drugs and monitor their stock levels and expiration dates.

The NICU pharmacist also plays a major role in solving clinical problems that arise in the ICU. On a daily basis, these roles involve the pharmacokinetic dosing of drugs in the case of patients with multiple system failure, the recognition of unusual adverse effects and unpublished drug interactions. Occasionally, clinical problems arise in which there are no specific guidelines for a solution, and published reports for reference are limited. When these problems involve drug therapy, the clinical pharmacist is asked to provide a possible solution. Examples of these problems include designing dosage regimens for newly developed drug therapy and recommending antibiotic instillation into brain empyema.

The first problem involved high-dose barbiturate therapy for refractory intracranial hypertension. This was a relatively new concept in the management of ICP; most published reports used pentobarbital.[45,49] It was felt, however, that thiopental might offer a therapeutic advantage over pentobarbital in head-injured patients because thiopental has a high lipid solubility and reaches rapid equilibrium between the plasma and the brain.[37] Although the use of thiopental for controlling ICP had been described, dosing recommendations were limited. The clinical pharmacist was then asked to develop a dosage regimen of thiopental for treating patients with intracranial hypertension. Because pharmacokinetic information on thiopental was limited to single-dose studies, a study was undertaken to characterize the pharmacokinetic properties of the continuous administration of thiopental. A dosage regimen was then designed to achieve rapidly and to maintain the therapeutic serum concentration.[50]

The critical care pharmacist was also asked for input on two cases involving antibiotic therapy for a brain empyema. This infection involved a collection of pus in the subdural space. In one case, the pus was attributable to a wound infection; in the other, to a para-nasal sinus infection. Both cases involved a Gram-negative organism, which was initially treated with systemic antibiotics; however, the infection was not improving. Because the empyema was thought to be multiloculated, it was decided to place multiple catheters in the subdural space to instill antibiotic therapy. The NICU pharmacist was asked to recommend the proper antibiotic and to formulate a dose of this drug. References on the management of a Gram-negative empyema were limited. Another problem involved calculation of the proper dose, because the antibiotic was not going to be diluted by plasma or CSF. This drug, thus, could potentially penetrate the brain tissue. A dose of preservative-free gentamicin was, therefore, calculated on the basis of references for the usual intraventricular dose, an estimation of its usual dilution of CSF, and the minimum inhibitory concentration of the organism.

Research

The NICU pharmacist is actively involved in research activities, especially those involving drugs. The pharmacist's role is to write research protocols, to coordinate the study design and activities, to collect appropriate data, and to monitor results. Research ideas and interests are initially developed at weekly research conferences held by the Neurosurgery Department, and the clinical pharmacist is often involved in these meetings. When there is interest in a study involving a pharmacologic agent, the pharmacist is asked to review the literature about this drug. The pharmacist pays particular attention to the approved indications and other applications of the drug, its pharmacokinetics and penetration into the CNS, and the drug's potential toxic effects.

At the next scheduled conference, the pharmacist presents a review of the drug, comments on the practicality of the study, and suggests a study design. If the research idea has scientific merit and potential therapeutic benefit, the Research Committee approves the study. A final protocol is then written by the pharmacist and other investigators for approval by the Neurosurgery Department. This protocol is then presented before the Human Research Committee of the hospital for formal approval.

Before a research protocol involving pharmacologic agents is begun, the pharmacist informs the nursing, pharmacy, laboratory, and other medical personnel about the study. In the study design, brief conferences are usually conducted about the rationale and the methodology for the study, as well as the role of these various departments. The pharmacist then enters patients into the study, writes medication and laboratory orders (which are later cosigned by the physician), and collects appropriate data. The pharmacist and other investigators of a particular protocol meet periodically to discuss the progress of the study and any changes that need to be made. Once the project has been completed, the pharmacist, along with the other researchers, presents the data at the appropriate conference and submits the results for publication.

Examples of research projects at HFH that involve the NICU pharmacist include barbiturate-induced coma for the treatment of patients with cerebral ischemia, mannitol versus glycerol for the treatment of cerebral edema, and the use of verapamil for the treatment of cerebral vasospasm. In the first project, a dosage regimen of thiopental was developed (as previously mentioned) for the treatment of intracranial hypertension.[50] A retrospective analysis was then made, and patients who received high-dose barbiturates were classified in an attempt to characterize differences in outcome and response to therapy.[51]

In the next study, intravenous glycerol was investigated, initially to determine its efficacy in reducing ICP, and then to compare its effects with mannitol in the treatment of cerebral edema. Verapamil was also studied in an attempt to determine its efficacy in preventing or treating cerebral vasospasm in patients with subarachnoid hemorrhage.

The future of research in the NICU will involve a number of neuropharmacologic agents and should improve the understanding and management of CNS disorders. There are many important areas of research in neurosurgery; most of these involve serious neurologic problems that have a high morbidity and mortality rate. Subarachnoid hemorrhage after rupture of an intracranial aneurysm has a high morbidity and mortality rate as a result of complications following the initial hemorrhage. One of the most serious complications is cerebral ischemia secondary to vasospasm.[20,52] Although a number of pharmacologic agents have been used, there is no universally effective regimen for preventing or treating this problem, and so cerebral vasospasm remains a therapeutic challenge.[20,53–55]

Future therapy of vasospasm includes the use of calcium antagonists, prostaglandins, and dimethyl sulfoxide (DMSO).[56–58] In vitro studies have shown that verapamil, nifedipine, and other calcium antagonists can counteract vasoconstriction produced by norepinephrine, serotonin, and blood in isolated human and animal cerebral arteries. Human clinical trials using calcium antagonists for cerebral vasospasm are also underway.[59,60] Not only are calcium antagonists being studied for the treatment of cerebral arterial spasm, but they are also being used investigationally for the management of postresuscitation brain injury. These drugs have been shown to protect cerebral blood flow and oxygen consumption during reperfusion after a 20-minute cardiac arrest in dogs.[61,62] Calcium channel blockers will play a major role in future neurologic research.

Prostacyclin (PGI_2), the prostaglandin, has also been studied in vitro to determine its ability to counteract cerebral arterial spasm. Prostacyclin is a potent vasodilator and inhibitor of platelet aggregation. This latter effect may prevent the development of histologic changes seen after a subarachnoid hemorrhage, which lead to smooth muscle necrosis and subsequent fibrosis.[63] The role of DMSO in treating arterial spasm is unclear. Proposed benefits of DMSO in treating this condition include increased cerebral blood flow, antiplatelet effects, and stabilization of membranes.[58,64] Perhaps research with these drugs or future studies will provide an effective regimen and thereby improve the prognosis of subarachnoid hemorrhage.

Recent studies have suggested that perfluorochemicals such as Fluosal-DA may be useful in treating cerebral ischemia.[65,66] Inasmuch as this emulsion enhances the oxygenation of whole blood and disposes of carbon dioxide in the lungs, Fluosal-DA has been used investigationally as an artificial blood substitute.[67,68] This agent may be beneficial in treating acute cerebral ischemia because its decreased viscosity, small particle size, and enhanced oxygen exchange may result in improved flow rheology in the vasculature despite decreased blood flow. Results from animal studies suggest that Fluosal-DA has a protective effect on acute focal cerebral ischemia and may improve neurologic outcome.[65,66] The use of these agents will definitely be an exciting area of future neurological research.

Intracranial hypertension is another neurologic problem associated with a high morbidity and mortality rate.[2] There have been many advances in the therapeutic management of this disorder. Two pharmacologic agents, lidocaine and DMSO, are currently being studied. DMSO has reduced the intracranial pressure in animal models as well as in a few human case reports; however, the mortality rate has remained high in this group.[69-71] Lidocaine has been used to control ICP intraoperatively and to prevent an increase in ICP during endotracheal suctioning.[72-74] Further research is necessary to define the role of these drugs in the treatment of intracranial hypertension. Although these investigational agents show some promise, continued research is necessary in the treatment of intracranial hypertension to improve the survival of these patients.

Another potential area for extensive research is pain control and the role of the recently discovered opiate peptides, endorphins, and enkephalins. These endogenous peptides are not only linked to pain but may also be involved in the development of tolerance and addiction, respiration, sleep, sexual activity, and endocrine function. The clinical application of the endorphins and enkephalins—and some of their synthetic analogs—is currently being investigated.[75-79] However, this vast area is only completing its first decade; extensive research is needed to understand and to utilize these substances fully.

There have been recent advances in the area of pain control. Opiate receptors have been identified in the brain and spinal cord as well as in the density of these receptors in specific areas.[75,80,81] This discovery led to intrathecal administration of opiates to produce analgesia in animals and humans. Intractable pain due to cancer has recently been treated with intrathecal or intraventricular morphine; however, these methods are still investigational.[82-84] This technique often uses an Ommaya reservoir inserted into the lumbar subarachnoid space or lateral ventricle for administration of morphine. A single injection of 2 to 4 mg of morphine has provided pain relief for up to 24 hours with no serious adverse effects.[47] Morphine has also been administered by the epidural route for chronic intractable pain.[82] A few patients have continued intrathecal or epidural morphine treatment at home after a responsible family member or—in at least one case—after the patient was taught to administer the drug himself.[47] These methods of opiate administration represent a challenge to the clinical pharmacist; however, much work is needed in this area to assure the safe administration of these drugs.

SUMMARY

The neurosurgery intensive care environment provides a unique opportunity for the clinical pharmacist's involvement. This specialized ICU is a relatively new concept in critical care that was introduced on the basis of advances in neurologic monitoring techniques and treatment modalities. The next decade in critical care will see further acceleration in the clinician's understanding of and ability to support the neurologic patient, and this support will involve a multidisciplinary team approach. The pharmacist's role on the NICU team will involve clinical, research, and teaching activities. The clinical aspects will present challenging problems that may involve developing new treatment regimens and pharmacokinetic parameters of new drugs, or formulating dosage forms or vehicles for drugs. Inservice lectures to physicians, nurses, and pharmacists will be a continual process, because our knowledge of acute neurologic problems and their management is rapidly increasing. Research in neurosurgery will involve many areas of CNS dynamics and pathology. Consequently, the pharmacist will play an important role investigating new drugs and developing new uses of drugs for treating neurologic problems.

REFERENCES

1. Marsh ML, Marshall LF, Shapiro HM: Neurosurgical intensive care. *Anesthesiology* 1977;17:149–163.

2. Marshall LF, Smith RW, Shapiro HM: The outcome with aggressive treatment of severe head injuries. Part I—The significance of intracranial pressure monitoring. *J Neurosurg* 1979;50:20–25.

3. McDowall DG: Monitoring the brain. *Anesthesiology* 1976;45:117–133.

4. Tindal S: Intensive care in the neurosurgical unit. *Can Anaesth Soc J* 1971;18:637–649.

5. Correll JW, Becker GL, Countee RW: Intensive care of the patient with central nervous system disease. *Med Clin North Am* 1971;55:1233–1248.

6. Overgaard J, Hvid-Hansen O, Land AM, et al: Prognosis after head injury based on early clinical examination. *Lancet* 1973;2:631–635.

7. Shapiro HM: Intracranial hypertension: Therapeutic and anesthetic considerations. *Anesthesiology* 1975;43:445–471.

8. Teasdale G, Jennett B: Assessment of coma and impaired consciousness. A practical scale. *Lancet* 1974;2:81–83.

9. Plum F, Posner JB: *The Diagnosis of Stupor and Coma.* Contemporary Neurology Series. Philadelphia, FA Davis, 1972.

10. Blaschke TF, Melmon KL: Antihypertensive agents and the drug therapy of hypertension, in Gilman AG, Goodman LS, Gilman A (eds): *The Pharmacologic Basis of Therapeutics.* New York, Macmillan, 1980, pp 793–818.

11. Carlston JA: Unilateral dilated pupil from scopolamine disk. *JAMA* 1982;248:31.

12. Verdier DD, Kennadell JS: Fixed dilated pupil resulting from transdermal scopolamine. *Am J Ophthalmol* 1982;93:803–804.

13. Thompson HS, Newsome DA, Loewenfeld IE: The fixed dilated pupil. Sudden iridoplegia or mydriatic drops? A simple diagnostic test. *Arch Ophthalmol* 1971;86:21–27.

14. Jaffe JH, Martin WR: Opioid analgesics and antagonists, in Gilman AG, Goodman LS, Gilman A (eds): *The Pharmacologic Basis of Therapeutics.* New York, Macmillan, 1981, pp 494–534.

15. Ong GL, Bruning HA: Dilated fixed pupils due to administration of high doses of dopamine hydrochloride. *Crit Care Med* 1981;9:658–659.

16. Dayla US, Chart GE, Fenton SSA: Gentamicin vestibulotoxicity. Long term disability. *Ann Otol Rhinol Laryngol* 1979;88:36–39.

17. Orth DN, Almeida H, Walsh FB, et al: Ophthalmoplegia resulting from diphenylhydantoin and primidone intoxication. Report of four cases. *JAMA* 1967;201:225–227.

18. Tyson RN: Simulation of cerebral death by succinylcholine sensitivity. *Arch Neurol* 1974;30:409–411.

19. Vesterhauge S, Peitersen E: Effects of some drugs on the caloric induced nystagmus, in Stable J (ed): *Advances in Oto-Rhino-Laryngology Base.* S Karger, 1979, pp 173–177.

20. Swan HJC: The role of hemodynamic monitoring in the management of the critically ill. *Crit Care Med* 1975;3:83–89.

21. Quandt CM, de los Reyes RA, Diaz FG, et al: Pharmacologic management of subarachnoid hemorrhage. *Drug Intell Clin Pharm* 1982;16:909–915.

22. Quandt CM, de los Reyes RA: Pharmacologic management of acute intracranial hypertension. *Drug Intell Clin Pharm* 1984;18:105–112.

23. Lundberg N: Continuous recording and control of ventricular fluid pressure in neurosurgical patients. *Acta Psychiatr Neurol Scand* 1960;36(suppl):149.

24. Vries JK, Becker DP, Young HF: A subarachnoid screw for monitoring intracranial pressure. *J Neurosurg* 1973;39:416–419.

25. Bruce DA: *The Pathophysiology of Increased Intracranial Pressure.* Kalamazoo, The Upjohn Company, 1978.

26. Mallett BL, Veall N: Measurement of regional cerebral clearance rates in man using Xenon-133 inhalation and extracranial recording. *Clin Sci* 1965;29:179–191.

27. Selman WR, Spetzler RF, Anton AH, et al: Management of prolonged therapeutic barbiturate coma. *Surg Neurol* 1981;15:9–10.

28. Astrup J, Symon L, Branston NM, et al: Cortical evoked potential and extracellular K^+ and H^+ at critical levels of brain ischemia. *Stroke* 1977;8:51–57.

29. Goff WR, Matsumiya Y, Allison T, et al: The scalp topography of human somatosensory and auditory evoked potentials. *Electroencephalogr Clin Neurophysiol* 1977;43:57–76.

30. Coward RB: Treatment of acute fractures and fracture dislocations of the cervical spine by vertebral-body fusion. *J Neurosurg* 1961;18:201–209.

31. Heffner JE, Sahn SA: Controlled hyperventilation in patients with intracranial hypertension. *Arch Intern Med* 1983;143:765–769.

32. Quandt CM, Diaz FG, de los Reyes RA: The pharmacists' role in the treatment of intracranial hypertension secondary to head injury. *US Pharmacist* 1981;6:H2–H10.

33. Trissel LA: *Handbook on Injectable Drugs.* Bethesda, American Society of Hospital Pharmacists, 1983, pp 271–272.

34. Bivins BA, Rapp RP, Griffen WO, et al: Dopamine-phenytoin interaction. A cause of hypotension in the critically ill. *Arch Surg* 1978;113:245–249.

35. Cooper PR, Moody S, Clark WK, et al: Dexamethasone and severe head injury. A prospective double-blind study. *J Neurosurg* 1979;51:307–316.

36. Gudeman SK, Miller JD, Becker DP: Failure of high-dose steroid therapy to influence intracranial pressure in patients with severe head injury. *J Neurosurg* 1979;51:301–306.

37. Harvey SC: Hypnotics and sedatives, in Gilman AG, Goodman LS, Gilman A (eds): *The Pharmacologic Basis of Therapeutics*, New York, Macmillan, 1980, pp 349–361.

38. Delgado-Escueta AV, Wasterlain C, Treiman DM, et al: Current concepts in neurology. Management of status epilepticus. *N Engl J Med* 1982;306:1337–1340.

39. Everett ED, Strausbaugh LJ: Antimicrobial agents and the central nervous system. *Neurosurg* 1980;6:691–714.

40. Allison RR, Stack PE: Intrathecal drug therapy. *Drug Intell Clin Pharm* 1978;12:347–358.

41. White RK: Aspects and problems of total parenteral alimentation in the neurosurgery patient, in Mayaline SI, Scarasio E (eds): *Total Parenteral Alimentation*. Amsterdam, Excerpta Medica, 1976, pp 208–214.

42. Benotti P, Blackburn GL: Protein and caloric or macro-nutrient metabolic management of the critically ill patient. *Crit Care Med* 1979;7:520–525.

43. Rapp RP, Young B, Twyman D: The favorable effects of early parenteral feedings on survival in head-injured patients. *J Neurosurg* 1983;58:906–912.

44. Pappas TN, Mironovich RO: Barbiturate-induced coma to protect against cerebral ischemia and increased intracranial pressure. *Am J Hosp Pharm* 1981;38:494–498.

45. Marshall LF, Smith RW, Shapiro HM: The outcome with aggressive treatment in severe head injury. Acute and chronic barbiturate administration in the management of head injury. *J Neurosurg* 1979;50:26–30.

46. DeNicola LK, Hayes DP: Phlebothrombosis as a complication of barbiturate-induced coma for neuroresuscitation. *Drug Intell Clin Pharm* 1981;15:601–602.

47. Leavens MF, Hill S, Cech DA, et al: Intrathecal and intraventricular morphine for pain in cancer patients: Initial study. *J Neurosurg* 1982;56:241–245.

48. MacDonald JT, Uden DL: Intravenous glycerol and mannitol therapy in children with intracranial hypertension. *Neurology* 1982;32:437–440.

49. Rea GL, Rockswald GL: Barbiturate therapy in uncontrolled intracranial hypertension. *Neurosurg* 1983;12:401–404.

50. Quandt CM, Bockbrader HN, Miller DA: Thiopental dosage regimen design for patients with intracranial hypertension, abstract No. 220. American Society of Hospital Pharmacists 15th Annual Midyear Clinical Meeting, San Francisco, December 7–11, 1980.

51. Quandt, CM, de los Reyes RA, Diaz FG: Barbiturate-induced coma for the treatment of cerebral ischemia: Review of outcome. *Clin Pharm* 1982;1:549–551.

52. Drake CG: Management of cerebral aneurysm. *Stroke* 1981;12:273–283.

53. Flamm ES: Treatment of cerebral vasospasm with aminophylline and isoproterenol, in Wilkins RH (ed): *Cerebral Arterial Spasm: Proceedings of the Second International Workshop*. Baltimore, Williams & Wilkins, 1980, pp 575–577.

54. Zervas NT, Candia M, Candia G, et al: Reduced incidence of cerebral ischemia following rupture of intracranial aneurysms. *Surg Neurol* 1979;11:339–344.

55. Giannotta SL, McGillicuddy JE, Kindt GW: Diagnosis and treatment of postoperative cerebral vasospasm. *Surg Neurol* 1977;8:286–289.

56. Cohen RJ, Allen GS: Cerebral arterial spasm: The role of calcium in in vitro analysis of treatment with nifedipine and morphine, in Wilkins RH (ed) *Cerebral Arterial Spasm: Proceedings of the Second International Workshop*. Baltimore, Williams & Wilkins, 1980, pp 527–532.

57. Boullin DJ, Bunting S, Blaso WP, et al: Responses of human and baboon arteries to prostaglandin endoperoxides and biologically generated and synthetic prostacyclin: Their relevance to cerebral arterial spasm in man. *Br J Clin Pharmacol* 1979;7:139–147.

58. Mullen S, Jafar J, Hanlon K, et al: Dimethyl sulfoxide in the management of postoperative hemiplegia, in Wilkins RH (ed) *Cerebral Arterial Spasm: Proceedings of the Second International Workshop*. Baltimore, Williams & Wilkins, 1980, pp 646–653.

59. Allen GS, Ahn HS, Preziosi TJ, et al: Cerebral arterial spasm—A controlled trial of nimodipine in patients with subarachnoid hemorrhage. *N Engl J Med* 1983;308:619–624.

60. Quandt CM, de los Reyes RA, Ausman JI: Verapamil for the treatment of cerebral vasospasm following subarachnoid hemorrhage, abstract No. 39. American Society of Hospital Pharmacists 17th Annual Midyear Clinical Meeting, Los Angeles, December 1982.

61. White BC, Gadzinski DS, Hoehner PJ, et al: Correction of canine cerebral cortical blood flow and a calcium antagonist. *Ann Emerg Med* 1982;11:118.

62. Turlapaty PD, Altura BM: Extracellular magnesium ions control calcium exchange and content of vascular smooth muscle. *Eur J Pharmacol* 1978;52:421–428.

63. Boullin DJ: Potential use of prostacyclin in the treatment of vasospasm, in Wilkins RH (ed) *Cerebral Arterial Spasm: Proceedings of the Second International Workshop*. Baltimore, Williams & Wilkins, 1980, pp 533–539.

64. Rosenblum WI, El-Sabban F: Dimethyl sulfoxide (DMSO) and glycerol, hydroxyl radical scavengers, impair platelet aggregation within and eliminate the accompanying vasodilation of injured mouse pial arterioles. *Stroke* 1982;13:35–39.

65. Peerless SJ, Ishikawa R, Hunter IG, et al: Protective effect of Fluosol-DA in acute cerebral ischemia. *Stroke* 1981;12:558–563.

66. Mizoi K, Yoskimoto T, Suzuki J: Experimental study of new cerebral protective substances—Functional recovery of severe, incomplete ischaemic brain lesions pretreated with mannitol and fluorocarbon emulsion. *Acta Neurochir (Wien)* 1981;56:157–166.

67. Honda K, Hoshino S, Shoji M, et al: Clinical use of blood substitute. *N Engl J Med* 1980;303:391–392.

68. Geyer RP: "Bloodless" rats through the use of artificial blood substitute. *Fed Proc* 1975;34:1449–1505.

69. Tsuruda J, James HE, Camp PE, et al: Acute dimethyl sulfoxide therapy on experimental brain edema. Part 2—Effect of dose and concentration on intracranial pressure, blood pressure, and central venous pressure. *Neurosurg* 1982;10:355–359.

70. de la Torre JC, Rowed DW, Kawanaga HM, et al: Dimethyl sulfoxide in the treatment of experimental brain compression. *J Neurosurg* 1973;30:345–352.

71. Runckel DN, Swanson JR: Effect of dimethyl sulfoxide on serum osmolality. *Clin Chem* 1980;26:1745–1747.

72. Donegan MF, Bedford RF, Dacey R: Lidocaine for prevention of intracranial hypertension. *Anesthesiology* 1979;51:S201.

73. Bedford RF, Persing JA, Poberiskin L, et al: Lidocaine or thiopental for rapid control of intracranial hypertension. *Anesth Analg (Cleve)* 1980;59:435–437.

74. Donegan MF, Bedford RF: Intravenously administered lidocaine prevents intracranial hypertension during endotracheal suctioning. *Anesthesiology* 1980;52:516–518.

75. Gringauz A, Mombach TA: The opiate peptides (endorphins). *US Pharmacist* 1983;8:53–65.

76. Bloom F, Segal D, Ling N, et al: Endorphins, profound behavioral effects in rats suggest new etiological factors in mental illness. *Science* 1976;194:630–632.

77. Kline NS, Li CH, Lehman HE, et al: Beta-endorphin-induced changes in schizophrenic and depressed patients. *Arch Gen Psychiatry* 1977;34:1111–1113.

78. Miller RJ, Cuartrecasas P: Neurobiology and neuropharmacology of the enkephalins. *Adv Biochem Psychopharmacol* 1979;20:187–225.

79. Oyama T, Matsuki A, Taneichi T, et al: Beta-endorphin in obstetric analgesia. *Am J Obstet Gynecol* 1980;137:613–616.

80. Bloom F, Battenberg E, Rossier J, et al: Neurons containing beta-endorphin in rat brain exist separately from those containing enkephalin: Immunocytochemical studies. *Proc Natl Acad Sci USA* 1978;75:1591–1595.

81. Rossier J, Vargo TM, Minick S, Ling N, Bloom FE, Guillemin R: Regional dissociation of beta-endorphin and enkephalin contents in rat brain and pituitary. *Proc Natl Acad Sci USA* 1977;74:5162–5165.

82. Behar M, Magora F, Olshwang D, et al: Epidural morphine in treatment of pain. *Lancet* 1979;1:527–529.

83. Wang JK, Nauss LA, Thomas JE: Pain relief by intrathecally applied morphine in man. *Anesthesiology* 1979;50:149–151.

84. Tung A, Maliniak K, Tenicela R, et al: Intrathecal morphine for intraoperative and postoperative analgesia. *JAMA* 1980;244:2637–2638.

Chapter 9

The Pharmacist in Coronary Care and Cardiovascular Surgery Intensive Care

David Angaran

United and Children's Hospitals, Incorporated, is a 700-bed private hospital that was formed from three hospitals—two adult (St. Luke's and Charles T. Miller) and St. Paul Children's—in the city of St. Paul. St. Luke's served as the nucleus of a $70-million renovation and expansion program that developed the current physical plant, housing all three hospitals. (For further information about the administration of the corporation, see Chapter 2.) United Hospitals is staffed by 550 private physicians and a house staff consisting of one rotating surgical resident from the University of Minnesota Surgical Program and five family practice residents from the University of Minnesota Family Practice Program. Family practice physicians have their own clinic, which is conducted under the supervision of a group of private practice physicians, and also make rounds with a selected group of private practice specialists in areas such as cardiovascular medicine, nephrology, and infectious disease.

One pharmacy department services both United and Children's Hospitals with a centralized unit dose distribution system and decentralized pharmacists. The department provides 24-hour service, with a decentralized service on a 18-hour basis, extending from 7 A.M. to 11:30 P.M. Ninety percent of the decentralized pharmacists are pharmacists who have the B.S. degree, and who have had primarily on-the-job clinical training. Although they are involved in distribution service activities and clinical activities, the majority of their time (60%–75%) is spent with the drug distribution system. The pharmacy department also provides a complete IV additive program, drug information service, poison control program, pharmacokinetic dosing service, investigational drug control service, Pharmacy and Therapeutics Committee (P&T) consultation, and formulary revision and development services.

The United Hospitals pharmacy department serves as an educational site for both pharmacists and pharmacy students. A program combining a Masters in Hospital Pharmacy and an ASHP-accredited residency through the University of

Minnesota College of Pharmacy has existed since 1977, with two students in each two-year program. There are also four to six undergraduate B.S. students receiving educational experience in the areas of internship and externship, in addition to two to five Pharm.D. clerkships in various clinical areas, such as internal medicine, pediatrics, oncology, and critical care.

DEMOGRAPHICS OF THE UNITS

The coronary care unit (CCU) is a ten-bed unit. United Hospitals admitted 168 myocardial infarction patients for the year 1982. The remaining beds were occupied by patients with primary cardiovascular disorders, such as severe congestive heart failure, hypertensive crisis, or intractable arrhythmias. The average occupancy rate is 70%.

The hospital provides a wide range of cardiovascular services, including coronary angiography and such current noninvasive techniques as MUGA, PYP scans, and 2D-Echo. Other available cardiovascular procedures include intracoronary streptokinase, electrophysiological studies, and percutaneous transluminal angioplasty. Both units commonly use pulmonary artery (Swan-Ganz®) catheters and intraaortic balloon pumps.

The majority of the CCU patients are seen primarily by or in consultation with a board-certified cardiologist. Nurse staffing is done on a one-to-one or one-to-two basis by a group of highly specialized nurses with considerable experience in electrocardiographic interpretation and cardiovascular assessment. Nurses are responsible for implementing several drug protocols without a physician's direct order or presence, including lidocaine therapy, cardiopulmonary resuscitation, and electrical defibrillation.

The cardiovascular surgery unit (CSU) is an 11-bed unit. Three hundred and forty aortocoronary bypass and 60 prosthetic valve procedures were conducted during 1982 at United Hospitals. The CSU serves as the ICU and the postanesthesia recovery unit, to which patients are brought directly from surgery. In uncomplicated cases the average length of stay is 1½ days. Patients are transferred to other ICUs if they develop complications (such as sepsis) or require dialysis. The CSU also cares for patients undergoing surgery for aortic aneurysms when they are hemodynamically unstable. The unit is equipped to treat patients requiring intraaortic balloon insertion. The nurse staffing ratio is 1:1 during the patient's first or second postoperative day and in the cases of unstable patients, but the ratio increases to 1:2 for more stable patients.

Patient care activities in the CCU and CSU are in rhythm with the usual activities of any private practice hospital without a significant house staff. Physicians arrive in the early morning to see their patients and, depending on how critical their patients' conditions are, come back in the afternoon or conduct further patient care by telephone. Some physicians take early morning (6 to 7 A.M.) calls to hear patients' laboratory results at home before leaving for the office. The cardiovascular surgeons usually make rounds between 7:30 A.M. and 8 A.M.—before surgery. After-office hours and patient care responsibilities occurring on days off are rotated between partners or other physician groups that share call.

One surgical resident and one family practice resident are in the hospital at all times to respond to emergencies. Staff physicians may be required for critically ill patients or for emergency surgeries.

DRUG RECORDS AND DATA COLLECTION

All drug administration records of the intensive care units (ICUs) are on a centralized sheet called a Medication Administration Record (MAR). Exhibit 9-1 depicts a sample copy of this record. This document provides a record of all drugs the patient receives while in the hospital. It also serves as the permanent nursing record for drug administration. The MAR is a multicopy carbon form that can be used for five days without necessitating recopy. Up-to-date carbon copies are placed in the charts. All intravenous solutions are documented on a separate IV record form (Exhibit 9-2), while TPN therapy is charted on another form (Exhibit 9-3).

Clinical laboratory data are provided by a computerized summary every 24 hours. Both intensive care units have a telex system that allows the laboratory to broadcast results stat to the units. A separate hemodynamic record (Exhibit 9-4), which includes temperature, blood pressure, heart and respiration rate, rhythm, pulmonary artery pressures, cardiac function, IV intake, output, and nursing notes, is maintained for each 24-hour period by nurses for each patient in the unit. There is no unified system that integrates physician notes, procedures, hemodynamic data and drug administration into one form. Currently a microcomputer is being placed in the ICU area, possibly to provide such a data base.

DRUG DISTRIBUTION SYSTEMS

Drug distribution to both ICUs is based on the hospital-wide system of a centralized unit-dose system with decentralized pharmacists. The drug delivery system is activated by a written order in the chart that produces a direct "pharmacy" copy. The pharmacy becomes aware of the order by being paged or by being informed during regular patient care rounds of the units. Assessment and interpretation of the drug order for accuracy and appropriateness before the initiation of the delivery process are the highest priorities.

Exhibit 9–1 Medication Administration Record

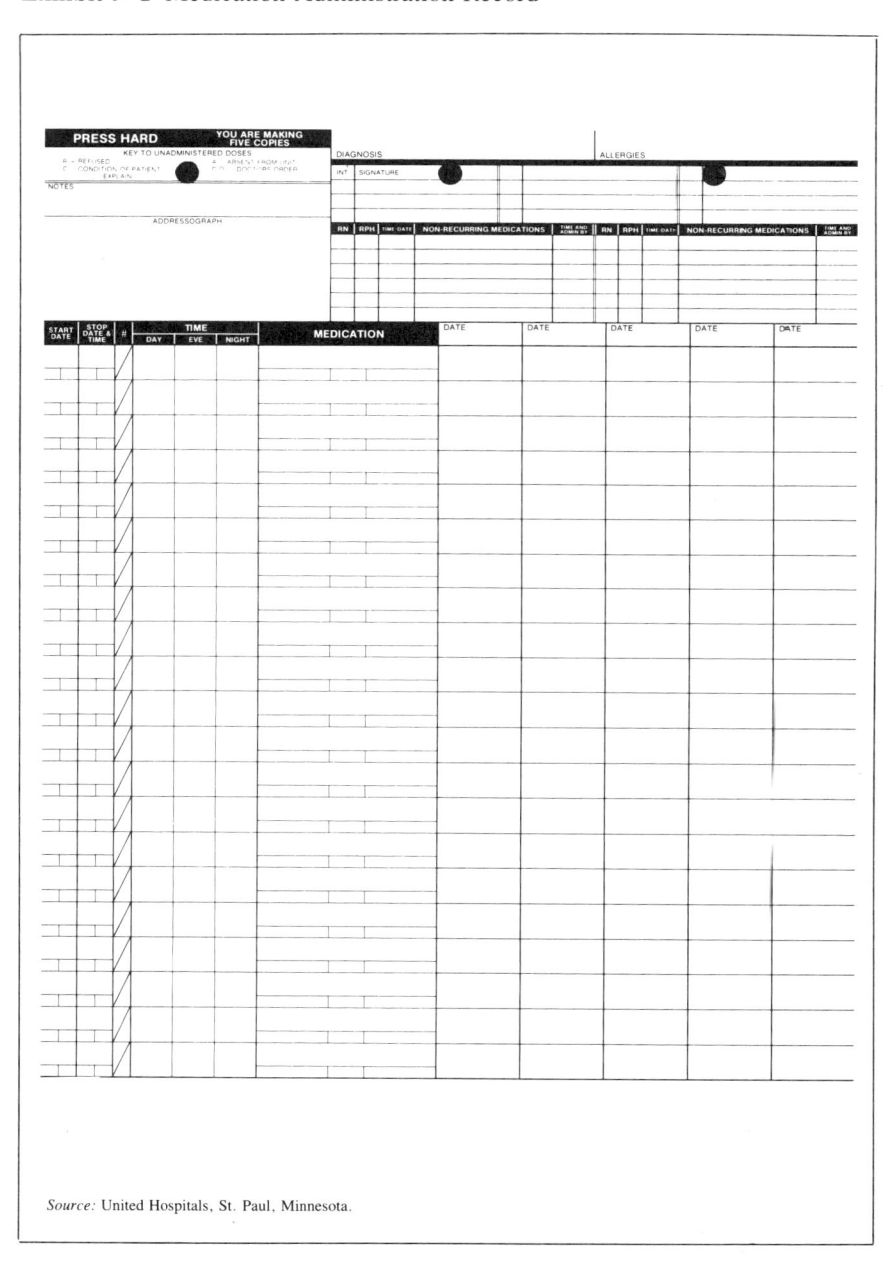

Source: United Hospitals, St. Paul, Minnesota.

Exhibit 9–2 IV Therapy Sheet

(SEE REVERSE SIDE FOR NOTES, DRIP RATES, ELECTROLYTE KEY, ETC.)

CURRENT I.V. ORDERS

ORDER DATE		DISCONT. DATE		I.V. ORDER			
RN	RPH	RN	RPH				

BOTTLE NO.	VOLUME / RATE	SOLUTIONS AND ADDITIVES	CHART EACH I.V. UPON HANGING: NEEDLE OR CATH. INSERTED/ CHANGED AND SITE	TUBE CHANGE / SITE CARE	DATE TIME STARTED / INITIALS	DATE TIME INFUSED / INITIALS	AMOUNT INFUSED	NOTES
	ml							
	ml/hr							
	ml							
	ml/hr							
	ml							
	ml/hr							
	ml							
	ml/hr							
	ml							
	ml/hr							
	ml							
	ml/hr							
	ml							
	ml/hr							
	ml							
	ml/hr							
	ml							
	ml/hr							
	ml							
	ml/hr							
	ml							
	ml/hr							
	ml							
	ml/hr							
	ml							
	ml/hr							
	ml							
	ml/hr							

INITIALS	SIGNATURES

Exhibit 9–2 continued

NOTES

RATE CONVERSION CHART

RATE IN ml/hour	RATE IN drops/minute For Tubing Delivering *10 drops/ml	*60 drops/ml	INFUSION TIME IN hours/liter
42	7	42	24
50	8	50	20
53	9	53	19
55	9	55	18
60	10	60	16½
63	10½	63	16
65	11	65	15
70	11-12	70	14
75	12	75	13
80	13	80	12½
83	14	83	12
90	15	90	11
100	17	100	10
110	18	110	9
125	21	125	8
140	23	140	7
150	25	150	6½
167	28	167	6

*TRAVENOL SETS WITH THE EXCEPTION OF "MINIDRIP" OR "PEDIATRIC SETS" DELIVER 10 DROPS/ML

NUMBERING OF INFUSIONS

MAINTENANCE: 1, 2, 3, 4, etc.

TPN: A, B, C, D, etc.

MEDICATION:
e.g. Lidocaine — I LIDO, II LIDO, III LIDO, etc.
Heparin — I HEP, II HEP, III HEP, etc.

MISCELLANEOUS:
e.g. Pressure Bags — I PB, II PB, III PB, etc.
Lipids — I LIPID, II LIPID, III LIPID, etc.
NG Replacement — I NG, II NG, III NG, etc.

ELECTROLYTE KEY (PER LITER)

	DEXT (g)	Na+ MEQ	K+ MEQ	Ca++ MEQ	Mg++ MEQ	Cl− MEQ	PHOS MM	ACET− MEQ	LACT− MEQ	INVERT SUGAR (g)
NaCl 0.2%		34				34				
NaCl 0.33%		56				56				
NaCl 0.45%		77				77				
NaCl 0.9%		154				154				
DEXTROSE 5%	50									
LACTATED RINGERS		130	4	3		109			28	
TRAVERTS 10%										100
ELECTROLYTE #2		56	25		6	56	6		25	
TPN (standard electrolytes)	35	30	5		5	35	15	TO BALANCE		
TRAVASOL 10%		40						87		

Source: United Hospitals, St. Paul, Minnesota.

Exhibit 9–3 TPN Therapy Sheet

CURRENT TPN ORDERS

ORDER DATE (RN / RPH)	DISCONT. DATE (RN / RPH)	AMINO ACID/ DEXTROSE SOLUTION	DEXT (g)	AMINO ACID (g)	NA+ (mEq)	K+ (mEq)	Ca++ (mEq)	Mg++ (mEq)	PHOS. (mM)	Cl− (mEq)	ACET.− (mEq)	MVI 12	VIT K	TRACE ELEM.	MISC	RATIO ADDED ANIONS Ac Cl	RATE	NOTES:
																	ml/hr	
																	ml/hr	
																	ml/hr	
																	ml/hr	
																	ml/hr	
																	ml/hr	

TPN CHARTING — **CHART EACH TPN UPON HANGING**

BOTTLE NO.	VOLUME / RATE	AMINO ACID/ DEXTROSE SOLUTION	DEXT (g)	AMINO ACID (g)	NA+ (mEq)	K+ (mEq)	Ca++ (mEq)	Mg++ (mEq)	PHOS. (mM)	Cl− (mEq)	ACET.− (mEq)	MVI 12	VIT K	TRACE ELEM.	MISC	NEEDLE OR CATH. INSERTED/ CHANGED AND SITE	TUBE CHANGE / SITE CARE	DATE TIME STARTED / INITIALS	DATE TIME INFUSED / INITIALS	AMOUNT INFUSED
	ml ml/hr																			
	ml ml/hr																			
	ml ml/hr																			
	ml ml/hr																			
	ml ml/hr																			
	ml ml/hr																			
	ml ml/hr																			
	ml ml/hr																			
	ml ml/hr																			
	ml ml/hr																			
	ml ml/hr																			
	ml ml/hr																			
	ml ml/hr																			
	ml ml/hr																			

INITIALS	SIGNATURE

Source: United Hospitals, St. Paul, Minnesota.

Exhibit 9–4 Hemodynamic Information

DATE: PAGE 1 **UNITED HOSPITALS CRITICAL CARE FLOW SHEET**

Addressograph

POST OP DAY

TODAY'S WT.

YESTERDAY'S WT.

PRE-OP WT.

	0800	0900	1000	1100	1200	1300	1400	1500		1600	1700	1800
104									104			
103									103			
102									102			
101									101			
100									100			
99									99			
98									98			
97									97			
RR / Vent									RR / Vent			
HR									HR			
BP									BP			
LAP									LAP			
PAS / MEAN									PAS / MEAN			
PAD / PWP									PAD / PWP			
CVP									CVP			
									8 HR TOTAL			
INTAKE: IV												
IV												
IV												
BLOOD												
ORAL/TUBE FEEDING												
								TOTAL 8 HR INTAKE				
OUTPUT: URINE												
CT												
NG												
								TOTAL 8 HR OUTPUT				
DU												
SG												

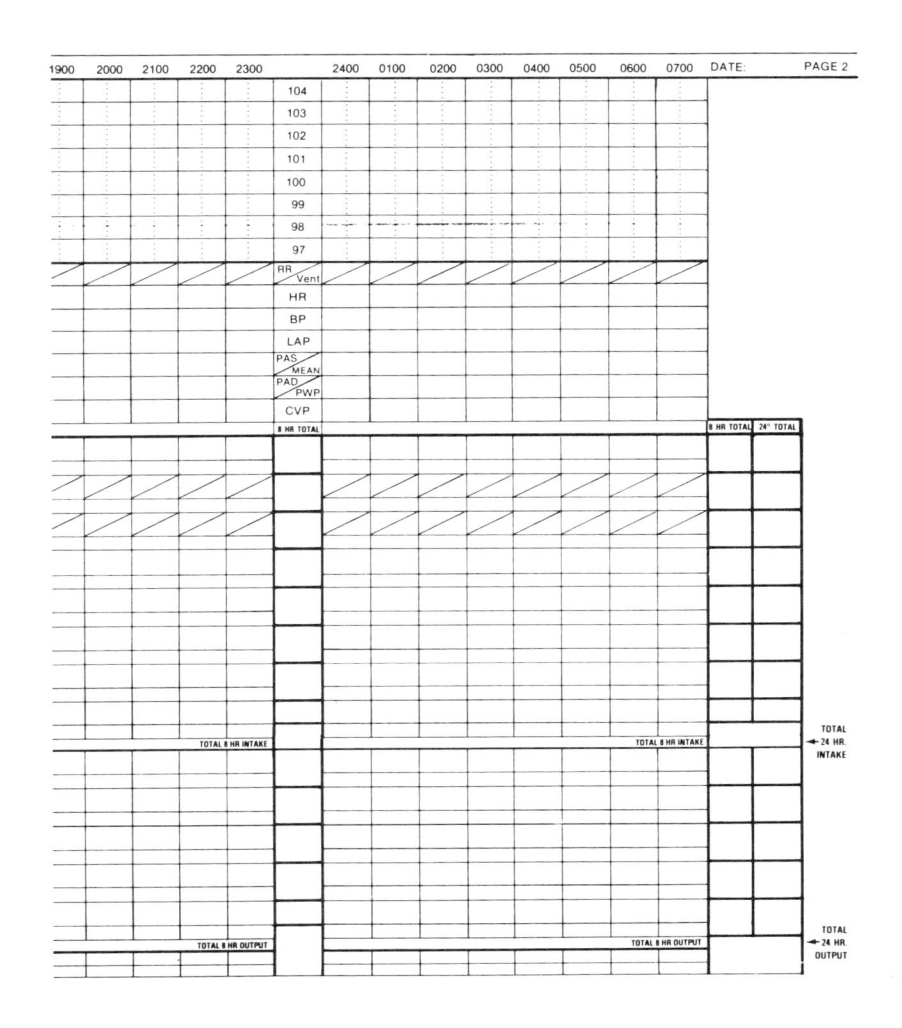

1900	2000	2100	2200	2300		2400	0100	0200	0300	0400	0500	0600	0700	DATE:		PAGE 2
					104											
					103											
					102											
					101											
					100											
					99											
					98											
					97											
					RR/Vent											
					HR											
					BP											
					LAP											
					PAS/MEAN											
					PAD/PWP											
					CVP											
					8 HR TOTAL									8 HR TOTAL	24" TOTAL	

TOTAL 8 HR INTAKE — TOTAL 8 HR INTAKE — TOTAL 24 HR. INTAKE

TOTAL 8 HR OUTPUT — TOTAL 8 HR OUTPUT — TOTAL 24 HR. OUTPUT

Exhibit 9–4 continued

LABORATORY DATA

DATE												
TIME												
NA												
K												
CL												
CO2												
PH												
PCO2												
HCO3												
BE												
PO2												
FIO2												
IMV/CMV												
PEEP												
TV/V.C.												
HGB												
HCT												
WBC												
PLATELETS												
PT												
PTT												
TT												
BS												

PAGE 3

	DATE	DATE	DATE	DATE
CPK/MB				
BUN				
CR				
ALB				
T. PROT				
CA				
MG				
PHOS				

CRITICAL CARE FLOW SHEET

Source: United Hospitals, St. Paul, Minnesota.

DATE		PAGE 4	
TIME	PROBLEM		PROGRESS NOTES

Seventy percent of the drug orders are filled from the central pharmacy. These orders are filled upon receipt of the original pharmacy copy or by a phone order from the decentralized pharmacist. All dosage forms, both sterile and nonsterile, are first prepared or obtained by a pharmacy technician and then checked for accuracy by a centralized pharmacist. Regularly scheduled orders are entered into the pharmacy computer. The unit-dose carts are filled with a 24-hour supply of drugs in individual doses. The carts are exchanged each morning between 6 A.M. and 7 A.M. The decentralized pharmacist checks the exchanged carts against the MAR each morning for accuracy. Furthermore, he makes such a check every time a new drug is requested for the patient.

The MAR is the joint responsibility of both nursing and pharmacy. Nurses are responsible for entering the order (drug, dose, route, frequency), and pharmacists check for the administration times and the start date. Nurses and pharmacists are required to check the order for its accuracy and appropriateness.

A new MAR is created when the five-day administration recording time has been exceeded or when all of the empty drug entries have been used up because of order changes or multiple drug use. Most patients in the ICUs require two drug MARs for the scheduled and PRN medications, in addition to the IV fluid MAR.

Time—response time and total time per patient—is the major problem of any drug delivery system in an ICU. The total pharmacy manpower committed to the ICU is dictated by the response time and intensity of care for a small number of patients. United Hospitals provides one decentralized pharmacist, covering a 16-hour time period (7 A.M. to 11 P.M.), for three ten-bed ICUs. These ICU pharmacists are also assigned the coverage of additional nursing units, depending on the hospital census, the day of the week, and the time of day. For example, on a Saturday evening shift (3 P.M.–11 P.M.), the ICU pharmacist has the responsibility for the ICUs and the two regular (30-bed) nursing units. There are, of course, times when floor-stock drugs must be used, and only a limited supply of key drugs may be available for use. (The content and quantity of these floor-stock supplies are decided jointly by pharmacists, nurses, and physicians.) The development of a quick, reactive system to process drug orders in the ICU is facilitated by the presence of the decentralized pharmacist and three modes of drug delivery: (1) a pneumatic tube system capable of transporting IV bags up to one liter capacity, (2) a dumbwaiter, and (3) an elevator system.

JUSTIFICATION, ORGANIZATION, AND IMPLEMENTATION OF THE SYSTEM

The discussion of the clinical position that was implemented will include a historical discussion of the original Pharm.D. positions. A brief overview of how the distribution pharmacist position was implemented is covered in Chapter 2.

The original Pharm.D. was hired in 1974 with the understanding that the responsibilities would be 20% clinical and 80% distributional. From that original commitment, a full-time clinical pharmacy position was developed. This position was funded by the hospital. The incumbent eventually became the Assistant Director for Clinical Services. The position was developed clinically by the implementation of a drug interaction monitoring system program. The idea was that the clinical pharmacist would monitor patients in St. Luke's Hospital (Miller and St. Luke's were geographically separated by one mile until 1980) and provide the physicians with notification, description, and evaluation of potential drug interactions in their patients. Physicians were asked to participate in a personal discussion about all pertinent or significant drug interactions that were apparently unrecognized. From these discussions, the physicians became educated about not only that drug interaction, but also about the capabilities and contribution of the clinical pharmacist. This was the beginning of clinical pharmacy services at United Hospitals.

Because of the initial favorable response to the drug interaction program, a second Pharm.D. was hired in 1975 with the understanding that the clinician's responsibilities would be 30% clinical and 70% distributional. This pharmacist, stationed at Miller Hospital, had responsibility for its 300 beds. Also during 1975, the first pharmacokinetic dosing program involving the aminoglycosides (gentamicin and tobramycin) was started. This service has grown to the point at which 80% to 90% of all aminoglycoside use receives a pharmacokinetic consultation, in addition to pharmacokinetic interpretations for drugs such as antiarrhythmics, anticonvulsants and theophylline. The second clinician was also soon relieved of dispensing functions and assumed full-time clinical duties.

In 1976, the Oncology Service requested a clinical pharmacist to take charge of the preparation of intravenous antineoplastic agents. Again, as in the previous two cases, this person quickly developed a full-time clinical service in the area of oncology, with antineoplastic agents being compounded in the centralized IV additive area.

St. Paul Children's Hospital's clinical program began in 1975 and brought a full-time pharmacy clinician with the merger of the three hospitals mentioned. United and Children's Hospitals' clinical pharmacy staff from 1979 to 1984 consists of four Pharm.D.s, one of whom is Assistant Director of Pharmacy Services.

During the developmental phase of clinical pharmacy services at United Hospitals, it quickly became apparent that the sickest patients with the most complex illnesses, requiring the greatest number of patient-monitoring hours, were located in the ICUs. The coming merger of the two hospitals meant a general upgrading of all services, but a particular impact was aimed at the ICUs. This upgrading resulted from an increase in the numbers and the acuity of patients because of the expanding cardiovascular surgery program and hemodialysis capabilities. Even though each of the four Pharm.D.s has a specialty interest, the 700-bed hospital was divided so that each clinician was responsible for providing clinical services for areas outside his/her specialties.

My involvement with United Hospitals began in 1979 through our joint interests, mine in critical care practice and theirs in expanding clinical services to the ICU. From the College of Pharmacy standpoint, in 1979, United was a progressive 700-bed hospital with four Pharm.D.s on staff, all very capable and former graduates of our program, all well known to the College. I was then an associate professor of pharmacy, serving in an administrative capacity as Director of the Clinical Practice Unit, but had decided to go back into clinical practice. My background was in the area of critical care from the University of Wisconsin. I had worked there in a trauma and life-support unit before leaving in 1976. Dean Larry Weaver approved my movement back into clinical practice, and we discussed where I might be sited to the greatest advantage, not only for my career but also for the College of Pharmacy.

The University of Minnesota Pharm.D. program clinical experience year, in 1979, was sited at the four major teaching hospitals throughout the Twin City area: two county hospitals, a veterans' hospital, and the University medical center. There was no exposure for the Pharm.D. student in the area of private medical practice and the private hospital clinical pharmacy practitioner. Twenty Pharm.D.s practiced clinical pharmacy in private hospitals in the Twin Cities. They were not supported by or associated with the College of Pharmacy. It seemed evident that United Hospitals would be an important addition to the curriculum and the experiences of our Pharm.D. students.

I began to develop a clinical practice at United Hospitals in July 1979. The agreement between the Director of Pharmacy and the College of Pharmacy was that I would continue as a fully paid member and as associate professor in the College of Pharmacy. I would provide clinical and educational services in the area of acute care medicine. In return for my services (I would be the fifth Pharm.D. clinician in the hospital), the College of Pharmacy would use the United pharmacy department personnel, clinicians, decentralized pharmacists, and administrative personnel to provide both didactic and clinical instruction for pharmacy students.

The lines of authority officially run between the Director of Pharmacy and the Dean of the College of Pharmacy. I report to the Dean. The functional lines of authority include the Assistant Director for Clinical Services, the Director of Pharmacy, and the Dean. Day-to-day discussions and planning concerning all areas of my involvement at United Hospitals (education, research and service) are conducted between me and the Assistant Director of Clinical Services.

Examples of how my activities and those of the pharmacy department are coordinated can be seen in the following:

- My patient care clinical activities are recorded on a Patient Care Unit (PCU) card—a mechanism to record work units by the clinical pharmacists—and entered into overall department workload statistics.
- I participated in gathering drug use data, such as antibiotic audits, and in suggesting and implementing cost control measures in the ICUs.
- Student scheduling is done by the assistant director because of its implications for patient care; it also reinforces in the students the understanding that they are part of the pharmacy department, no matter how short their stay.
- Pharmacy department personnel are closely involved in college program development through committee work and student evaluation.
- I am on clinical pharmacy call for the entire hospital two nights per week.
- The pharmacy department personnel and resources are involved in current clinical research projects. These resources are paid for by research grants.
- Clinical pharmacy coverage for my practice areas and students is provided by the other clinicians during weekends and absences.
- A clinical pharmacy research fellowship has existed under my direction since 1980. This position has been filled by a Pharm.D. and was funded earlier through a mixture of research, hospital, and physician monies, but now it is funded entirely through research money. The fellow provides coverage for my clinical service and student responsibilities during my absence and, therefore, contributes to pharmacy department activities.

DESCRIPTION OF ACTIVITIES

The activities of the clinical pharmacist in the CCU and the CSU include providing pharmacokinetic dosing services, drug monitoring, investigational drugs, drug interactions, research, formulary evaluation, parenteral nutrition, and general problem solving.

The daily routine starts at 6 A.M. with personal rounds and review of the night's activities in the two ICUs. Information on all old patients is reviewed, and the new admissions are evaluated. From 7 to 7:30 A.M., the clinical pharmacist attends nursing reporting in the CSU and that of the Pharm.D. student in the CCU. The time from 7:30 to 9 A.M. is divided between rounds with the cardiovascular surgeons and the Pharm.D. student in the CCU. These morning rounds with the Pharm.D. student are directed toward identifying which therapeutic problems must be acted upon that morning, new patient evaluation, and possible afternoon activities.

If everything is quiet in the ICU, the time from 9 A.M. to 3:30 P.M. is divided between research projects, college of pharmacy activities, and pharmacy department objectives.

A second teaching and service round is conducted between 3:30 P.M. and 5:30 P.M. by the clinical pharmacist and the Pharm.D. student. At that time, all kinetic consultations are completed, the day's activities reviewed, and plans for the next morning are made.

Therapy-Planning Activities

One of the most interesting aspects of this service in a private hospital, in both intensive care units, is the opportunity to plan with the nurse two important aspects of therapy. One aspect is the phone call to the physician to obtain an answer to a patient problem. This requires cooperation to insure that all pertinent data are organized in an understandable fashion. These data should provide the optimum amount of information in the minimum amount of time. This procedure sounds simple, but it is not. It takes a lot of practice to learn how much information to give over the phone, by what method, and in what order so that an informed decision can be reached.

The second aspect of planning with the nurses is the procedure for initiating and administering a drug order in a safe and reasonable manner. This aspect is one of the most exciting and interesting parts of the day's work. Many medication orders are vaguely written and leave a certain amount of discretion to the nurse or the pharmacist as to how they are to be implemented. This implementation process may include starting time, titration schedule, therapeutic end-points, and side-effect detection as just representative examples. This prospective process develops a strong bond between pharmacists and nurses because it is a cooperative effort.

The decentralized pharmacist also has a role in the clinical care of the patient. It obviously involves ensuring that all drug orders are accurately and promptly filled. In addition to making sure that the distribution system works, the decentralized pharmacist in the critical care area answers many questions about IV drugs, such as their incompatibilities, dilutions, and rates of administration. The pharmacist also serves as a primary screen for drug-related problems that he detects, but may not have the time to pursue in depth. This interchange may work both ways as the students and I coordinate our work to ensure an efficient use of the distribution system. A common example is the notification of the decentralized pharmacist of potential TPN changes so that wastage may be reduced. As the decentralized pharmacists gain more experience, plans call for their increased involvement in the clinical decision process.

Educational Activities

A second area of clinical activity is education. The educational effort includes not only Pharm.D. students, but also physicians, nurses, laboratory technologists, dietitians, and other hospital personnel.

The most interesting and fruitful education, in this writer's view, is the one-on-one or one-on-two teaching that takes place at the patient's bedside; there, a patient's problem can be solved and used as a brief educational example. Seeing something and using the understanding that accompanies it has no substitute.

Pharm.D. students receiving their clinical education at United Hospitals are placed in the position of identifying drug-related problems, responding to questions, and developing a therapeutic strategy—all under close supervision. Once a satisfactory plan has been developed, however, the students are charged with the responsibility of communicating, implementing, and monitoring this plan. Making prospective decisions under supervision is the key to clinical education.

The education of pharmacy students in the hospital for practical experience that is clinical and nonclinical is now a universal reality. The attitude of nonuniversity teaching centers toward their involvement in such programs varies from enthusiasm to active antagonism. I must be considered suspect because of my affiliation, but I would offer my 15 years' experience and expect that students return as much as they receive. In fact, what they return most often reflects what they receive—not every student, but the majority. They are maturing professionals looking for guidance and example, a role model. Provide that and they will return your effort.

What do the students actually return for your efforts? The students can extend your ability to follow patients by gathering data into a concise interpretable format. They may not know what to gather in the beginning, but once you point out what is needed, they will follow through. Students ask both very simple and very complex questions. Nothing you do should be beyond question. Lastly, in the system at United Hospitals, students rotate among hospitals in the Twin City area and serve as a means of communication and transporters of ideas between hospitals.

Research Activities

Research activities in a private hospital and CCU provide both opportunities and problems that can differ from those in the traditional university setting.

How do you get started? We evaluated the ICUs for the largest group of homogeneous patients under the control of a small group of physicians who had a positive attitude toward research. Just after my arrival at United Hospitals, a cardiovascular surgery team was leaving the University of Minnesota to continue work in private practice. The original group was composed of three surgeons, three pump technicians, and two nurse practitioners. It has grown to a group that includes five surgeons and four pump technicians.

The original group of cardiovascular surgeons were all veteran academic faculty with numerous publications and who were interested in continuing clinical investigation into patients undergoing cardiovascular surgery.

Because my experience in cardiovascular surgery was limited, I first became involved with daily patient care activities by making rounds on a daily basis six days a week. The first six months were a time of becoming familiar with other personnel. Soon thereafter we began our first research project involving me, the surgeons, and a Pharm.D. student who was on a one-month project. This original effort has now expanded to include a six-member cardiology group, a full-time Pharm.D. clinical pharmacy research associate, a high-pressure liquid chromatography (HPLC) technologist, and various part-time Pharm.D. and Ph.D. students doing special projects.

The beginning research money was supplied by the Research and Education Committee of United Hospitals. (The hospital was obviously less interested in supporting a clinical pharmacist than in supporting a surgical group that brought 400 bypass patients a year to the hospital.) The United Hospitals Education and Research Committee provided money for two small research projects and, in 1981, matched funds with the cardiovascular surgeons for a clinical pharmacy research associate. The 1983–1984 research associate was funded without hospital money, being supported by surgery, cardiovascular, and research funds.

The United Hospitals clinical laboratory has been a source of great cooperation for both the research effort and the clinical activities. A drug assay laboratory (DAL) was funded through medical staff research funds as a joint effort by the clinical laboratory and me. The DAL currently consists of an HPLC and one technologist funded for two years, but the other drug assay equipment, such as the TDX equipment, is used at reduced rates for research.

A representative sample of our investigations includes the influence of cardiopulmonary bypass on the pharmacokinetics and pharmacodynamics of drugs, the influence of antibiotics on oral anticoagulation in the prosthetic valve patient, the prevention of arrhythmias in the postaortocoronary bypass period, and the phase III study of a new short-acting beta blocker.

One of the major differences between a university training center and the private hospital is not only the lack of house staff, but the attitude toward research. Staff and patients expect a university center (but not a private hospital) to be on the cutting edge of science and knowledge. We could not conduct our investigations without the complete cooperation of the nursing staff, because they are directly involved in a number of our investigations. My evaluation is that the key to nursing cooperation has been clinical practice, communication, and applied research topics.

The clinical practice of pharmacy is the primary factor that serves as the basis for better communication and identification of major patient problems for clinical investigation. In my experience, there is no substitute for being there together while trying to solve a patient care problem that builds a bond of trust and understanding between nursing and pharmacy. Not just I, but the entire group representing pharmacy, the decentralized pharmacist, other clinical practitioners, and the research associate, contribute to this positive atmosphere.

Communication is an obvious and well-worn word. The key is not only quality and quantity; the key is inclusion of nursing in the early planning and implementation process of a research project. It is important to accomplish projects without disrupting the delivery of good patient care.

The research topics have all been aimed at applied areas of clinical care. We have joint discussions about the problem and how our investigation could possibly lead toward better patient care.

A cooperative effort with the clinical laboratory is also necessary. Again, clinical practice and the pharmacokinetic dosing service provided the process of joint problem solving that naturally extended into the research area. As an example, we performed a study involving the accuracy of coagulation studies obtained from arterial lines. This work eliminated the need for venipuncture in cold, vasoconstricted postoperative cardiac surgery patients—a time-consuming and frustrating practice.

The cooperation of the pharmacy department is also imperative and has been exemplary. Our success was similar to that obtained by the nurses' early involvement and their feeling of participation. I have used the excellent decentralized unit-dose system as a selling point to pharmaceutical companies about drug control and patient identification.

The pharmacist, independent of his pharmacotherapy expertise, has something to offer in clinical therapeutic research. Drug companies are looking for people to conduct studies on many patient populations. The major problem they face is the assurance that projects will be completed in a timely manner and with adequate data collection. By assuring that things get done in an efficient, accurate, and complete manner, you do not even have to construct your own protocols.

We have kept the pharmaceutical companies that make drugs used in our patient population appraised of our interest through letters and telephone calls about current or future investigations. We inform the company about what clinical problem we are interested in, how their drug fits in, the numbers of patients seen with this problem per year, and which physicians are involved.

The physician-pharmacist interaction is also best based on this anticipatory planning. Even though there are hundreds of practicing physicians at United Hospitals, the majority of the patients in the acute care areas are seen by a select number of specialists. My approach has been to determine how each specialist uses his drugs and to assist in assuring that they are administered as expected. Any differences of opinion we might have about choice of drug, dose, route, regimen, and so forth are discussed in an open manner. This type of interchange creates an understanding between physician and pharmacist that is absolutely essential to caring for any patient.

SUMMARY

Given the assumption that I have been relatively successful in establishing a critical care practice in both a university and private hospital setting, how would I analyze the reasons for that success?

Competence. In both critical care settings I started at a low level of understanding about trauma and heart surgery patients. I reviewed the literature and asked many questions of the nurses and the physicians. Although this procedure sounds simple, it includes careful observation of patients, with an emphasis on drug-related problems, how they are treated now, and how they might be treated better. I try to establish a norm for each situation and, when something happens outside that norm, I try to find a reason why—a Bayesean approach to patient care. I am not sure what prompts people to trust your judgment when faced with the unknown. It is that intangible combination of knowing the theory, knowing what others have done, and knowing how that information influences the problem you are faced with at that moment; and then devising an approach that has defined goals for identifying success and failure.

Visibility. I am in the hospital early; often, I stay late. I call back frequently. There is no substitute for being there on the scene when help is needed. It is a hundred times better to participate in an anticipatory manner than to correct a poor decision after the fact.

Reliability. Be honest, accurate, and dependable. Patient care comes first.

Pharmacy Department. I have always been associated with an aggressive and progressive pharmacy department. The establishment of a clinical practice can be done in the absence of, or even in spite of, an inadequate pharmaceutical service, but it is much more difficult.

Communication. No one likes to be the last to know. Therefore, an endless amount of time must be taken for informing, reminding, explaining, and exploring. Because everything we do requires cooperation, there is no substitute for communication.

Chapter 10

The Pharmacist in Medical Intensive Care

Joyce B. Comer

DEMOGRAPHICS

The position to be discussed in this chapter is located at Hartford Hospital, a 1,000-bed community hospital that has a teaching affiliation with the University of Connecticut Medical School. The hospital has over 200 house officers and offers educational programs in medicine, surgery, obstetrics-gynecology, and subspecialty areas (e.g., radiology, infectious disease, and cardiology).

Hartford Hospital has three primary buildings, which house a variety of services (see Exhibit 10–1). These services include six intensive care units (ICUs), a recovery room, and an emergency room.

The general medical floor houses 120 beds as well as a separate 11-bed medical intensive care unit (MICU). The majority of patients on this floor are cared for by house officers. The internal medicine house officers serve as junior and senior residents; interns are from various programs within the hospital, including internal medicine, psychiatry, and obstetrics-gynecology. In addition, most patients have private physicians and subspecialty consultants who are responsible for their care.

The MICU is staffed by a senior internal medicine resident and two internal medicine interns. The interns rotate every six weeks, and the residents rotate every four weeks. These house officers are directly responsible for any ward medicine patients in the MICU. They are also responsible for private medical patients. Because Hartford Hospital has several ICUs, the general types of patients admitted to the MICU are determined by the following primary indications:

- diabetic ketoacidosis
- acute respiratory failure or decompensation
- gastrointestinal bleeding (variceal and nonvariceal)
- septic shock

Exhibit 10–1 Geographic Description of Hartford Hospital

South building
    Gynecology
    Outpatient clinics

Continuing care building
    Hemodialysis unit
    Inpatient psychiatry
    Physical medicine

Main building (each line represents a separate patient floor)
    Cardiology and cardiac intensive care unit
    Private medical and surgical units
    Ophthalmology, urology, and general surgery
    General medicine and medical intensive care unit
    Neurology-orthopedics and neurosurgical intensive care unit
    Pediatrics and obstetrics with pediatric and neonatal intensive care units
    Surgery and surgical intensive care unit
    Operating Room and Recovery Room
    Emergency Room

Source: Hartford Hospital, Hartford, Connecticut.

- drug overdose or ingestion
- overwhelming sepsis (e.g., meningicoccal meningitis)
- massive pulmonary embolism
- ventilator dependent patients (e.g., Guillian-Barré Syndrome)
- uncontrollable status epilepticus
- acute respiratory distress
- postcardiac arrest

Occasionally, when the cardiac or neurosurgical intensive care units do not have an available bed, the MICU has patients with cardiogenic shock, acute myocardial infarction, or subarachnoid hemorrhage. In addition to diagnosis, the MICU is required for the performance of several procedures and the administration of several medications (Table 10–1).

POSITION DEVELOPMENT

Clinical pharmacy services and a drug information center have been available to medical personnel at Hartford Hospital since 1974. At that time, routine clinical pharmacy services were provided to the department of pediatrics. At present, the staff has grown, and now full-time clinical pharmacy services are provided to cardiology, infectious disease, pediatrics, surgery, and medicine. The department of pharmacy services drug distribution is provided by a floor-stock system, which is currently being converted to a decentralized unit-dose system with an intravenous admixture program.

The author's responsibility as the clinical pharmacist at Hartford Hospital is to provide clinical pharmacy services to the Department of Medicine. When the position was originated in 1978, it became apparent that it would be difficult to provide an adequate clinical service on a daily basis to 120 patients on five different nursing units, plus an 11-bed MICU. It then became necessary to identify those patients who would require the services of a clinical pharmacist. Thus, over the following one to two years, several revisions were undertaken to accommodate the situation.

First, the clinical pharmacist identified the patients in the MICU who were critically ill and thus in need of routine coverage on a daily basis (this concept will be expanded later). In this manner, the majority of the pharmacist's time could be devoted to the most critically ill patients on the medical service. Also, inasmuch as all internal medicine house officers rotate through the MICU, they would there be exposed to the services and information the clinical pharmacist had to offer, and would therefore be more likely to contact this pharmacist when there were drug-related patient problems on the medical floor, outside the MICU.

Second, the clinical pharmacist also provided monthly inservices to the members of each nursing unit. This function enabled the nurses to identify this person

Table 10–1 Procedures and Medications Requiring the MICU

Outside MICU Setting	Requires MICU
Procedures	
Central venous catheters	Swan-Ganz® catheters
Femoral catheters	Ventilators
Peritoneal dialysis	Arterial lines
	Continuous ECG monitoring
Medications	
Heparin	Parenteral antiarrhythmics
Thrombolytics	Sympathomimetics (e.g., dopamine)
Aminophylline	Nitroprusside
	Intravenous nitroglycerin
	Intravenous vasopressin
	Intravenous pentobarbital infusion

Source: Hartford Hospital, Hartford, Connecticut.

as a problem-solver for drug-related patient problems. These inservices helped to amplify the services the pharmacist had to offer and to maintain good public relations and visibility with the nurses.

Third, the pharmacist would touch base with each nursing unit every day. Again, this contact provided the nurses with an opportunity to discuss drug-related problems with the pharmacist.

Last, the clinical pharmacist provided a consultation service. Patients were seen in consultation for pharmacokinetic evaluation, pain control, or evaluation of adverse drug reactions or drug interactions. A consultation for a patient could be requested by a physician or nurse.

Therefore, the position evolved from that of a clinical pharmacist on a medical service to that of a clinical pharmacist of an MICU who then saw non-MICU medical patients by consultation or referral from a physician or a nurse. Table 10–2 illustrates the evolution and the progression of the clinical pharmacist in the MICU. As stated earlier in this chapter, the hospital is presently changing from a floor-stock drug distribution system to a decentralized unit-dose system. Thus, the unit-dose pharmacists now receive problems and identify patient problems, which they refer to the clinical pharmacist. This restructuring also resulted in an increase in the use of the pharmacist by the MICU and to an increase in consultations outside the MICU.

This position is totally funded by the hospital. The position involves an academic appointment with the School of Pharmacy (University of Connecticut). However, the school does not fund this position.

Table 10–2 Evolution of Pharmacist Role in MICU

Service	1978	Present
Clinical service	To 120 medical patients	To 11 MICU patients
	To 11 MICU patients	To non-MICU patients on consultation by physician or nurse referral
		To see all medical nursing units daily
Education	To physicians	To physicians
	To nurses	To medical nurses
	To University of Connecticut Pharmacy students in Clinical Clerkship	
Research	Projects in conjunction with the Departments of Medicine and Pharmacy	

Source: Hartford Hospital, Hartford, Connecticut.

SERVICE DEVELOPMENT

Pharmacist's Introduction to Department Structures

When establishing the service, one must identify the department structures of medicine and nursing. Although the pharmacist may not work with these people on a daily basis, it is important to identify them and to explain to them what a clinical pharmacist offers and does. These initial introductions can help the pharmacist in the development of the position and in the promotion of good public relations. In the Department of Medicine, it is important to meet the director (or chief), the associate director, the director for the MICU, and the chief medical resident. Each year the clinical pharmacist should be included in the house officers' orientation and should be introduced accordingly. Meeting the house officers and attending staff can be accomplished by providing lectures at the Department of Medicine's teaching conferences (e.g., medical grand rounds). In addition, the pharmacist can become involved with the care of patients in the MICU and can then meet additional physicians. The Department of Nursing should also be introduced to the clinical pharmacist, including the director, the assistant director for medical nurses, the clinical coordinator or the supervisor for medical nurses, and the head nurse and assistant head nurse for each nursing unit. It is important that the pharmacist has a thorough understanding of each nurse's role in order to work more effectively and efficiently. It is also essential to have the nurses' support so that projects and changes can be successful.

Pharmacist's Time Commitment

When establishing a clinical service in an MICU, the pharmacist must make a significant time commitment. As the pharmacist—as well as the nurses and physicians—becomes comfortable with this new role, the commitment and activities change, allowing the pharmacist to improve his efficiency and to increase activities in other areas, such as research. Table 10–3 illustrates how the general daily activities of the pharmacist in the MICU have changed. Morning work rounds were and are an essential activity for this person. These rounds are conducted with the senior medical resident (SMR), two medical interns, head nurse (or nurse in charge) of the MICU, and the pharmacist. It is not possible for the pharmacist to follow every patient's drug therapy in detail or with flowsheets. The patients in the MICU are critically ill. Their conditions change hourly. Any attempt to monitor the patient's drug therapy in detail serves only to make the pharmacist a bookkeeper and heighten frustration. Instead, the pharmacist should review the patient medication record before rounds and make notes of issues or questions to address while on morning work rounds. Calculations, adjustments in dosage, and so forth, can all be handled during rounds and can be followed briefly

Table 10–3 Daily Activities of the Pharmacist in the MICU

Initial	Present
½–1 h before rounds, review patient's drug therapy	½ h before rounds, review patient's drug therapy
1–2 h attending morning work rounds	1–2 h attending morning work rounds
1–2 h attending teaching rounds	Midday check with the senior medical resident and charge nurse
Midday check with the senior medical resident and charge nurse	Evening check with the senior medical resident and charge nurse
Midafternoon check with the senior medical resident and charge nurse	
Evening check with the senior medical resident and charge nurse	
Attend teaching conferences, review of x-rays, etc., with medical resident and interns	

Source: Hartford Hospital, Hartford, Connecticut.

on a 3 × 5 index card, rather than in detail on an extensive monitoring sheet. The pharmacist can update information during the day as to changes in patient drug therapy by reviewing the patient medication record or by speaking with the SMR or charge nurse. If the pharmacist has a question concerning this change, he may address the question at that moment by getting in touch with the physician or may simply make a note of the question and speak with the physician at their next meeting. So that this system may work, the pharmacist must have a thorough understanding of the diseases seen and drugs commonly prescribed for patients in an MICU.

There are three keys to success for a clinical pharmacist in an MICU: (1) visibility and accessibility, (2) nursing personnel, and (3) the ability to identify a need or problem.

Pharmacist's Visibility and Accessibility

Visibility is an essential component of any clinical pharmacist's position. Initially, my visibility to the MICU comprised about 75% of my total day (see Table 10–3). The pharmacist must attend all departmental conferences, teaching rounds, physician work rounds, and so forth; the pharmacist must be a shadow who actively participates. What is difficult and time-consuming about critical care is the rapidly changing nature of each patient. To be an active, contributing member on morning work rounds, the pharmacist must know each patient's events from the previous evening and night. Thus, the pharmacist must review the patient's therapy before attending the morning work rounds, so that there are no surprises. The pharmacist can then have an active, as opposed to a passive, role in the patient's therapy. When the visibility component is high, accessibility is not a problem.

Once the physicians and nurses learn and understand the type of service and information that a clinical pharmacist provides in an MICU, then the pharmacist's visibility may be decreased to about 25% each day. Under these conditions, nurses and physicians can identify concerns regarding patient drug therapy and present them to the pharmacist, so that the issue can be addressed before it evolves into a problem. There is no point in providing a service if the provider of the service cannot be reached. Once visibility is decreased, accessibility must be guaranteed. The clinical pharmacist should have an office in or adjacent to the MICU; however, if this is not possible, the pharmacist must have a beeper or pager, so that he or she may be reached without difficulty.

Pharmacist's Relationship to Nursing Personnel

The nursing personnel are vital to the physician's as well as to the pharmacist's success in an MICU. Basically, the nurses in an MICU "run the show." These nurses all have had nursing experience before their employment in an MICU. They are highly trained, competent, motivated individuals who have the interest, desire, and time to provide the patient with ideal medical and nursing care. The pharmacist must develop an excellent rapport with the nursing staff.

Initially, the pharmacist should attend the change-of-shift report in the morning (nights to days) and the afternoon (days to evenings). This practice allows the pharmacist to meet most of the nurses in a quick and efficient fashion. If there is no formal change of shift report, the pharmacist should try to meet briefly with the nurse in charge of the shift and see if there are any patient problems in which he may be of assistance. Because each nurse is caring for one to two patients and is with that patient for a complete 8- to 12-hour shift, she can provide the pharmacist with current and thorough information about a patient's response to drug therapy. For example, a frequent problem in an MICU is agitation in ventilator-dependent patients. The nurses may report that they have been administering morphine 5 mg IV q 1 hour, alternating with diazepam 5 mg IV q 1 hour to control agitation, and the medication has not helped. This is the pharmacist's opportunity to review the patient's chart, to eliminate medications that may cause agitation, and to develop a drug therapy regimen to control the patient's agitation. In time, the nurses will learn the type of services the pharmacist can provide. Then the pharmacist will no longer find it necessary to attend change-of-shift report, because the nurses will contact him. By working closely with the nurses, the pharmacist is able to maximize the impact on patient care.

Another service to initiate for the nurses is bimonthly inservices in the MICU. As previously stated, these nurses are highly motivated persons who are always eager to learn. These inservices allow the nurses to associate the pharmacist directly with patient drug therapy and so provide good public relations. It is especially important to provide the nurses with an inservice when a drug-related patient problem occurs—for example, a patient who is being managed with hemoperfusion because of a theophylline overdose is admitted to the MICU. This would be an excellent opportunity to teach the nurses about theophylline toxicity, serum theophylline levels, and hemoperfusion. It should be noted that the pharmacist must also be motivated and flexible, so that an inservice can be provided with limited time to plan or prepare.

It is also important to learn whether a hospital has a training or orientation program for ICU nurses. Generally, nurses are the educators in these programs and provide lectures on ICU drug therapy. Most nurses welcome a pharmacist into such a program; thus, the pharmacist should volunteer and offer to teach this aspect of the program. An additional benefit to teaching an ICU program is that many of the nurses in attendance are also nurses working in the pharmacist's ICU.

Pharmacist's Ability To Identify a Need or Problem

Identifying problems is generally easier than identifying a need, inasmuch as problems always manage to find the person.

Fortunately, no major drug distribution problems have arisen. The MICU at Hartford Hospital is a participant in an intravenous admixture program and has a floor-stock distribution system. The clinical pharmacist may be helpful by alerting the pharmacy to an unusual dosage of medication, or perhaps note that an infrequently used medication is being prescribed (e.g., the use of doxapram as a respiratory stimulant).

Clinical problems that have arisen can be divided into three groups: physician problems, nursing problems, and pharmacist problems.

Physician-Related Problems

The physician-related problem is one common to all clinical pharmacists. Time and patience are required for pharmacists to explain to physicians the role and the service a clinical pharmacist provides. This explanation must be completed in a nonthreatening manner. A problem for all newly hired clinical pharmacists is their unfamiliarity with the physicians. As was stated previously, the pharmacist must be visible at all departmental conferences and, in addition, should offer to present several departmental teaching conferences. The types of patient problems most physicians are apt to present to the pharmacist involve pharmacokinetic evaluations, dosage calculation, and evaluation of drug-induced adverse effects. A key to the pharmacist's success with physicians is credibility. The pharmacist must establish himself as a person who provides information and solutions to problems. One favorable interaction with a physician can establish a good physician-pharmacist relationship for many years.

Nursing-Related Problems

The nursing-related problems are similar to that of the physician. Nursing inservices can provide the pharmacist with a format to meet nursing personnel effectively and efficiently. The patient problems that nursing personnel present to the pharmacist generally involve patient comfort. Frequently, the pharmacist is asked to develop a sedation or pain control regimen for patients in the MICU. An evaluation of this nature requires close work between the pharmacist and the nurse if it is going to be of benefit to the patient. The need for good communication between nurses and the pharmacist cannot be overemphasized.

Pharmacist-Related Problems

The pharmacist's problems are of two types. First, the pharmacist must address the daily activities of providing a clinical service. The pharmacist must develop a work schedule that allows him or her to answer drug information requests in a timely fashion, to adjust dosages relative to serum drug concentrations, or to intervene when a patient's drug therapy is not being maximized. The second problem is that the pharmacist must realize that he cannot follow the patient's daily drug therapy in detail. (This problem was addressed earlier in this chapter.) Instead, the pharmacist must rely on colleagues—namely, physicians and nurses—to fact-gather and to enable him or her to assimilate the information and make decisions and recommendations about patient drug therapy. Additionally, the pharmacist must develop a work schedule that establishes several times during the day to report or check on the MICU. Again, because of the dynamic nature of ICU patients, the pharmacist may feel that enough time is never devoted to the MICU. Failure to develop an efficient and workable schedule can lead to frustration and a feeling of inadequacy on the part of the pharmacist. Good communication with physicians and nurses should enable the pharmacist to spend no more than 25% of the work day physically in the MICU.

Identifying a need is equally important to problem solving, because it is essentially problem prevention. A frustration experienced with the MICU at the Hartford Hospital was the failure of personnel to refer to all drug dosages in terms of milligrams per hour or micrograms per minute. To alleviate the frustration and to improve the delivery of care, the pharmacist developed charts for determining the dosages for bretylium, dobutamine, dopamine, lidocaine, nitroglycerin, nitroprusside, norepinephrine, and procainamide in mg/min and µg/kg/min. Originally, each drug dosage was given on an 8 × 12 sheet of paper (Table 10–4).

Table 10–4 Dobutamine Hydrochloride for Injection (Dobutrex®)

mL/h	1 amp 250 mg/1000 mL	2 amps 500 mg/1000 mL	4 amps 1000 mg/1000 mL
10	41.6 μg/min*	83.3 μg/min	166.6 μg/min
20	83.3 μg/min	166.6 μg/min	333.3 μg/min
30	125.0 μg/min	250.0 μg/min	500.0 μg/min
40	166.6 μg/min	333.3 μg/min	666.6 μg/min
50	208.3 μg/min	416.6 μg/min	833.3 μg/min
60	250.0 μg/min	500.0 μg/min	1000.0 μg/min

	250 mg/500 mL	500 mg/500 mL	1000 mg/500 mL
10	83.3 μg/min	166.6 μg/min	333.3 μg/min
20	166.6 μg/min	333.3 μg/min	666.6 μg/min
30	250.0 μg/min	500.0 μg/min	1000.0 μg/min
40	333.3 μg/min	666.6 μg/min	1333.3 μg/min
50	416.6 μg/min	833.3 μg/min	1666.6 μg/min
60	500.0 μg/min	1000.0 μg/min	2000.0 μg/min

Notes: 1 amp of dobutamine = 250 mg dobutamine

*The dose is given in μg/min. To obtain the dose in μg/kg/min, divide the dose given in μg/min by the patient's lean body weight (kg):

Lean body weight = 50 kg
$$\frac{83.3 \; \mu g/min}{50 \; kg} = 1.6 \; \mu g/kg/min$$

If the dose is ordered in μg/kg/min, multiply by the patient's lean body weight (kg) to obtain the infusion rate in μg/min or mL/h:

Give 20 μg/kg/min of a 250 mg/500 mL solution.
Patient weight = 50 kg
(20 μg/kg/min) (50 kg) = 1000 μg/min
According to the chart this would be 120 mL/h

Average dose = 2.5–10 μg/kg/min

Eventually the format was reduced to a single 3 × 5 foldout pocket-sized card. Thus, the physicians' and the nurses' aggravation, caused by the need to perform a mathematical calculation, was eliminated by a convenient chart.

Another need that was identified was to develop drug protocols or guidelines for infrequently prescribed medications. For example, each time vasopressin was prescribed for the treatment of bleeding esophageal varices the same questions arose: What was the dose? What was the concentration? What were the adverse effects?

To alleviate these questions, a protocol was designed that addressed all of these questions; thus, personnel are provided with consistent information that is easily obtainable and can be used each time they choose to prescribe vasopressin. At present, we are planning protocols for hydrochloric acid, propranolol, and verapamil continuous infusions.

Another need that was identified was that of developing a file of references concerning drug overdose or ingestions. A file of current references was compiled and placed in the MICU. In this way, it was easily accessible to physicians at any time of day. The file has been received so favorably that a copy will soon be placed in the residents' on-call room and in the emergency room.

Several other needs that were identified were beneficial to the entire medical floor as well as to the MICU. One of these needs was for the development of an intravenous compatibility chart the nurses could use on the nursing units. A frequent concern of nurses is the compatibility of two different intravenous medications. This chart provided the nurses with an easy format—on the nursing unit—to determine whether two intravenous medications were compatible. Another need that was recognized was that some medications carried a greater risk of potential morbidity or mortality. In an effort to minimize potential morbidity or mortality, guidelines were developed for heparin, aminophylline, and thrombolytics. These guidelines were designed to assist the practitioner in prescribing these medications and to minimize the risk to the patient. In addition, the guidelines provided the nurses with information concerning adverse effects and nursing parameters while the patients were receiving the medication.

The nursing personnel of the MICU have developed two flowsheets that are of benefit to the pharmacist. One flowsheet is for arterial blood gases and the other is for stat blood work. The stat sheet is useful to the pharmacist who does not work with computerized laboratory data. The sheet allows the pharmacist to review quickly and efficiently many of the laboratory studies that are used to monitor a patient's drug therapy. The pharmacist must learn to use these supplemental tools to improve his or her overall efficiency.

RESEARCH

The research activities that are undertaken may involve physicians or nurses. The opportunity to conduct research in an MICU is good, inasmuch as a wide variety of projects may be initiated. Projects may involve subjective elements (e.g., the incidence of erythromycin-induced thrombophlebitis) or they may be very technical (e.g., aminoglycoside pharmacokinetics in MICU patients). Again, to ensure the success of the project, the nurses must be included in the development of the protocol as well as in the completion of the project.

CONCLUSION

The MICU is an area in which a pharmacist can have a superb clinical impact on patient care. To highlight some of the points discussed in this chapter concerning the service, the following summary is given:

- Meet with the departments of medicine and nursing.
- Provide inservices to physicians and nurses to acquire visibility as well as credibility.
- Initially, make a significant time commitment to the MICU. Attend all rounding activities and nursing reports. When the nurses and physicians learn how to use your service effectively, you may decrease your specific time commitment.
- Do not undertake detailed measures for monitoring patients. Instead, review the patient's medication record and develop a technique for identifying what should be addressed with the physicians and nurses on morning work rounds.
- Initially, offer your services, repeatedly. With time, once credibility is established and the pharmacist is accepted, nurses and physicians will ask for input and will seek out the pharmacist.

Remember, identifying a need (problem prevention) is more important than solving a problem. However, preventing and solving problems require the pharmacist to be visible and easily accessible.

Chapter 11

The Pharmacist in Pediatric and Neonatal Intensive Care

Gary C. Cupit

HISTORICAL PERSPECTIVE

The development of intensive care units for the treatment of newborns, infants, and children has grown rapidly over the last 20 years. Newborn intensive care units were first developed in the early 1960s. The impact of former President John F. Kennedy's interest in newborn survival cannot be ignored. During his term in office, President Kennedy lost a child to "diseases of prematurity." It is not coincidental that one of the first newborn units was developed at the Children's Hospital of Philadelphia in 1964.

Tracing the origins of older infants' and children's intensive care units is more difficult. For many years the joint care of children and adults in the same intensive care unit was a standard of care in the United States. During the late 1960s the inadequacy of this approach to the treatment of critically ill children was recognized. The shortcomings of joint care of infants and adults include difficulty in training medical and nursing personnel to render care to both age groups, logistical problems in the provision of equipment and supplies to meet all needs, frequent medication administration errors due to preparation ambiguities, and inadequate social-psychological support to deal with the families and relatives of patients hospitalized within the unit.

NEONATAL INTENSIVE CARE UNIT

Description

The neonatal intensive care unit (NICU) at the Children's Hospital of Philadelphia is a 22-bed unit (see Figure 11–1). The unit consists of 21 acute care beds and one isolation room. In addition, there are 30 "step-down" beds in an infant transitional unit for infants who no longer require critical care but need nutrition

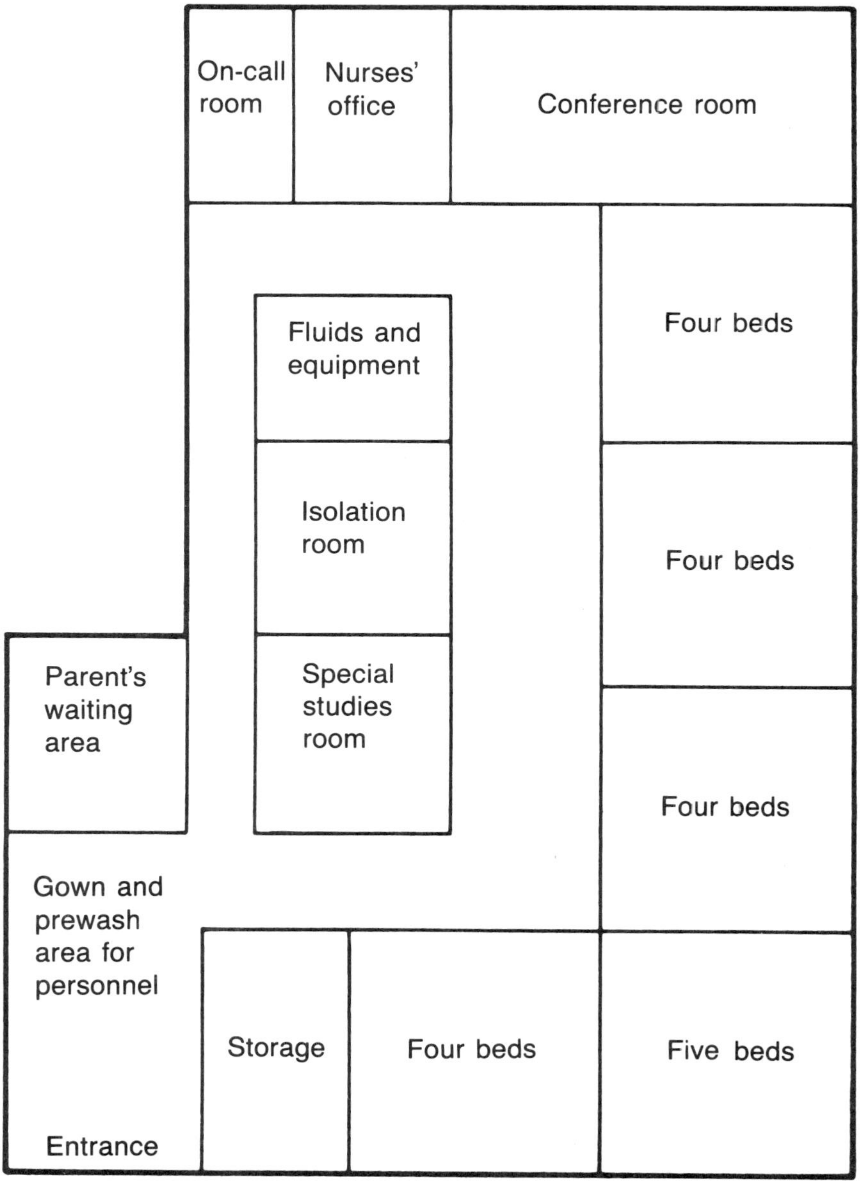

Figure 11-1 Neonatal Intensive Care Unit at Children's Hospital of Philadelphia

support, monitoring for disorders such as apnea, or training of parents for home care of an infant with a chronic disorder. Infants admitted to this unit no longer require ventilators or blood-gas monitoring. The NICU at present admits approximately 650 infants yearly with a distribution of 500 medical admissions and 150 surgical admissions. A listing of the most frequent causes for admission to the NICU is provided in Table 11–1. The occupancy rate is at present over 90%.

Unit Staffing

The unit is presently staffed by six on-site neonatologists who assume primary responsibility for patients referred from outlying hospitals. The rounding team for the NICU consists of an attending neonatologist, a neonatal fellow, three house officers, one or two medical students, a pharmacist, and the head nurse. Rounds are conducted daily in the morning; a briefer rounding period is scheduled for the late afternoon.

During morning rounds, the team completely reviews each patient. The problem list includes not only the patient's disease states but each monitoring parameter that is being used to assess progress. (A sample patient monitoring sheet is shown in Exhibit 11–1.) All current medications are listed, and each major organ system of the patient is reviewed. At the completion of the patient review, all team members are aware of the plans and the reasons for those plans for that day.

Rounds are a dynamic interchange that reflect the medical opinions of the attending fellow and resident physicians, the respiratory therapist, the nurse, and

Table 11–1 Most Frequent Causes for Medical Admission in 1982, NICU, Children's Hospital of Philadelphia

Admitting Diagnosis	Percentage
Respiratory distress syndrome	42
Cardiac disorders	11
Severe prematurity	5
Meconium aspiration	5
Necrotizing enterocolitis	4
Asphyxia	4
Pneumonia	4
Multiple congenital anomalies	3
Seizures	2
Sepsis	2
Hyperbilirubinemia	2
Other	14

Source: NICU, Children's Hospital of Philadelphia, Pennsylvania.

Exhibit 11-1 Infant Intensive Care Flowsheet

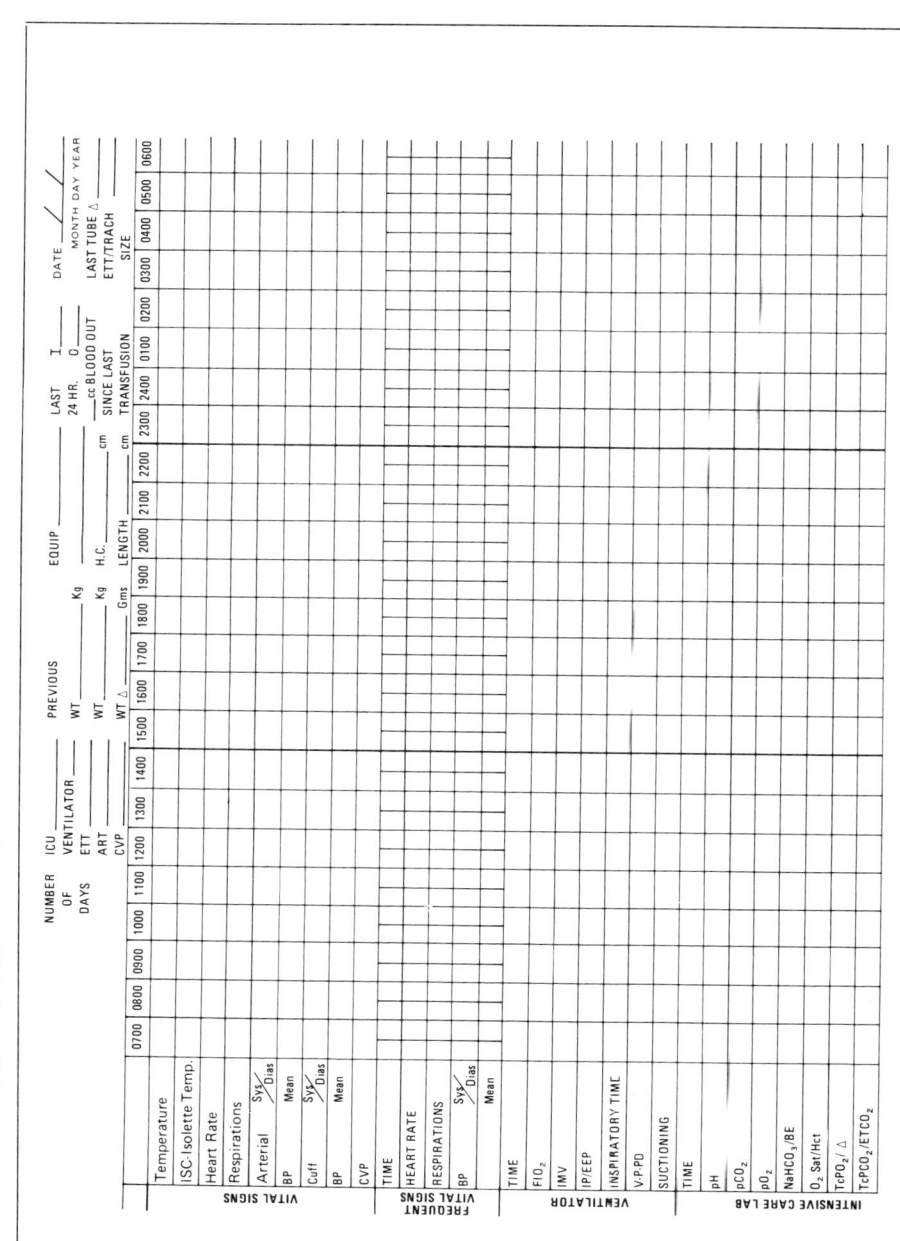

Pediatric and Neonatal Intensive Care 223

Na/K		
TP/Ca/on		
SERUM OSM		
GLUCOSE REAGENT STRIPS		
ABD. GIRTH		
ETT RETAPED		
BILI RADIOMETER		
APNEA/BRADYCARDIA	SPECIAL MONITORING	
Solution IMED		
Sol H VOL/INFUSED/CUM		
Solution IMED		
Sol H VOL/INFUSED/CUM		
Solution IMED		
Sol H VOL/INFUSED/CUM	IV, TPN, BLOOD PRODUCTS	
U/A-I/A-CVP-U/V VOL/INFUSED/CUM		
p̄ ABG VOL/CUM		
MED		
HEPARIN LOCK	FLUSHES	
INFUSION		
INFUSION		
OTHER FLUIDS		
PO-N/G-N/J-GT-OG FORMULA cc/	FEEDS	

Exhibit 11-1 continued

INTAKE TOTALS				
URINE				
STOOLS HEM/CLIN				
N/G-T-EMESIS ASPIRATE q STR. DRAINAGE		24°		
BLOOD OUT				
CUM FROM LAST TRANSFUSION				
CT. DRAINAGE				
LEVEL/DRAIN/CUM				
CT. DRAINAGE				
LEVEL/DRAIN/CUM				
CT. DRAINAGE				
LEVEL/DRAIN/CUM				
OUTPUT TOTALS				
Specific Gravity/pH		24°		
GLUCOSE/KETONES				
BLOOD/PROTEIN				
CLINETEST/ACETONE				
Hgb/Hct				
WBC				
PLATELETS				
PT/PTT				
Na/Cl				
K/CO$_2$				
Ca/GLUCOSE				
BUN/CREAT				
BILIRUBIN				
SIGNATURE & INITIAL				

Source: NICU, Children's Hospital of Philadelphia, Pennsylvania.

the pharmacist. The interchanges that occur during this time period are tremendous opportunities for improved patient care and teaching of the unit staff. The attending physician, however, makes the final decision.

Drug Distribution Services

The NICU is served by a decentralized satellite on the same floor. This satellite is also responsible for the pediatric intensive care unit (PICU), the operating rooms, the day surgery, and the recovery room. It is staffed 24 hours a day by personnel in three shifts. The satellite is covered from 7 A.M. to 3 P.M. by one pharmacist and one technician, from 3 P.M. to 11 P.M. by two pharmacists and two technicians, and from 11 P.M. to 7 A.M. by one pharmacist and one technician. The satellite is responsible from 7 A.M. to 3 P.M. for only the fourth floor. After 3 P.M., it serves all 207 beds of the hospital. Daily, at 3 P.M., medications prepared by the unit dose method are distributed in a 24-hour supply. The satellite is equipped with "picking bins" and a small horizontal laminar airflow hood in an area of 400 square feet. Any medications for patients being discharged are handled by the satellite only from 4:30 P.M. to 8:30 P.M. The outpatient pharmacy prepares discharge medications from 8:30 A.M. to 4:30 P.M.

Functions completed in the central pharmacy are routine IV admixtures, parenteral nutrition solutions, chemotherapy medications under a vertical laminar airflow hood, and routine narcotic orders. In a stat situation, the satellite can complete these functions, but the volume prohibits the performance of these functions on a routine basis.

The patient's medications are monitored by using a pharmacy generated patient medication profile. (See Exhibits 11-2 and 11-3.) The information gathered is transferred to a computer for billing, checking interactions, and preparing labels.

The importance of establishing unit dose distribution services to the critical care environment cannot be overemphasized. This patient care area is associated with a high risk of medication errors ranging from calculations of doses[1-3] to confusion from look-alike, commercial labels.[4] Such errors can result in patient morbidity. Previous studies have shown that the average infant receives 150 drug administrations during its stay in the NICU. Based on an 8% error rate previously reported,[2] the average infant is potentially overmedicated or undermedicated 12 times during hospitalization.

Clinical Activities and Services

Clinical services are provided by the decentralized pharmacy personnel and the clinical faculty member from the College of Pharmacy. The services offered include drug information, pharmacokinetic monitoring and consultation, nutrition consultation (a pharmacist is a member of the Nutrition Support Team), and

226 Practice of Critical Care Pharmacy

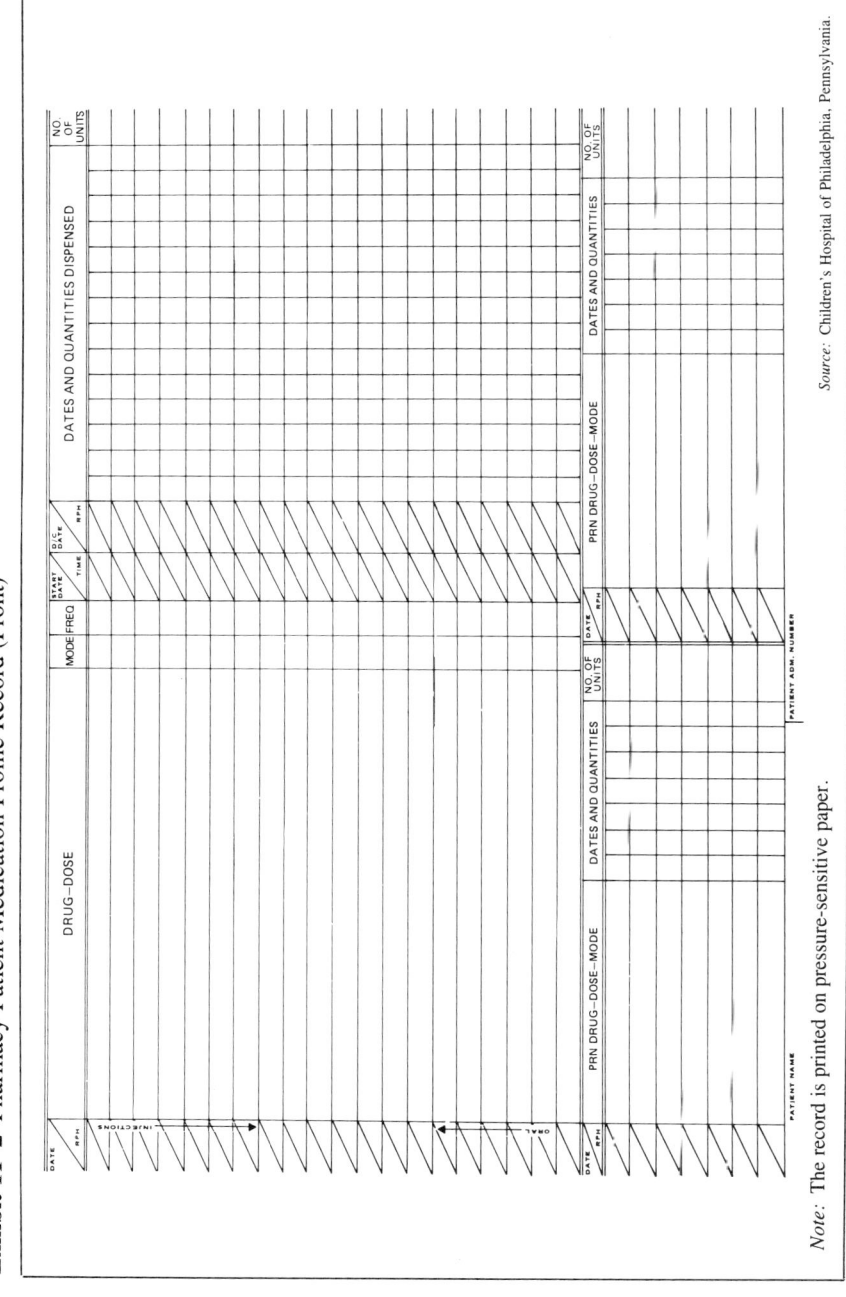

Exhibit 11–2 Pharmacy Patient Medication Profile Record (Front)

Note: The record is printed on pressure-sensitive paper.

Source: Children's Hospital of Philadelphia, Pennsylvania.

Exhibit 11-3 Pharmacy Patient Medication Profile Record (Back)

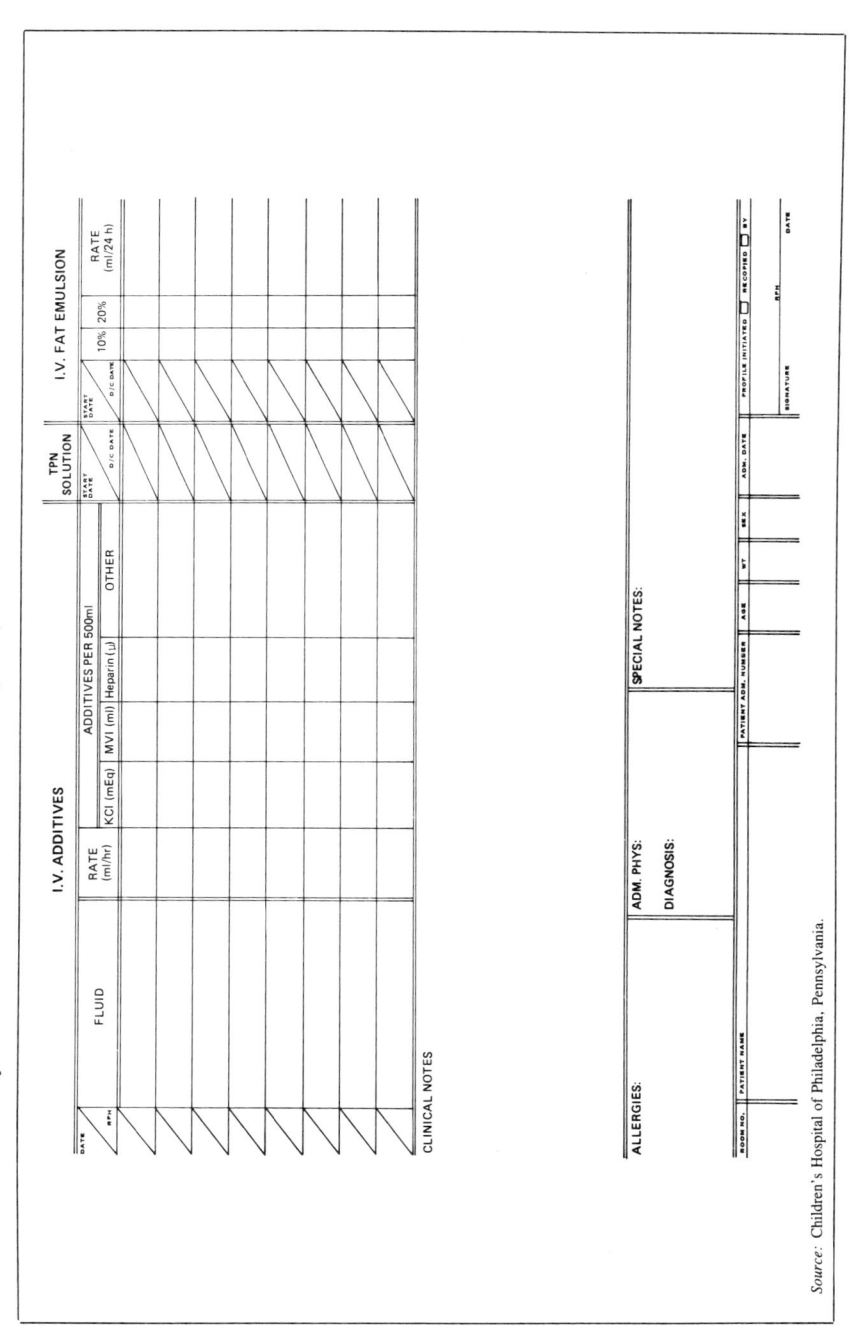

Source: Children's Hospital of Philadelphia, Pennsylvania.

assistance during resuscitation by the preparation of stat drugs. A pharmacist makes rounds with the team members on a scheduled rotation to provide input to the team and to assure adequate record keeping in the satellite pharmacy.

Developing Skills in Neonatal Therapeutics

The provision of a role on the team by the pharmacist requires that this newest member be versed in the medical, surgical, and pharmacologic care of newborn infants. A good place to begin this understanding is by electing clerkship rotations in pharmacy school, when such rotations are offered. Another method is to complete a postgraduate residency in pediatric pharmacy practice. These residencies presently are offered in pediatric hospitals and are usually affiliated with schools of pharmacy. (A current listing of these residencies-fellowships may be obtained from the Chairman, Pediatric Special Interest Group, American Society of Hospital Pharmacists, Washington, DC.) The training offered can usually be directed to a particular area of specialization, for example, neonatology or critical care. If specialty residencies are not available, pharmacists may obtain expertise by working with a functioning unit. These units are most receptive to the additional input, and the on-the-job training is valuable for the pharmacist.

Once the decision has been made to provide clinical expertise to the unit, practicing pharmacists may seek ways to upgrade their data base in neonatology. It is this author's opinion that this goal is best accomplished by the RAP method—Read, Attend, and Participate. Reading material on the pathophysiology and treatment of the disease states mentioned in Table 11–1 would provide an excellent starting point. A listing of select journals that focus on the problems of neonates and selected textbooks that provide good pathophysiology discussions is provided in Table 11–2. Through a regimen of regular reading of this material, the pharmacist can achieve an adequate baseline to begin to develop this new area of practice.

The next step is the attendance of neonatal conferences at the local, regional, and national level. Local conferences (e.g., weekly pediatric staff conferences, grand rounds, research, and patient care conferences) are usually available within the hospital. Institutions that provide fellowships in neonatology provide regular seminars on many areas of interest to the pharmacist.

After reading basic material and attending conferences, the pharmacist is prepared to begin the next area of involvement—participation. Initially, this process is often passive. During rounds and conferences there may be a period, often seeming interminable, during which the pharmacist is absorbing information at a level above the point at which his ability to contribute has been developed. A good forum for discussion is a journal club. Each person's contribution to the analysis of an article or study is based on not only that person's areas of interest but also the common goal of good communications and methodology. From this

Table 11-2 Recommended Journals for Topics in Neonatal-Pediatric Care

Journal	Neonatal Topics	Pediatric Topics
American Journal of Diseases in Children	X	X
American Journal of Obstetrics and Gynecology	X	O
Annals of Emergency Medicine	O	X
Archives of Diseases of Childhood	X	X
Biology of the Neonate	X	O
Clinics in Perinatology	X	O
Critical Care Medicine	O	X
Journal of the American Medical Association	O	X
Journal of Infectious Diseases	X	X
Journal of Parenteral and Enteral Nutrition	X	X
Journal of Pediatrics	X	X
Journal of Trauma	O	X
New England Journal of Medicine	X	X
Obstetrics and Gynecology	X	O
Pediatric Alert	X	X
Pediatric Clinics of North America	X	X
Pediatric Infectious Disease	X	X
Pediatric Notes	X	X
Pediatric Research	X	X
Pediatrics	X	X
Seminars in Perinatology	X	O

point, the pharmacist participates on rounds. Next, he contributes as a member of the audience at conferences and eventually as a presenter at one of the specialty conferences.

Once the ice has been broken, many pharmacists develop their role in the NICU. Basic involvement with the NICU should include service, education, and research. Service should combine the assurance of the provision of clinical and distributive functions. Services should be provided in the areas of drug monitoring, pharmacokinetics, consultations, drug selection, and the management of adverse reactions. If this information is provided on a regular basis, it may be beneficial to develop a syllabus of references for use by the unit staff. Examples of material to be included are information on the transfer of drugs into breast milk,[5] the osmolality of medications for oral and intravenous use,[6,7] dosage guidelines for medication administration in neonates,[8] and neonatal drug withdrawal.[9]

Through experience and spending time in the neonatal environment, the pharmacist is exposed to many additional areas of concern in neonatology. Issues in the bioethics of procedures (e.g., circumcision,[10,11] treatment of critically ill prematures,[12-19] and the economic-social issues of survival) begin to make an impact on the pharmacist. These and other areas continue to evolve and to provide areas of input for the pharmacist as a health care provider and as a person concerned about human life.

Educational Activities

Educational opportunities in the NICU begin with pharmacy staff conferences. Pharmacists specializing in neonatology may educate fellow pharmacists, so that coverage of the unit may be improved on evenings and weekends. This opportunity may then be extended to pharmacy students who may wish to complete an elective rotation in neonatal pharmacotherapy.

The members of the nursing staff of the NICU are always interested in increasing their knowledge and awareness of pharmacology in the neonate. Of particular interest are the rationale for dosage and selection of antibiotics,[20] diuretics, anticonvulsants, and other medications. This material may be coordinated for presentation with the head nurse. Increased communication between nurses and pharmacists fosters good relationships that are vital to the pharmacist's function in the intensive care environment.

Units responsible for the training of medical students and the house staff offer frequent opportunities for the presentation of educational material. These lectures, presented on a regularly scheduled basis, offer the opportunity for interaction with many of the physicians-in-training. These educational interfaces provide invaluable opportunities to initiate the next component of the role—research.

Research

In view of today's technology, research opportunities in the NICU are abundant. The utilization of micro assays in performing plasma drug concentration measurements and electrolyte assessments is a welcome addition to the neonatal researcher. Projects involving pharmacokinetics, therapeutic response, and toxicology are at present fertile areas. As new drugs and devices are developed for adults, their safety and efficacy must be assessed for neonates and children.[21] At present, the areas of antibiotic therapy, opioid antagonism, and prostaglandins are the most active areas of research. The development of noninvasive monitoring techniques (e.g., transcutaneous pO_2) has facilitated this research.

PEDIATRIC INTENSIVE CARE UNIT

Description

The PICU at the Children's Hospital of Philadelphia is a 31-bed unit that conforms to recognized guidelines for pediatric intensive care units.[22] (The most frequent causes for admission to the PICU are listed in Table 11–3.) The unit consists of 15 acute care beds in a single unit (PICA), 6 acute care isolation beds in a smaller unit (PICS), and 10 intermediate care beds (PICI) (Figure 11–2). Patients with diseases that are not communicable (e.g., trauma, asthma, and ingestions) are admitted to the acute care beds. The isolation unit is responsible for patients requiring treatment for a communicable disease (e.g., bacterial diarrhea or infectious hepatitis) or those patients who require reverse isolation as a result of cancer chemotherapy or organ transplant. Responsibilities of the intermediate care unit are for those children who require chronic ventilator support or are in the process of being weaned or who require parents'/guardians' education in the home care of these patients. A valuable addition to the unit is the provision of a separate stat lab that is responsible only for samples from the NICU, PICU, and the OR. This laboratory provides the use of rapid monitoring capabilities. Again, noninvasive techniques of monitoring (e.g., end-tidal pCO_2) have reduced the frequency of many laboratory assessments.

Unit Staffing

The PICUs are staffed with a nurse-to-patient ratio of 1:2. A medical team consisting of a critical care attending physician, three critical care fellows, an attending pediatrician, three pediatric second-year residents, a pharmacist, and a respiratory therapist functions for all three units. (An additional critical care attending physician functions to provide continuity of care for the PICI, inasmuch

Table 11–3 Most Frequent Causes for Medical Admission in 1982, PICU, Children's Hospital of Philadelphia

Admitting Diagnosis	Percentage
Meningitis	13.0
Pneumonia	10.7
Sepsis	8.6
Seizures	7.8
Ingestions	7.8
Asthma	7.5
Epiglottitis	7.0
Respiratory distress	6.1
Diarrhea and dehydration	4.9
Congestive heart failure	3.5
Reye's	2.9
SIDS	2.3
Other	17.9

Source: NICU, Children's Hospital of Philadelphia, Pennsylvania.

Figure 11–2 Pediatric Intensive Care Unit (PICU) at the Children's Hospital of Philadelphia

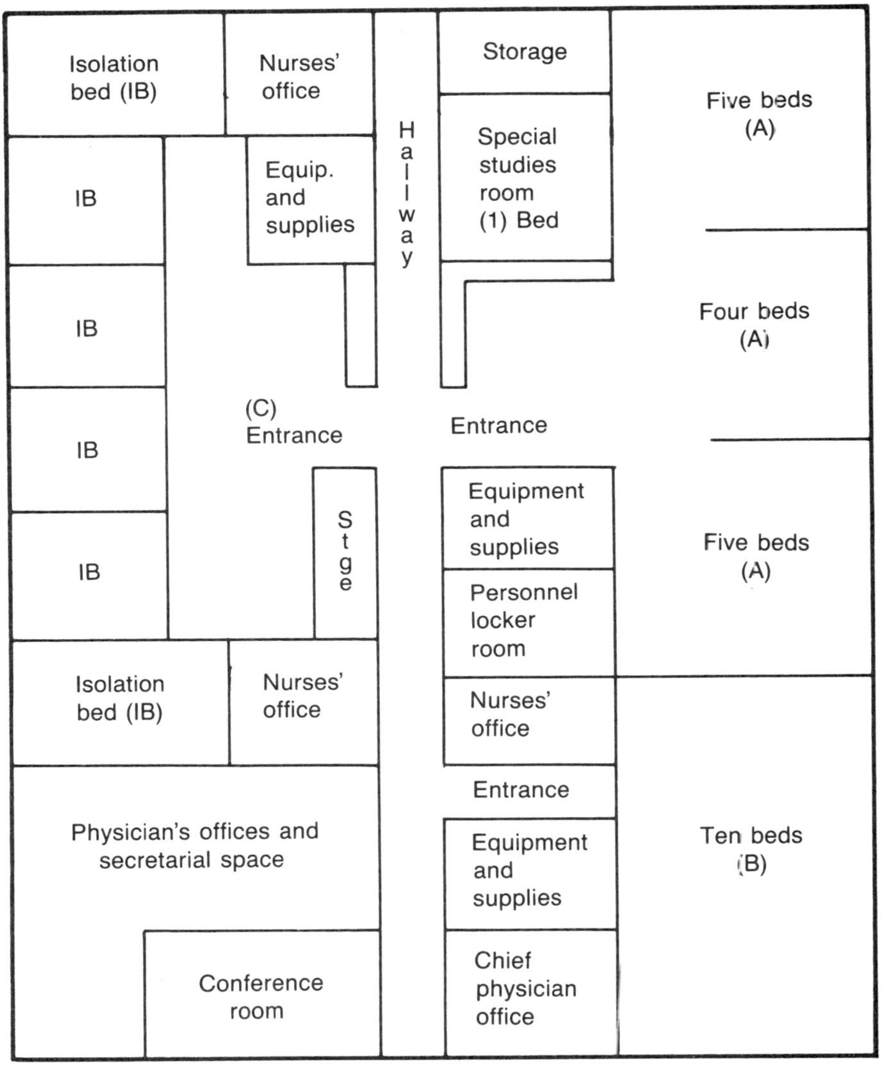

Isolation bed (IB)	Nurses' office	Hallway	Storage	Five beds (A)
IB	Equip. and supplies		Special studies room (1) Bed	
IB				Four beds (A)
IB	(C) Entrance		Entrance	
IB	Stge		Equipment and supplies	Five beds (A)
			Personnel locker room	
Isolation bed (IB)	Nurses' office		Nurses' office	
Physician's offices and secretarial space			Entrance	Ten beds (B)
			Equipment and supplies	
	Conference room		Chief physician office	

Notes: (*A*) Pediatric intensive care acute (PICA), (*B*) Pediatric intensive care intermediate (PICI), and (*C*) Pediatric intensive care sterile (PICS).

as these patients are hospitalized for weeks to months.) Morning rounds begin at 7:30 A.M. and consist of presentations of each patient's problems and therapy. An ICU monitoring sheet is used to review each case (Exhibit 11-4). Assignments for the day, changes in treatment plans, and patient dispositions are decided at this time. Another set of sign-off rounds is held from 4 P.M. to 5:30 P.M. daily.

Drug Distribution Services

Drug distribution units are covered by the satellite pharmacy responsible for the NICU. These services have been discussed in that section of this chapter.

Developing Skills in Pediatric Acute Care

As with neonatal care, pediatric intensive care pharmacy requires a strong data base in critical care therapeutics and a continuing commitment to keep abreast of developments (see Table 11-2). This goal can be accomplished by involvement in a journal club, attendance at acute care conferences, and participation in ongoing research projects.

Clinical Activities and Services

Pharmacy involvement in the PICU was initiated among the Department of Anesthesia and Critical Care, the Department of Pharmacy, and the College of Pharmacy. This joint venture centered on improving drug distribution to the unit and providing technical services. From this interest, a clinical faculty member was recruited by the College of Pharmacy and began working with the acute care unit.

One of the most pressing clinical problems was the pharmacological management of patients with cerebral edema, because this unit serves as a regional head trauma unit for children in a population area of approximately 5 million people. Additional patients who develop cerebral edema include those with hypoxic brain damage, Reye's Syndrome, and postoperative neurosurgical cases. Previous management of these cases had been done with fluid restriction, elevation of the head to 30 degrees, diuretics, osmolar therapy, and hypothermia. Barbiturate coma had been tried on a sporadic basis but with equally sporadic results.

Upon the arrival of the clinical pharmacist, a meeting of the critical care unit physicians, the neurosurgery division, and the pharmacist was held to discuss the utility of barbiturate coma in the management of cerebral edema. This conference resulted in a prospective evaluation of the therapeutic benefit and pharmacokinetics of pentobarbital in the treatment of elevated intracranial pressure.[23]

While this protocol was being evaluated, the opportunity to participate in daily rounds, to establish a consulting service, and to begin educational conferences was realized.

Exhibit 11-4 Pediatric Intensive Care Daily Record Sheet

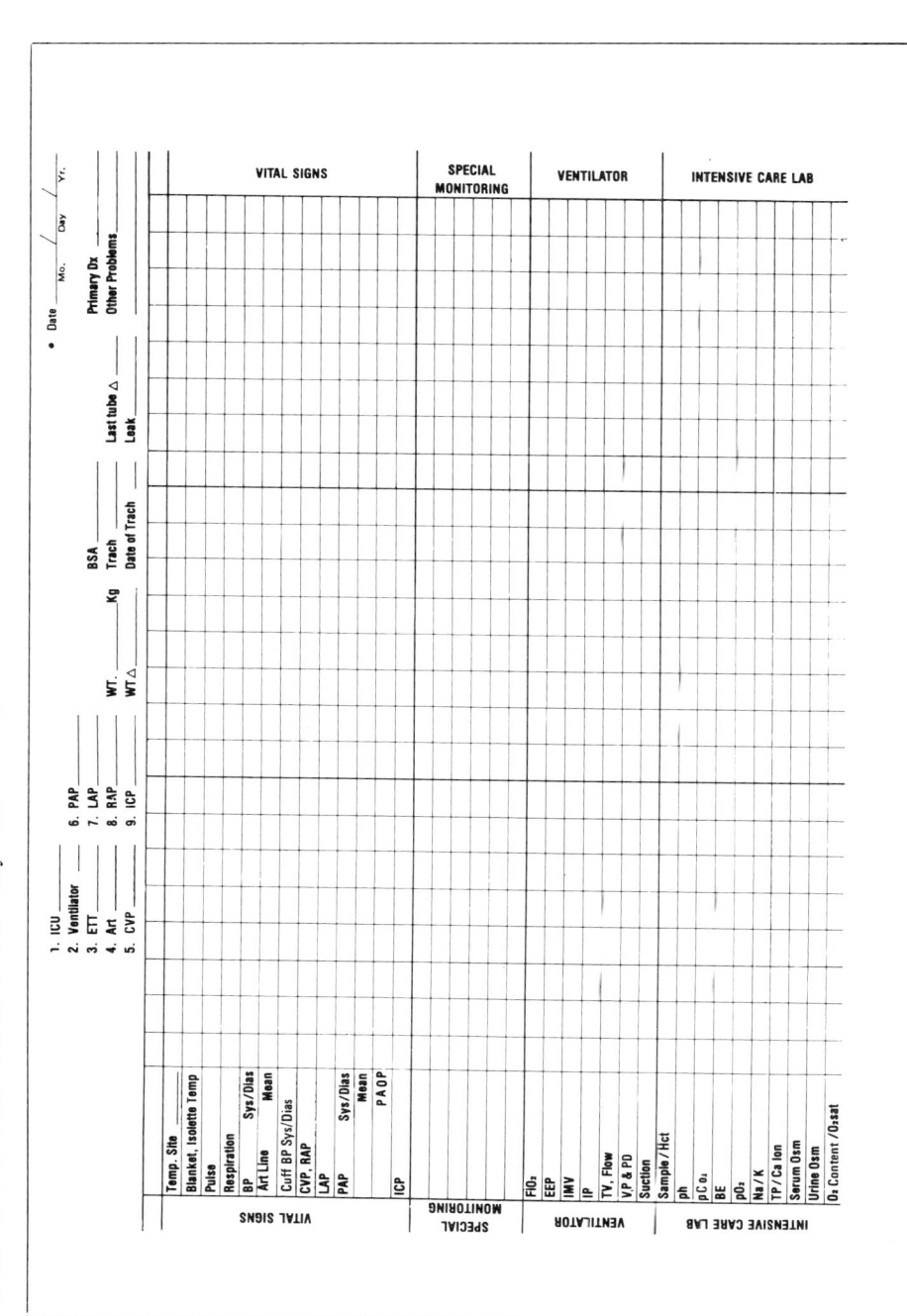

IV, TPN, BLD PRODUCTS				INFUSIONS			FLUSHES		FEEDS		OUTPUT					
Stk _#_ Rate / Pump Setting / Vol/Infused/Cum	Stk _#_ Rate / Pump Setting / Vol/Infused/Cum	Stk _#_ Rate / Pump Setting / Vol/Infused/Cum	Stk _#_ Rate / Pump Setting / Vol/Infused/Cum	Medication / Vol/Infused/Cum	Medication / Vol/Infused/Cum	Medication / Vol/Infused/Cum	Soln / Vol/Infused/Cum	Soln / Vol/Infused/Cum	PO, NG, GT, NJ / Hrly/Cum / Solids	INTAKE TOTALS	Urine / Hrly/Cum	Stool	NG/GT / Hrly/Cum	Emesis	CT, Hemovac, Drains / Hrly/Cum	CT, Hemovac, Drains / Hrly/Cum	CT, Hemovac, Drains / Hrly/Cum	OUTPUT TOTALS

Exhibit 11-4 continued

URINE	HEME	CHEMISTRY	PUPILS	EYE OPENING	VERBAL RESPONSE	MOTOR RESPONSE	STAT. PRN MEDS
Sp. Gr/ph Glucose/Ketones Blood/Protein	Hgb/Hct WBC Platelets PT/PTT	Na/K Cl/CO₂ Ca/Glucose BUN/Creat Bilirubin	Size R/L Reaction R/L	Spontaneous To Verbal Stim To Painful Stim None	Oriented Confused Inappropriate Incoherent None	Obeys Command Localizes Pain Withdraws from Pain Flexion to Pain Extension to Pain Flaccid Other	

Source: Children's Hospital of Philadelphia, Pennsylvania.

Educational Activities

Educational conferences to the acute care staff and fellows are of great value in a teaching hospital. Because housestaff rotate through the units on a monthly basis, it is most useful to give the same topics on a regular schedule to assure continuity and uniformity of treatment regimens. Topics that have been well received include management of drug overdose, therapeutic use of anticonvulsants, drug dosing in renal failure, selection of inotropes, approach to practical pharmacokinetics, and the drug therapy of asthma.

A particularly successful conference for pharmacy involvement has been the "Transport Conference." This conference is devoted to the initial assessment, stabilization, and transport of patients from outlying hospitals to the ICUs. One of the most frequent issues that arise is the selection of a therapeutic agent to manage the clinical situation initially. This selection may also include alteration of a dose due to impairment of organ function. For these reasons, pharmacy input is extremely valuable. (It should be noted that any recommendation instituted on a hospital-wide basis should be made in conjunction with the appropriate specialty services.)

Research

Research opportunities in pediatric intensive care are similar to those available in adult critical care. Working with larger patients than in an NICU, the clinician has a much easier task of using existing adult monitoring methodology (e.g., Swan-Ganz® catheters, adult drug assays).

Research and advances in the management of meningitis, asthma, cerebral edema, and seizures offer exciting areas for development. The critical care pediatric patient is particularly challenging because of the frequent changes in hemoglobin and hematocrit, serum proteins, and fluids and electrolytes. These conditions, superimposed on failures of organ systems, offer many challenges.

SUMMARY

The development of critical care services for the management of neonates and children has been evolving over the last decade. A parallel, though delayed, evolution of pharmacy services to these areas has been occurring. The initial emphasis has been the maturation of distribution functions to the neonatal and pediatric intensive care units. Now is the time for pharmacists to assume clinical roles with these units. It is hoped that the material presented here can provide the encouragement, information, and direction to fulfill this new role.

REFERENCES

1. Bleyer WA, Koup JR: Medication errors during intensive care. *Am J Dis Child* 1979; 133:366–367.
2. Perlstein PH, Callison C, White M, et al: Errors in drug computations during newborn intensive care. *Am J Dis Child* 1979;133:376–379.
3. Simons FER, Friesen FR, Simons KJ: Theophylline toxicity in term infants. *Am J Dis Child* 1980;134:39–41.
4. Solomon SL, Wallace EM, Ford-Jones EL, et al: Medication errors with inhalant epinephrine mimicking an epidemic of neonatal sepsis. *N Engl J Med* 1984;310:166–170.
5. Committee on Drugs of the American Academy of Pediatrics: The transfer of drugs and other chemicals into human breast milk. *Pediatrics* 1983;72:375–383.
6. Ernst JA, Williams JM, Glick MR, et al: Osmolality of substances used in the intensive care nursery. *Pediatrics* 1983;72:347–352.
7. Glasgow AM, Boeckx RL, Miller MK, et al: Hyperosmolality in small infants due to propylene glycol. *Pediatrics* 1983;72:353–355.
8. Howry LB, Bindler RM, Tso Y: *Pediatric Medications*. Philadelphia, JB Lippincott, 1981.
9. Committee on Drugs of the American Academy of Pediatrics: Neonatal drug withdrawal. *Pediatrics* 1983;72:895–902.
10. McCracken GH, Nelson JD: *Antimicrobial Therapy for Newborns: Practical Application of Pharmacology to Clinical Usage*. New York, Grune & Stratton, 1977.
11. Warner E, Strashin E: Benefits and risk of circumcision. *Can Med Assoc J* 1981;125:967–992.
12. Committee on Fetus and Newborn and Committee on Drugs of the American Academy of Pediatrics: Benzyl alcohol: Toxic agent in neonatal units. *Pediatrics* 1983;72:356–358.
13. Herrera AJ, Trouern-Trend JBG: Routine neonatal circumcision. *Am J Dis Child* 1979;133:1069–1070.
14. Rothberg AD, Maisels MJ, Bagnato S, et al: Infants weighing 1,000 grams or less at birth: Developmental outcome for ventilated and nonventilated infants. *Pediatrics* 1983;71:599–602.
15. Ruiz MPD, LaFever JA, Hakanson DO, et al: Early development of infants of birth weighing less than 1000 grams with reference to mechanical ventilation in the newborn period. *Pediatrics* 1981;68:330–335.
16. Knobloch H, Malone A, Ellison PH, et al: Considerations in evaluating changes in outcome for infants weighing less than 1501 grams. *Pediatrics* 1982;69:285–295.
17. Cohen RS, Stevenson DK, Malachowski W, et al: Favorable results of neonatal intensive care for very low-birth weight infants. *Pediatrics* 1982;69:621–625.
18. Britton SB, Fitzhardinge PM, Asby S: Is intensive care justified for infants weighing less than 801 grams at birth? *J Pediatr* 1981;99:937–943.
19. Hirata T, Epcar JT, Walsh A, et al: Survival and outcome of infants 501 to 750 grams: A six-year experience. *J Pediatr* 1983;102:741–748.
20. Committee on Bioethics of the American Academy of Pediatrics: Treatment of critically ill newborns. *Pediatrics* 1983;72:565–566.
21. Strain JE: The decision to forgo life-sustaining treatment for seriously ill newborns. *Pediatrics* 1983;72:572–573.
22. Committee on Hospital Care of the American Academy of Pediatrics and the Pediatric Section of the Society of Critical Care Medicine. *Pediatrics* 1983;72:364–372.
23. Schaible DH, Cupit GC, Swedlow DB, et al: High-dose pentobarbital pharmacokinetics in hypothermic brain-injured children. *J Pediatr* 1982;100:655–699.

Appendix 11-A
Selected Bibliography

Neonatology

Respiratory Distress Syndrome

Aranda JV, Turmen T: Methylxanthines in apnea of prematurity. *Clin Perinatol* 1979;6:87–108.

Ballard PL, Ballard RL: Corticosteroids and respiratory distress syndrome: Status 1979. *Pediatrics* 1979;63:163–165.

Hallman M, Gluck L: Respiratory distress syndrome—Update 1982. *Pediatr Clin North Am* 1982;29:1057–1073.

Harris MC, Baumgart S, Rooklin AR, et al: Successful extubation of infants with respiratory distress syndrome using aminophylline. *J Pediatr* 1983;103:303–305.

Mathew OP, Roberts JL, Thach BT: Pharyngeal airway obstruction in preterm infants during mixed and obstructive apnea. *J Pediatr* 1982;100:964–968.

Roberts JL, Mathew OP, Thach BT: The efficacy of theophylline in premature infants with mixed and obstructive apnea and apnea associated with pulmonary and neurologic disease. *J Pediatr* 1982;100:968–970.

Stahlman M, Hedrall G, Lindstrom D, et al: Role of hyaline membrane disease in production of later childhood lung abnormalities. *Pediatrics* 1982;69:572–576.

Cardiac Disorders

Bell EF, Warburton D, Stonestreet BS, et al: Effect of fluid administration on the development of symptomatic patent ductus arteriosus and congestive heart failure in premature infants. *N Engl J Med* 1980;302:598–604.

Bendayan R, McKenzie MW: Digoxin pharmacokinetics and dosage requirements in pediatric patients. *Clin Pharm* 1983;2:224–235.

Gersony WM, Peckham GJ, Ellison RC, et al: Effects of indomethacin in premature infants with patent ductus arteriosus: Results of a national collaborative study. *J Pediatr* 1983;102:895–906.

Jacob J, Gluck L, DiSessa T, et al: The contribution of PDA in the neonate with severe RDS. *J Pediatr* 1980;96:79–87.

Johnson GL, Desai NS, Pauly TH, et al: Complications associated with digoxin therapy in low-birth weight infants. *Pediatrics* 1982;69:463–465.

Kearin M, Kelly JG, O'Malley K: Digoxin "receptors" in neonates: An explanation of less sensitivity to digoxin than in adults. *Clin Pharmacol Ther* 1980;28:346–349.

Nyberg L, Wettrell G: Digoxin dosage schedules for neonates and infants based on pharmacokinetic considerations. *Clin Pharmacokinet* 1978;3:453–461.

Roehl S, Townsend RJ: Alprostadil. *Drug Intell Clin Pharm* 1982;16:823–832.

Sacksteder S, Gildea JH, Dassy C: Common congenital defects. *Am J Nurs* 1978;78:266–278.

Thalji AA, Carr I, Yeh TF, et al: Pharmacokinetics of intravenously administered indomethacin in premature infants. *J Pediatr* 1980;97:995–1000.

Valdes R, Graves SW, Brown BA, et al: Endogenous substance in newborn infants causing false positive digoxin measurements. *J Pediatr* 1983;102:947–950.

Vert P, Bianchetti G, Marchal F, et al: Effectiveness and pharmacokinetics of indomethacin in premature newborns with patent ductus arteriosus. *Eur J Clin Pharmacol* 1980;18:83–88.

Meconium Aspiration

Cassin S: Role of prostaglandins and thromboxanes in the control of the pulmonary circulation in the fetus and newborn. *Semin Perinatol* 1980;4:101–107.

Drummond WH, Gregory GA, Heymann MA, et al: The independent effects of hyperventilation, tolazoline, and dopamine on infants with persistent pulmonary hypertension. *J Pediatr* 1981;98:603–611.

Hegyi T, Hiatt MI: Tolazoline and dopamine therapy in neonatal hypoxia and pulmonary vasospasm. *Acta Pediatr Scand* 1980;69:101–103.

Hyman AL, Mathe AA, Lippton HL, Kadowitz PJ: Prostaglandins and the lung. *Med Clin North Am* 1981;65:789–808.

Stevenson DK, Kasting DS, Darnall RA, et al: Refractory hypoxemia associated with neonatal pulmonary disease: The use and limitations of tolazoline. *J Pediatr* 1979;95:595–599.

Truog WE, Lyrene RK, Standaert TA, et al: Effects of PEEP and tolazoline infusion on respiratory and inert gas exchange in experimental meconium aspiration. *J Pediatr* 1982;100:284–290.

Necrotizing Enterocolitis

Brown EG, Sweet AY: Neonatal necrotizing enterocolitis. *Pediatr Clin North Am* 1982;29:1149–1170.

Kliegman RM: Neonatal necrotizing enterocolitis: Implications for an infectious disease. *Pediatr Clin North Am* 1979;26:327–344.

Wilson R, del Portillo M, Schmidt E, et al: Risk factors for necrotizing enterocolitis in infants weighing more than 2,000 grams at birth: A case control study. *Pediatrics* 1983;71:19–22.

Sepsis

Harris MC, Polin RA: Neonatal septicemia. *Pediatr Clin North Am* 1983;30:243–258.

Philip AGS, Hewitt JR: Early diagnosis of neonatal sepsis. *Pediatrics* 1980;65:1036–1041.

Siegel JD, McCracken GH: Sepsis neonatorum. *N Engl J Med* 1981;304:642–647.

Seizures

Gal P, Boer HR: Early discontinuation of anticonvulsants after neonatal seizures: A preliminary report. *South Med J* 1982;75:298–300.

Lockman LA, Kriel R, Zaske D, et al: Phenobarbital dosage for control of neonatal seizures. *Neurology* 1979;29:1445–1449.

Painter MJ, Pippenger C, MacDonald H, et al: Phenobarbital and diphenylhydantoin levels in neonates with seizures. *J Pediatr* 1978;92:315–319.

Painter MJ, Pippenger C, Wasterlain C, et al: Phenobarbital and phenytoin in neonatal seizures: Metabolism and tissue distribution. *Neurology* 1981;31:1107–1112.

Pitlick W, Painter M, Pippenger C: Phenobarbital pharmacokinetics in neonates. *Clin Pharmacol Ther* 1978;23:346–350.

Hyperbilirubinemia

Brodersen R: Bilirubin treatment in the newborn infant: Reviewed with relation to kernicterus. *J Pediatr* 1980;96:349–356.

Harper RG, Sia CG, Kierney CMP: Kernicterus 1980: Problems and practices viewed from the perspective of the practicing clinician. *Clin Perinatol* 1980;7:75–89.

Pediatric Intensive Care

Ingestions

Henretig FM, Cupit GC, Temple AR: Toxicologic emergencies, in Fleisher G, Ludwig S (eds): *Textbook of Pediatric Emergency Medicine.* Baltimore, Williams & Wilkins, 1983, pp 489–531.

Epiglottitis/Croup

Cherry JD: The treatment of croup: Continued controversy due to failure of recognition of historic, ecologic, etiologic and clinical perspectives. *J Pediatr* 1979;94:352–354.

Faden HS: Treatment of haemophilus influenzae Type B epiglottitis. *Pediatrics* 1979:63:402–407.

Leipzig B, Oski FA, Cummings CW, et al: A prospective randomized study to determine the efficacy of steroids in treatment of croup. *J Pediatr* 1979;94:194–196.

Tunnessen W, Feinstein AR: The steroid-croup controversy: An analytic review of methodologic problems. *J Pediatr* 1980;96:751–756.

Zack BG: Managing croup and epiglottitis: A clinical challenge. *Drug Therapy* 1983;January:153–168.

Diarrhea/Dehydration

Cupit GC, Serrano VA: Pediatric therapy, in Katcher BS, Young LY, Koda-Kimble MA (eds): *Applied Therapeutics: The Clinical Use of Drugs.* San Francisco, Applied Therapeutics, 1983, pp 1489–1492.

George WL: Antimicrobial agent-associated colitis and diarrhea. *West J Med* 1980;133:115–123.

Reye's Syndrome

Frewen TC, Swedlow DB, Watcha M, et al: Outcome in severe Reye's syndrome with early pentobarbital coma and hypothermia. *J Pediatr* 1982;100:663–665.

Committee on Infectious Disease of the American Academy of Pediatrics: Aspirin and Reye Syndrome. *Pediatrics* 1982;69:810–812.

Mutchie KD, Burkhart GD: Drug therapy of Reye's Syndrome. *Am J Hosp Pharm* 1979; 36:767–773.

Nahata MC, Kerzner B, McClung HJ, et al: Variations in glycerol kinetics in Reye's Syndrome. *Clin Pharmacol Ther* 1981;29:782–787.

Raphaely RC, Swedlow DB, Downes JJ, et al: Management of severe pediatric head trauma. *Pediatr Clin North Am* 1980;27:715–727.

Reye's Syndrome Working Group of the Aspirin Foundation of America: Reye Syndrome and salicylates: A spurious association. *Pediatrics* 1982;70:158–160.

Shaywitz SE, Cohen PM, Cohen DJ, et al: Long-term consequences of Reye Syndrome: A sibling-matched, controlled study of neurologic, cognitive, academic, and psychiatric function. *J Pediatr* 1982;100:41–46.

Wilson JT, Brown RD: Reye Syndrome and aspirin use: The role of prodromal illness severity in the assessment of relative risk. *Pediatrics* 1982;69:822–825.

Chapter 12

The Pharmacist in Emergency Medicine

Robert M. Elenbaas

EMERGENCY MEDICINE

During the last 30 years, patient visits to emergency rooms in the United States have increased more than 300%. In 1981 alone, more than 83 million Americans were treated within emergency facilities. Despite pleas from third party payers, patient visits to emergency departments continue to increase. This marked increase in emergency department use undoubtedly arises from several factors; however, the availability of physician services 24 hours a day, seven days a week, makes the hospital emergency department easily accessible and attractive to the patient with an acute medical problem or to the patient without a family physician. This chapter provides an overview of the medical specialty of emergency medicine and describes some avenues for expanding pharmacy practice within the emergency department.

Not all patient visits to the emergency room (ER) represent immediate, life-threatening illnesses or injuries. The emergency medicine practitioner must, therefore, be knowledgeable and skilled in the assessment and treatment of an extremely wide variety of medical problems.[1] The discipline of Emergency Medicine saw its most rapid growth between 1970 and 1980; during this time, the federal government actively supported the development of emergency medical service (EMS) programs for prehospital care, as well as physician and nurse training programs leading to specialization in emergency medicine. In 1979, emergency medicine was recognized as a formal medical specialty by the American Board of Medical Specialties. Approximately 15,000 physicians and 60,000 nurses currently practice within emergency departments of hospitals in the United States; over 43,000 emergency medical technicians (EMTs) deliver prehospital care; and over 5,000 hospitals have functioning emergency departments. It is quite natural that the increased utilization of emergency departments and the increased organization of emergency medicine as a discipline have drawn the attention of other health professions.

Pharmacy has only recently begun to view the emergency department as a practice locale, encompassing the drug distribution and the clinical practice activities of pharmacists.[2-8] Relatively little has been done to document drug use trends within emergency medicine. It has been estimated, however, that an average of 1.4 drugs are given or prescribed per patient visit to the emergency department, and that almost 50% of the patients receive at least one medication (Table 12–1).[9] It can be conservatively estimated that in excess of $500 million is spent annually on medications administered in US hospital emergency departments.

An interesting parallel has existed over the preceding decade in the evolution of emergency medicine and clinical pharmacy as health care specialties. Both have been striving for recognition as legitimate practice specialties and academic disciplines; both have faced the struggles of introducing change into established patterns of health care. Although early attention was placed on the development of sound practice concepts and the formation of education and training programs,

Table 12–1 Drugs Given or Prescribed in Emergency Departments

Drug Class	Percent of Total Prescriptions	Rate Per 1000 Visits
Antitetanus	24.5	168.0
Narcotics	17.5	120.0
Anti-infectives	16.9	116.0
Aspirin, other nonnarcotic analgesics	13.8	94.7
Barbiturates, other sedatives and tranquilizers	9.3	64.0
Antihistamines	5.3	36.3
Adrenergics, anticholinergics	3.8	25.8
Antacids, antidiarrheals, antiemetics	2.5	17.4
Steroid hormones	1.5	10.2
Diuretics, other antihypertensives	1.1	7.4
Emetics	0.8	5.4
Muscle relaxants	0.7	4.9
Cocaine derivatives	0.6	4.1
Cardiac glycosides, other antiarrhythmics	0.4	2.7
Anticonvulsants	0.3	2.3
Antidiabetics	0.2	1.2
Antidotes	0.2	1.7
Cholinergics, antiadrenergics	0.2	1.5
Serums, vaccines, globulins	0.2	1.4
Antidepressants, amphetamine derivatives	0.1	0.6

Source: Hosmer RR, Waldman ML: Drugs given or prescribed in the emergency department. JACEP 1976;5:908–909.

subsequent emphasis has been focused on research activities and the development of new knowledge in the discipline.

EMERGENCY MEDICINE AT TRUMAN MEDICAL CENTER

Truman Medical Center, the principal teaching hospital of the University of Missouri–Kansas City (UMKC) health professions schools, is a 310-bed acute care general hospital. It serves as the city and county hospital for Kansas City, Missouri. Truman Medical Center is affiliated with other institutions that provide pediatric, mental health, and long-term care for the same patient population.

The Department of Emergency Health Services occupies about 5000 square feet on the hospital's first floor (Figure 12–1). It includes general treatment beds for 14 patients, two major trauma rooms, and a 10-bed observation unit.[10] About 40,000 patients are seen annually; approximately 15% of those treated within the department are admitted to the hospital, accounting for about 30% of all hospital admissions (Table 12–2). Pediatric patients are not routinely treated in the emergency department of Truman Medical Center.

The Department of Emergency Health Services has a core faculty of five physicians and one clinical pharmacist. The department offers an accredited residency in emergency medicine for physicians wishing to specialize in the field. In addition to postgraduate training of physicians from other specialties and clinical pharmacy residents, members of the department conduct required clerkship or didactic courses for all students in the Schools of Medicine and Pharmacy. Truman Medical Center is a Level I trauma center, and faculty from the emergency department provide medical supervision for the prehospital care system of Kansas City, Missouri. The pharmacy department provides 24-hour services, unit-dose, intravenous additives, and parenteral nutrition from a central area and three inpatient decentralized units.

CLINICAL PHARMACY WITHIN EMERGENCY MEDICINE

Clinical pharmacy services were established within the emergency department of Truman Medical Center in 1974. The need for a clinical pharmacist was seen when the department's emergency medicine residency was established. Clinical pharmacists had been an integral component of the practice and teaching activities of the Department of Medicine,[11,12] and extension of the role to emergency medicine seemed both natural and potentially beneficial to the department's programs. Furthermore, the site would open a new avenue for pharmacy education and training. The clinical pharmacy position was originally funded by the UMKC School of Pharmacy; funding is now provided jointly by the School of Pharmacy and the Department of Emergency Health Services.

Figure 12–1 Department of Emergency Health Services, Truman Medical Center

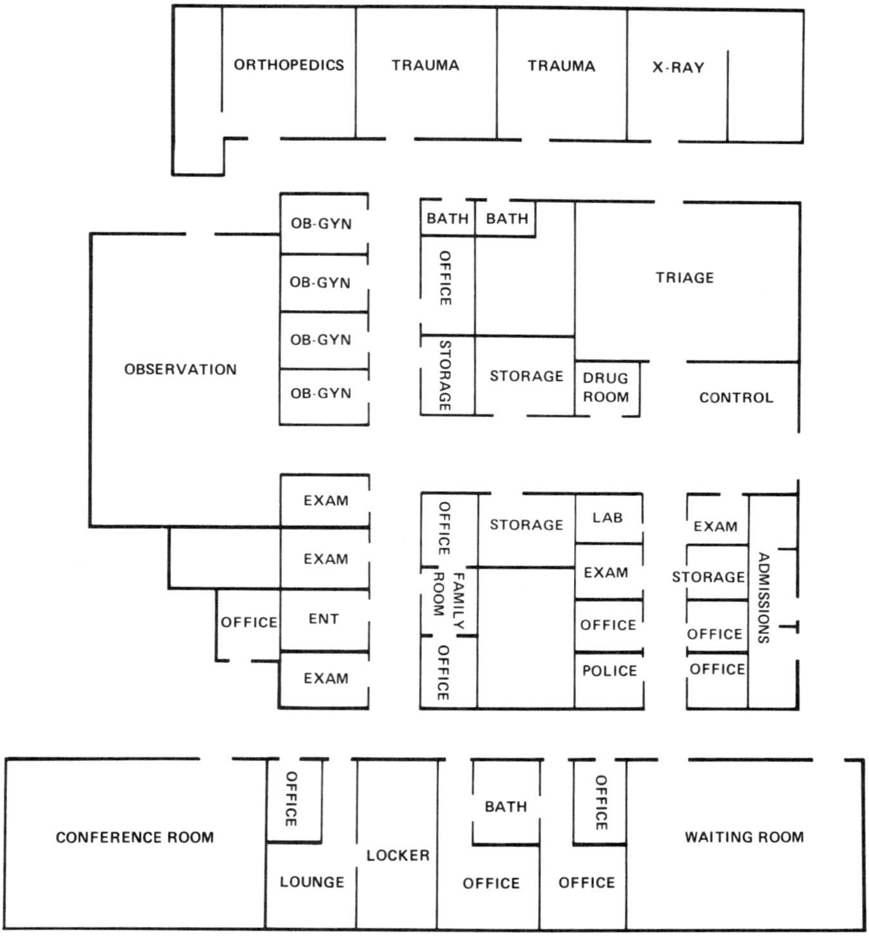

Source: Truman Medical Center, Kansas City, Missouri.

General Activities

A reasonable question about the pharmacy's relationship to the emergency department is whether sufficient clinical material exists to warrant the assignment of a pharmacist to the area. As a general rule, the input of a pharmacist is appropriate and necessary at any place in which patients and drugs interface. The

Table 12–2 Stratification of Patients Treated in Emergency Department

		Percent of Patients	
ICD-9-CM*	Description	Treated and Discharged	Admitted to Hospital
001–139	Infections and parasitic diseases	2.73	0.40
140–239	Neoplasms	0.10	1.46
240–279	Endocrine, nutritional and metabolic diseases, immunity disorders	0.26	3.72
280–289	Diseases of the blood and blood-forming organs	0.26	2.26
290–319	Mental disorders	2.89	4.12
320–389	Diseases of the nervous system and sense organs	1.96	1.26
390–459	Diseases of the circulatory system	2.37	10.7
	Hypertension	0.67	0.8
	Ischemic heart disease	0.10	1.99
	Arrhythmias	0.46	1.4
	Heart failure	0.10	2.92
	Cerebrovascular disease	0.01	2.06
460–519	Diseases of the respiratory system	9.63	9.57
	Acute respiratory infections	4.84	0.47
	Pneumonia and influenza	0.82	2.72
	Asthma/COPD	3.04	7.64
520–579	Diseases of the digestive system	6.70	8.90
580–629	Diseases of the genitourinary system	11.03	7.64
630–676	Complications of pregnancy, childbirth and the puerperium	1.03	2.99
680–709	Diseases of the skin and subcutaneous tissues	3.66	1.99
	Infections	1.80	1.66
710–739	Diseases of the musculoskeletal system and connective tissue	4.84	1.46
780–799	Symptoms, signs, and ill-defined conditions	14.27	20.07
	Convulsions	1.18	3.92
800–999	Injury and poisoning	36.48	19.93
	Musculoskeletal injuries	9.38	7.18
	Intracranial injuries	1.70	1.26
	Lacerations	12.16	6.45
	Burns	0.57	0.40
	Poisoning	0.82	1.00

Note: *International Classification of Diseases, 9th Revision, Clinical Modification.

Source: Department of Emergency Health Services, Truman Medical Center, Kansas City, Missouri.

level and type of input are what must be determined, and are undoubtedly location-dependent. The following discussions outline clinical pharmacy activities within the emergency department of Truman Medical Center and comment on their general transference to other institutions.

The principal goal of clinical pharmacy services is to promote and to assure rational pharmacotherapeutics within all aspects of health care offered by the Department of Emergency Health Services. To meet this goal, the activities of the pharmacist can be divided into the three areas of (1) clinical practice, (2) education, and (3) research.

Clinical Practice

The emergency department predictably is the busiest between 2 P.M. and 2 A.M., with variable activity taking place during the rest of the day. To maximize pharmacy's contribution, therefore, the clinical pharmacist staffs the emergency department chiefly during the afternoon and evening hours. Residents in clinical pharmacy also assist in providing evening and night coverage as a component of their on-call responsibilities. Key clinical practice activities include—

- bedside consultation with physicians and nurses to design, to implement, and to monitor a patient-specific therapeutic plan using the most efficacious, least toxic, and most economical drugs available;
- patient education directed toward increasing understanding of medication-use and thus maximizing the chance of therapeutic success;
- assistance in maintaining emergency department compliance with pharmacy procedures and in developing an appropriate formulary of medications in the emergency room. (See Table 12–3; drug distribution activities, per se, are not part of the clinical pharmacist's activities.)

Education

The Department of Emergency Health Services has a heavy commitment to the education of physicians, pharmacists, and nurses. Recognizing that a pharmacotherapeutic consultation is also an educational session, the clinical pharmacy activities involve a variety of formal and informal educational programs. The department conducts didactic conferences covering the emergency medicine core curriculum[13] and other pertinent topics, morbidity and mortality discussions, and a monthly journal club. Many of these conferences are conducted by or include the clinical pharmacist (Table 12–4). Nursing inservice education is scheduled to discuss pharmacologic topics of particular importance to the emergency nursing staff.

Table 12–3 Chargeable Drug Items Routinely Stocked in Truman Medical Center Emergency Department

Item	Inventory Level
Oral	
Acetaminophen 350 mg	100
Activated charcoal (30 g)	4
Aminophylline (100 mg)	10
Ampicillin (3.5 g)	4
ASA (350 mg)	100
Diphenhydramine (50 mg)	10
Gelusil liquid	2
Ipecac syrup (30 mL)	10
Lasix (40 mg)	5
Lidocaine, viscous	2
MOM (30 mL)	5
Phenytoin (100 mg)	20
Potassium chloride (25 mEq)	5
Probenecid (50 mg)	16
Theophylline elixir (80 mg/15 mL)	1 pt
Trimethoprim-sulfamethoxazole (double strength)	9
Rectal	
Prochlorperazine (25 mg)	5
Topical	
Silver sulfadiazene (20 g)	12
Parenteral	
Aminophylline (250 mg/10 mL)	6
Aminophylline (500 mg/20 mL)	6
Ampicillin (1 g)	4
Atropine (0.4 mg)	8
Benzathine Penicillin G (1.2 mU)	5
Benzquinamide (50 mg)	6
Bretylium (500 mg)	3
Calcium chloride (1 g)	5
Calcium gluconate (1 g)	5
Cephapirin (1 g)	2
Clindamycin (600 mg)	5
Cyanide antidote kit	1
Dexamethasone (4 mg)	5
Dextrose 50% (50 mL)	6
Diazoxide (300 mg)	2
Digoxin (0.5 mg/2 mL)	4
Diphenhydramine (50 mg)	8
Dopamine (200 mg)	4
Edrophonium (10 mg/mL; 10 mL)	1
Epinephrine 1:1000 (1 mL)	10

Table 12-3 continued

Item	Inventory Level
Epinephrine 1:10,000 (10 mL)	20
Furosemide (20 mg)	5
Furosemide (40 mg)	5
Gentamicin (80 mg)	4
Haloperidol (5 mg)	4
Hydrocortisone (250 mg)	2
Hydrocortisone (500 mg)	2
Hydroxyzine (100 mg)	10
Immune Serum Globulin	5
Insulin U-100: regular	1
NPH	1
Lente	1
Semi-Lente	1
Isoproterenol (1 mg/5 mL)	5
Levarterenol (4 mg/4 mL)	5
Lidocaine (100 mg syringe)	10
Lidocaine (2 g vial)	5
Magnesium sulfate 50% (2 mL)	10
Mannitol (12.5 g/50 mL)	10
Metaraminol 10 mg/mL; 10 mL)	2
Methylprednisolone (40 mg)	2
Methylprednisolone (125 mg)	2
Multivitamin	2
Naloxone (0.4 mg)	15
Nitroprusside (50 mg)	2
Oxacillin (1 g)	2
Oxytocin (10 U)	4
Pralidoxime (1 g)	6
Penicillin G aqueous (1 mU)	2
Penicillin G aqueous (5 mU)	2
Phentolamine (5 mg)	2
Phenytoin (250 mg/5 mL)	8
Physostigmine (2 mg/2 mL)	5
Potassium chloride (40 mEq)	5
Potassium phosphate (15 mL)	2
Procainamide (100 mg/mL; 10 mL)	2
Procaine Penicillin G (2.4 mU)	20
Propranolol (1 mg)	10
Sodium bicarbonate (44.6 mEq)	20
Spectinomycin (2 g)	2
Tetanus immune globulin (250 U)	5
Tetanus/diphtheria toxoid (0.5 mL)	20
Thiamine (200 mg/2 mL)	6
Verapamil (5 mg/2 mL)	4

Note: Table does not include ENT, crash cart items, or nonchargeable floor stock.

Source: Truman Medical Center, Kansas City, Missouri.

Table 12–4 Representative Pharmacology Lectures

Curriculum Area	Title
Allergy	Anaphylaxis
Cardiology	Antiarrhythmic drugs Bretylium in ventricular fibrillation Catecholamines Dopamine vs dobutamine Hypertension in the ER Hypertensive emergencies Hypothermia and bretylium Nitroprusside vs nitroglycerin Pulmonary edema Supraventricular tachycardia Vasopressors Verapamil
Endocrine	Diabetic ketoacidosis Insulin
General	Autonomic pharmacology Biostatistics Drug-induced skin eruptions Drugs in pregnancy and breast feeding General anesthetics Local anesthetics Narcotic analgesics Neuromuscular blocking agents Nonsteroidal anti-inflammatory drugs Techniques of literature evaluation The placebo Review of the ER prescribing
Infectious disease	New antibiotics New cephalosporins Prophylactic antibiotics in the ER Prophylactic antibiotics in bite wounds Septic shock Topical antibiotics Urinary tract infections
Neurology	Alcohol-induced seizures Cerebral edema Extrapyramidal side effects of antipsychotics Phenytoin Treatment of seizures
OB-Gyn	Problems with oral contraceptives

Table 12–4 continued

Curriculum Area	Title
Pulmonary	Management of asthma
	Pulmonary aspiration
	Theophylline pharmacokinetics
	Theophylline pharmacology
Rheumatology	Treatment of acute gout
Toxicology	Acetaminophen overdose
	Alcohol withdrawal
	Alcohol intoxication
	Alkaline diuresis in acute salicylism
	Amanita poisoning
	Antabuse reactions
	Antidotes
	Barbiturate overdose
	Carbon monoxide poisoning
	Charcoal hemoperfusion
	Cocaine
	Digitalis toxicity
	Drug-induced alcohol intolerance
	Drug-withdrawal syndromes
	Hallucinogens
	Herbicide poisoning
	Iron poisoning
	Lead intoxication
	Management of drug overdose
	Narcotic overdose
	Organophosphate poisoning
	PCP
	Pesticide poisoning
	Petroleum distillates
	Phenothiazine overdose
	Salicylism
	Tricyclic antidepressant overdose
	Vitamin toxicity

Research

Although certain aspects of the practice of clinical pharmacy and emergency medicine have advanced tremendously in the preceding ten years, both are only beginning to realize their potential as academic disciplines. The need for a strong academic and research base upon which to build clinical practice, and the need to link effectively the basic and clinical sciences, have been editorialized upon within both pharmacy and emergency medicine.[14,15] Formalization of emergency medicine as a practice specialty has allowed recognition that many unanswered questions exist in the evaluation and treatment of problems encountered in the emergency department. Considering the large number of patients treated in emergency facilities, this knowledge void may assume a special significance. An organized campaign of clinical pharmacy research within emergency medicine has thus begun.

GENERAL IMPLEMENTATION OF PROGRAM

Physicians and nurses have accepted clinical pharmacy services within emergency medicine.[5] A survey not only found overwhelming support for the activities of the clinical pharmacist at Truman Medical Center, but also suggested the ease with which such services could be transferred to other institutions. Ninety-five percent of physicians surveyed felt that the activities of the pharmacist were transferable to other hospitals.

A three-tiered approach can be suggested for the implementation of pharmacy services within the emergency department: administration, drug distribution, and clinical-educational.

Administrative Approach

Administrative relationships between the pharmacy and emergency departments almost certainly exist already in all hospitals. However, are these relationships loosely structured, or do they demonstrate a real interest in the emergency department by pharmacists? Are they dispersed among a number of persons or centralized in one pharmacist who has a genuine interest in emergency medicine?

The hospital's committees on cardiopulmonary resuscitation (CPR), disaster preparedness, pharmacy and therapeutics (P&T), or medical audit at one time or another deal with matters of importance to the emergency department. Such a type of administrative relationship does not require actually stationing a pharmacist in the emergency room but opens useful routes of communication for subsequent activities with physicians and nurses. Additionally, periodic pharmacy inspections, as required by the Joint Commission on Accreditation of Hospitals (JCAH), provide an opportune occasion for the pharmacist to extend his or her activities in the emergency department.

Drug Distribution

Drug distribution responsibilities in the emergency department may be structured in such a way that they require either the periodic presence only of the pharmacist or his continuous presence. Periodic activities might include the following:

Emergency Department Formulary. All emergency rooms require the maintenance of at least some floor stock items within the department. The variety and level of inventory are determined by the type of patients treated and the pharmacy services available for general support of the emergency room. The general criteria for maintaining a supply of given medication in the ER should be either that it is needed immediately when prescribed (e.g., lidocaine for treating premature ventricular contractions), or that it is prescribed so commonly that efficiency is gained by keeping a supply. The availability of 24-hour pharmacy services should allow a smaller inventory to be maintained in the emergency department. The department at Truman Medical Center has found that those medications listed in Table 12–3 provide for more than 95% of the drug needs.

Inventory Levels. Concurrent with establishing an ER formulary, one should set inventory levels for each drug item. A natural tendency of emergency department personnel is to overstock. Only the pharmacist has an interest in maintaining inventory at its appropriate level. (See Table 12–3 for inventory levels established at Truman Medical Center.)

Crash Cart Content. The drug and supply items maintained on hospital emergency carts are generally determined by the P&T or CPR committees or by some multidisciplinary group with a similar working authority. These items should be uniform in content and design throughout the institution; the drugs maintained should generally adhere to American Heart Association guidelines for advanced cardiac life support (ACLS). The drug items stocked on crash carts at Truman Medical Center are indicated in Table 12–5.

Discharge Medications. Unless the institution provides 24-hour outpatient pharmacy services, the physicians and nurses of most emergency rooms normally request a method of discharging patients with medication to initiate follow-up treatment. This procedure generally should present a problem only during the late evening and early morning, when community pharmacies will not open for several hours. Unless pharmacy input is available to those designing a system for discharge medications, the result may be an irrational (and possibly illegal) dispensing of unlabeled pharmaceutical samples.[2] A reasonable solution seems to be to develop a small cadre of medications in unit-of-use packaging, prelabeled with drug name, quantity, and hospital name. Emergency room personnel can complete the label with the date, the patient and physician names, and the instructions for use at the time of discharge. Information cards, supplied by the pharmacy, could be used by nurses in counseling patients at the time of discharge about medication usage.

Table 12–5 Crash Cart Drug Contents at Truman Medical Center

Drug	Inventory Level
Atropine Sulfate (0.4 mg/mL; 1-mL vial)	6
Bretylium (500-mg ampule)	2
Calcium Chloride 10% (1 g/10-mL vial)	2
Dextrose 50% (50 mL)	1
Diphenhydramine (50-mg injection)	2
Dopamine (200 mg/5-mL ampule)	2
Epinephrine 1:10,000 (1 mg/10-mL syringe with intracardiac needle)	5
Isoproterenol 1:5,000 (1 mg/5-mL ampule)	2
Levarterenol (4 mg/4-mL ampule)	2
Lidocaine (20 mg/mL; 5-mL syringe [100 mg])	3
Lidocaine 4% (2 g/50-mL vial)	1
Naloxone (0.4 mg/mL ampule)	4
Phenytoin (250 mg/5-mL ampule with syringe)	4
Procainamide (100 mg/mL; 10-mL vial)	1
Sodium Bicarbonate (44.6 mEq/50-mL syringe)	8
Sodium Chloride 0.9% bacteriostatic for inj. (30 mL)	1

Source: Truman Medical Center, Kansas City, Missouri.

A periodic presence of the pharmacist, however, cannot meet all the needs; rather, a continuous, or scheduled, presence must exist if drug distribution responsibilities are to extend significantly beyond those outlined above. Fortunately, it is probably not necessary to schedule a pharmacist in the ER on a 24-hour basis. An evaluation of workload patterns in the emergency department may suggest the optimal shift for pharmacy coverage. Most likely, however, this shift will involve the evening hours, when patient encounters peak and the pharmacist can most easily extend the basic services of the pharmacy department. Such an extension would involve at least two areas of service: (1) discharge prescriptions and (2) comprehensive pharmaceutical services.

Discharge Prescriptions. Programs of decentralized pharmaceutical services functioning in the emergency department have been described in various publications.[6,8] At the University of Nebraska Medical Center, for example, a mobile medication cart stocked with a limited inventory of prepackaged medications was capable of meeting more than 90% of the discharge prescription needs.[6] The revenue generated by filling these prescriptions (previously lost because the outpatient pharmacy was closed during the evening hours) easily provided for the pharmacist's salary. Importantly, the time required to provide these prescription services was not thought to interfere with the provision of clinical services.

Comprehensive Pharmaceutical Services. The provision of all pharmaceutical services by a decentralized emergency room pharmacy requires a commitment exceeding that described thus far. As described by Beaty and Puckett[8], working from a central area within the emergency department, the pharmacist is able to perform traditional dispensing functions and to serve actively as a drug information consultant.

Clinical-Educational

Clinical pharmacy or educational responsibilities within the emergency department may also be structured so that they require either the periodic or the continuous presence of the pharmacist. The choice, of course, depends upon resource availability and the programmatic needs of the pharmacy and emergency departments. Clinical or educational activities the pharmacist can provide on an episodic basis might include the following:

Cardiac Arrest Team. The responsibilities of pharmacists as members of the cardiac arrest team have been described.[16,17] All pharmacists should become certified in basic CPR, and those participating as members of the cardiac arrest team should also pursue the advanced certification provided by ACLS. Participation on the cardiac arrest team would certainly extend the pharmacist's responsibilities to hospital areas other than the emergency room.

Poison Information. Without attempting to duplicate the resources or activities of a regional poison control center, the pharmacist can serve as a natural source of inhouse information on poisoning and drug overdose. Through basic training in pharmacology and toxicology, supplemented by participation in continuing education in clinical toxicology, a pharmacist can readily develop the data base to serve as an effective consultant in this area.

Inservice Education. Providing inservice education programs for emergency department physicians, nurses, or paramedics can serve as an entree to the clinical environment. While demonstrating his capabilities and interest in being of assistance, the pharmacist is also building communication links likely to lead to requests for consultation or regular participation in patient care and education programs.

Going beyond the provision of periodic clinical or educational services like those described above requires a significant resource commitment. Except in institutions with an active teaching and research program based on emergency medicine, it is probably most reasonable to tie these ongoing clinical responsibilities to a drug distribution commitment.[6,8]

Cost Justification

Future changes in methods of hospital reimbursement for emergency room services could alter the following comments. Nevertheless, cost justification for developing ongoing pharmaceutical services in the ER has generally been achieved to date by demonstrating either increased revenue[6,8] or a reduction of costs, and both of these are affected by three factors—inventory control, revenue loss, and decentralization.

Inventory Control. Developing an effective emergency department formulary and inventory levels can probably reduce the total drug stock maintained in the emergency department. This reduction can be directly transferred into dollar savings. Before the initiation of clinical pharmacy services in the emergency department of Truman Medical Center, about 350 different drug items were stocked in the ER. This stock has now been reduced to that shown in Table 12–3.

Lost Revenue. It is well known that a ward-stock system of drug distribution, such as is typically found in most ERs, is inherently associated with lost revenue because of failure to charge for medications administered. It has been suggested that busy ER personnel do not place a high priority on pharmaceutical control[3] and, further, that a unit-of-use drug distribution system[3] or a decentralized pharmacy may markedly reduce this area of lost revenue.[8]

Decentralized Pharmacy. Extending the hours of outpatient prescription services into the evening by placing a pharmacist in the ER may not only provide a patient service not previously available, but also may create a new revenue source. It has been found in at least two settings, for example, that revenue from filling discharge prescriptions was sufficient to cost-justify the pharmacist's activities.[6,8]

CONCLUSIONS

In most respects, establishing clinical pharmacy services in the emergency department is no different from doing so in other areas of the hospital. Although many persons may not see the ER as a prime area in need of comprehensive pharmaceutical services, their belief is probably caused by an inappropriately narrow view of the scope of patient care delivered. As mentioned in the opening paragraphs of this chapter, the number of patients treated in ERs is large, and a considerable amount of money is spent on drugs administered in this setting.

Pharmacists initially venturing into the emergency department may be anxious because of the broad range of patient problems encountered there (see Table 12–2). Unfortunately, no textbook of emergency medicine clinical pharmacy exists to provide a convenient, comprehensive source of pharmacotherapeutic information specifically relative to this area. However, textbooks of emergency medicine written for physician audiences, the emergency medicine core curriculum,[13] a bibliography of critical care,[18] or textbooks on clinical toxicology can identify pertinent topics for study. If available, knowledge about drug-use patterns or data describing the emergency department's patient population can be used to identify areas the pharmacist may need to review before entering the clinical environment.

REFERENCES

1. Definition of emergency medicine. *Ann Emerg Med* 1981;10:385–388.

2. Maudlin RK, Owyang E: Emergency department drugs. *Hospitals* 1971;45:88–92.

3. Mar DD, Hanan ZI, LaFontaine R: Improved emergency room medication distribution. *Am J Hosp Pharm* 1978;35:70–73.

4. Schiavone JD: Developing a unit-of-use drug distribution system for the hospital emergency room. *Hosp Pharm* 16:208–209, 214–215, 219–221.

5. Elenbaas RM, Waeckerle JF, McNabney WK: The clinical pharmacist in emergency medicine. *Am J Hosp Pharm* 1977;34:843–846.

6. Spigiel RW, Anderson JR: Comprehensive pharmaceutical services in the emergency room. *Am J Hosp Pharm* 1979;36:52–56.

7. Carmichael JM, Hak SH, Edgman SM, et al: Emergency room services for a community health center. *Am J Hosp Pharm* 1981;38:79–83.

8. Beaty S, Puckett W: Expanding pharmacy services in the emergency room. Abstracts, American Society of Hospital Pharmacists, Midyear Clinical Meeting. New Orleans, December 1981.

9. Hosmer RR, Waldman ML: Drugs given or prescribed in the emergency department. *JACEP* 1976;5:908–909.

10. Landers GA, Waeckerle JF, McNabney WK: Observation ward utilization. *JACEP* 1975;4:123–125.

11. Noback RK: The full time doctor of pharmacy in health care and education. *Greater KC Medical Bulletin* 1978;73:(Apr.):10.

12. Covinsky JO, Hamburger S, Twin EJ: A look at the educational responsibilities and cost impact of the docent clinical pharmacist. *Drug Intell Clin Pharm* 1980;14:266–271.

13. Tintinalli J (ed): *A Study Guide in Emergency Medicine*. Dallas, American College of Emergency Physicians, 1978, vol. 1–4.

14. Romankiewicz JA: Spanning the gap—clinical research. *Drug Intell Clin Pharm* 1975;9:324.

15. McNabney WK: On being academic. *Ann Emerg Med* 1981;10:117.

16. Schwerman E, Schwartau N, Thompson CO, et al: The pharmacist as a member of the cardiopulmonary resuscitation team. *Drug Intell Clin Pharm* 1973;7:299–308.

17. Ludwig DJ, Abramowitz PW: The pharmacist as a member of the CPR team: Evaluation by other health professionals. *Drug Intell Clin Pharm* 1983;17:463–465.

18. Elenbaas RM, Cerra FB, Curtis RA, et al: Therapeutic bibliograpy of critical care. *Drug Intell Clin Pharm* 1983;17:722–725.

Chapter 13

The Pharmacist in the Trauma Center

Thomas C. Majerus

The cost of trauma to society exceeds that of other major illnesses, such as cancer and heart disease. Trauma, ranking third to heart disease and cancer as a killer, predominantly affects the young. Trauma is the greatest killer of Americans between the ages of 1 and 44, and accidents are responsible for four times more children's deaths than is any other cause. Beside the cost of the initial emergency care, the total cost of trauma includes the loss of productivity and earnings in families not cared for by a principal provider, the loss of a productive member of society, and the prolonged cost of rehabilitation and therapy for the trauma victim. The cost of accidental trauma in terms of lost wages is estimated at more than $63 million per day.[1] The total annual cost of accidental trauma is approximately $50 billion.

TRAUMA CENTER ENVIRONMENT

The system under which a trauma center works is dedicated to complete preparedness for any life-threatening injury. The trauma center, in its entirety, is dedicated to the care of the critically injured patient. Whether the patient has minor or severe injuries, the center is ready to care for that patient in a way similar to a standard emergency department in any hospital; nevertheless, a trauma center is more than an emergency department. The major difference between an emergency department and a trauma center is the trauma center's capability of a more definitive management than any outpatient clinic.[2] A trauma center could be classified as a combination emergency department and intensive care unit (ICU), except that most of the patients treated in ICUs have had their illnesses diagnosed previously. A patient entering an emergency system dedicated to the treatment of trauma victims is undiagnosed, and so immediate and definitive resuscitation and treatment of their clinical condition are the first requirements. Trauma patients are treated first and diagnosed second. This order is the reverse of conventional emergency care.

In fiscal year 1983, the Maryland Institute for Emergency Medical Services Systems (MIEMSS) had a total of 1,692 admissions with 54% of the admissions resulting from motor vehicle related accidents. The other accident classifications were pedestrian accidents, motorcycle accidents, industrial accidents, farm accidents, home accidents, recreational accidents, assaults, and other minor accident classifications.[3]

ORGANIZATION OF EMERGENCY MEDICAL SERVICES SYSTEM

Approximately 5% of people injured in traumatic events in the United States require the techniques offered by an organized trauma center. Nearly 85% of injured patients can be managed at the local level; another 10% require care at areawide trauma centers. Not included in this latter group are patients who require specialized treatment in one of the state's designated specialty referral centers.

As the coordinating agency for the statewide emergency medical system in Maryland, MIEMSS has been given the task to coordinate treatment facilities throughout the state, to coordinate the transportation of the injured, to organize and to apply all communications equipment, and to train the emergency medical services (EMS) personnel responsible for prehospital care. A seemingly minor but important function of the operations section is the handling of public affairs and information, which keeps the citizens of Maryland informed of EMS activities and progress.

The state is divided into regions, each of which is governed by a regional administrator and a volunteer advisory council. The council is composed of medical care providers, institutional personnel, consumers, representatives of local and state government, and professionals in the EMS system.

As in any system that is widespread and complex, communications are critical. The Maryland EMS system is linked together by a statewide EMS communications system. One major component of this system is the Systems Communication Center (SYSCOM), located at MIEMSS. SYSCOM is staffed 24 hours a day by communicators who are trained emergency medical technicians (EMTs). SYSCOM coordinates Med-Evac helicopter missions, notifies the receiving hospital of patient information and arrival time, establishes consultations between prehospital care providers in the field and physicians in hospitals, and provides communications during disasters. Another major component of the system is the Emergency Medical Resource Center, which establishes medical communications between prehospital care providers in the field and medical personnel at hospitals in the Baltimore metropolitan area.

Transportation of the patient to a trauma center, in which definitive emergency care is provided, is another critical component of the EMS system. During fiscal year 1983, over 69% of the total admissions to MIEMSS came directly from the scene of the trauma. Approximately 79% of the direct admissions to MIEMSS were by Med-Evac helicopter, with an average response time of 63 minutes. (Response time is defined as the interval between the time of the accident and the time of arrival at the Shock Trauma Center.)[3] Although the Maryland State Police Med-Evac helicopter system transports most of the patients taken to the Shock Trauma Center, ambulance and rescue companies—made up of paid and volunteer personnel—serve the citizens of Maryland well.

ECHELONS OF CARE

The system for providing highly specialized trauma care is called the Maryland echelons of trauma care, which consists of five basic levels: (1) MIEMSS, (2) specialty referral centers, (3) cardiac surgery centers, (4) areawide trauma centers, and (5) the local hospital emergency rooms and coronary care units (Figure 13-1).

Victims of severe multiple injuries, cardiac and major vessel injuries, cardiogenic shock, multiple injuries with complications, gas gangrene, carbon monoxide intoxication, scuba accidents, drowning, and smoke inhalation are admitted to the MIEMSS Shock Trauma Center.[4] Areawide trauma centers are designated throughout the state to care for patients with combinations of trauma injury, crush or blunt trauma, penetrating trauma, injury with severe hemorrhage, one or more extremities paralyzed as a result of trauma, and traumatic amputations. A poison control center serves the statewide system 24 hours a day from the University of Maryland School of Pharmacy. They give advice to physicians—as well as to the lay public—concerning poisoning, toxicology, and related subjects.

The specialty referral centers include pediatric trauma centers, burn centers, neonatal ICUs, a hand center, eye trauma centers, and a center for patients with brain or spinal cord injuries.

PREHOSPITAL CARE

The immediate management of the multiple trauma patient has a great impact on patient survival. The prehospital phase of the management of the trauma patient is integrated into the total clinical care of the patient. Basic life support performed by EMTs is available throughout the country. A higher level of care is provided through advanced life support programs, in which EMTs are trained to perform invasive medical techniques, such as central venous access line insertion and endotracheal intubation. These prehospital care personnel represent an extension

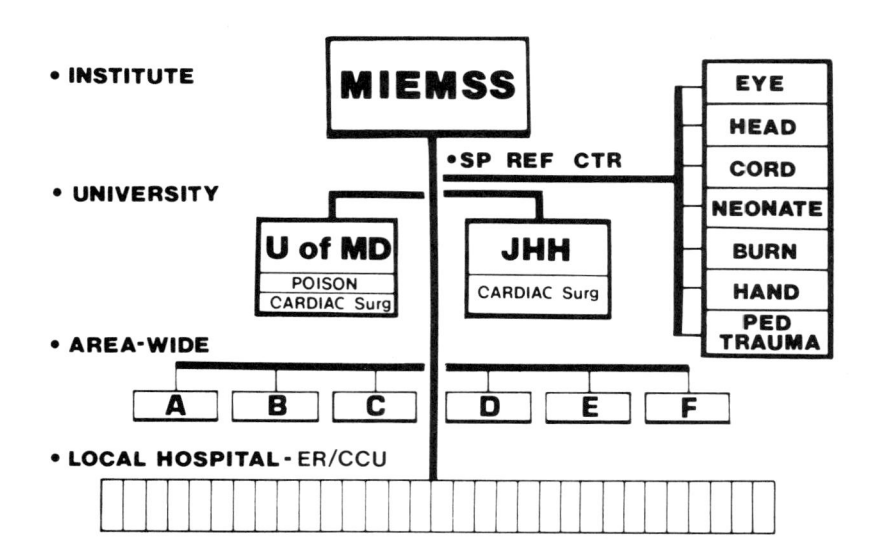

Figure 13-1 Echelons of Care in Maryland

- **INSTITUTE**
- **UNIVERSITY**
- **AREA-WIDE**
- **LOCAL HOSPITAL** - ER/CCU

MIEMSS — SP REF CTR

U of MD (POISON, CARDIAC Surg) — JHH (CARDIAC Surg)

EYE, HEAD, CORD, NEONATE, BURN, HAND, PED TRAUMA

A B C D E F

Source: Cowley RA, Dunham CM (eds): *Shock Trauma/Critical Care Manual—Initial Assessment and Management*. Baltimore, University Park Press, 1982, p 565.

---

of the physician and the patient care that will be provided in the receiving hospital. Different therapeutic modalities are performed by the technicians, either by protocol or through radio communication with a physician at a resource center.

Prehospital protocols address the medical care provided by field personnel before consultation with a physician. These protocols define the immediate management of the multiple trauma patient. The immediate care provided by field personnel allows stabilization and information exchange to take place. There are protocols for routine patient care, care for unconscious patients, care for patients with multiple or severe trauma, treatment of patients with burns, treatment of pediatric emergencies, care and treatment of patients with respiratory distress, treatment and stabilization of patients in varying types and degrees of shock, and treatment of patients with spinal cord and other central nervous system (CNS) injuries.[5] Also included are protocols that address the initial patient assessment and triage and a system to allow ongoing assessment of the efficacy of prehospital protocols and prehospital care. Only through a concerted belief in the importance of prehospital care can the benefit of proper training and the application of paramedic skills be realized. The system undergoes constant revision, fine tuning, and improvement because the importance of prehospital personnel is appreciated.

CLINICAL SIDE OF THE SYSTEM

The team charged with caring for the trauma patient is undoubtedly unique in medicine or surgery. The environment of the trauma center is dynamic.[6] The specialists on the staff in a trauma center are on duty 24 hours a day with a senior surgeon specializing in traumatology present at all times. In addition to the traumatologist, the specialists include anesthesiologists, orthopedic surgeons, neurosurgeons, cardiovascular and thoracic surgeons, plastic surgeons, oral maxillofacial surgeons, radiologists, urologists, nephrologists, internists, intensivists, and multiple paramedical and parasurgical personnel. In addition to working with the specialists mentioned, clinical pharmacists work with respiratory therapists, physical therapists, biomedical engineers, social workers, and chaplains. All efforts are integrated so that each team member contributes his much needed input for total patient care.

In a trauma center, as in critical care in general, the key element for the day-to-day care of a patient is the nursing personnel. The one person who is with a patient continuously is the nurse; the care provided by the nurse is largely responsible for the successful outcome of a critically ill or injured patient's treatment. The singular effects of the nursing efforts in a trauma center are based on postgraduate training in critical care medicine and a solid knowledge base in physiology and pathophysiology applicable to the multiple trauma patient.

All members of the team work together toward a common goal in a way unlike that of specialists in other hospital settings. The care of the severely injured patient is beyond the capabilities and experience of any individual physician.[2] Within the system, the multidisciplinary staff works to provide the best possible care for the critically ill or injured patient from admission to discharge. Specialty barriers do not exist; they have been replaced by active participation and open communication.

As was mentioned previously, prehospital care is governed by a protocol system. In a similar fashion, hospital-based care is dictated by protocols that cover practices involving protocol studies, as well as special studies for all facets of care. Included are clinical laboratory protocols and protocols for addressing trauma-induced death. Protocols play a part in ensuring unhesitant treatment. Protocols are guidelines, but they do not obviate clinical judgment in the art of medicine. Indeed, they allow a standardization of treatment so that no critical points will be omitted during the care of the patients.[2] While specialists interact in providing patient care, the surgical team's primary responsibility for the patient and its overall responsibility for patient care rest on the shoulders of the team leader. Just as the primary team must know treatment protocols, other specialists, including the clinical pharmacist, must be aware of treatment protocols and take part in continuous, effective communication with the team. Continuous interaction among all of the clinicians involved in the care of the patient is necessary.

THE CLINICAL PHARMACIST

The clinical services provided by pharmacists in the trauma center are as variable as the clinical picture is changeable. Pharmacokinetic application of drug dosing continues as one of the most frequent services offered by pharmacists. Nutritional support of the trauma patient is also an important part of the therapy as the patient begins posttrauma convalescence.

Basic to adequate clinical pharmacy services in the trauma center is an efficient drug distribution system.[7] Moreover, an efficient drug distribution system entails audits, formulary management, and an adequate inventory of required drugs. Likewise, an ongoing quality assurance program to monitor pharmacologic therapy is necessary. Other therapy offered in the center must also be monitored. Continuous monitoring of physiologic systems and of the effects of therapy on those systems is thus a regular feature in the daily work load of a pharmacist in a trauma center. This program requires monitoring drug therapy, then, as well as knowing the physiology and the pathophysiology of the basic disease state.

Similarly, a general working knowledge of toxicology and drug overdose is required of the clinical pharmacist because of varied patient histories, which involve recreational and therapeutic drugs ingested before the admission. Drug interactions are an ever-present threat to the smooth pharmacologic support needed in the care of the critically ill patient. Physical and chemical incompatibilities with a variety of pharmacological therapies have the potential of complicating therapy.

Taken together, these variables suggest that an efficient and readily available drug information center is most advantageous for the entire staff. If such a center is not available, however, the pharmacist in the trauma center must develop a reference system that serves the needs of the clinical pharmacy and the remainder of the staff.

PHARMACOKINETIC APPLICATIONS

The application of pharmacokinetic principles for drug dosing has been responsible for the introduction of pharmacists into many clinical areas. Pharmacokinetic dosing is an active part of logical and safe patient care. Yet, except where computer-based programs are available for general use, pharmacokinetics has, for the most part, remained a patient care tool used exclusively by the pharmacist.

Mathematically applied, pharmacokinetics is an exact science. However, in the case of the critically ill patient, the utility of such a seemingly inflexible science requires tempering with clinical acumen and knowledge of the pathophysiology of the critically ill patient. Drug recommendations for the trauma patient are greatly simplified through the application of these pharmacokinetic and pathophysiologic principles. To apply the mathematics properly, however, a pharmacist must balance knowledge of the disease with the calculated parameters. The pharmacist must be able to think as a kinetically-oriented clinician rather than as a clinically-oriented kineticist.

In the case of the trauma patient, there is no preferred method of drug dosing. Rather, a combination of assessment techniques must be called upon. Many drugs with narrow therapeutic indices are used in the trauma center. Using serum drug concentration data, the pharmacist may calculate proper dosages. At times, a clinically useful serum assay may not be available, and so one must rely upon recommendations in the medical literature—possibly the use of nomograms and, most importantly, clinical judgment.

Pharmacokinetic services are complex and, once utilized within a center, are irreplaceable. The pharmacist must ensure a method to guarantee accurately timed serum concentrations and an assay system upon which everyone may rely. Once the data obtained have been determined to be reliable, recommendations from pharmacokinetic analysis are more useful. Anyone who has studied pharmacokinetics knows that the greater the number of samples the more predictable and useful the science is. However, the pharmacist must judge the number of samples so that the maximum amount of information may be obtained with the smallest number of samples. Once the serum concentration data have been determined, they must be put into perspective relative to the patient's renal and hepatic function, therapeutic response, and possible drug and drug-laboratory interactions.

Flowsheets may be utilized and inserted into the patient's chart; however, the addition of new forms into a hospital's record-keeping system is not instantaneous. The medical records committees of hospitals decide which forms are to be retained in a patient's chart. If a pharmacokinetic flowsheet is added to the patient's chart while the patient is hospitalized, it may be discarded when the patient is discharged. The chart is then retrieved by Medical Records for organization and storage. At MIEMSS, drug concentration data are listed on the clinical data sheet on which all other clinical information about the patient is recorded (Figure 13-2). Ideally, the pharmacist should enter recommendations in the progress notes, where they are most likely to be available for reference.

Routine pharmacokinetic analysis and serum drug concentration determinations are performed with many antibiotics, cardiotonic agents, antidysrhythmic agents, anticonvulsants, and bronchodilating agents. Although the pharmacokinetic principles and mathematical manipulations in trauma patients are no different from those basically applied to other hospitalized patients, trauma patients may show physiological parameters different from those of other patients. A prime example of this common physiological variance is plasma protein binding.

Plasma protein binding is changed drastically in trauma patients because of their decreased plasma protein level. The prime example in which this change has an

Figure 13–2 Clinical Data Sheet

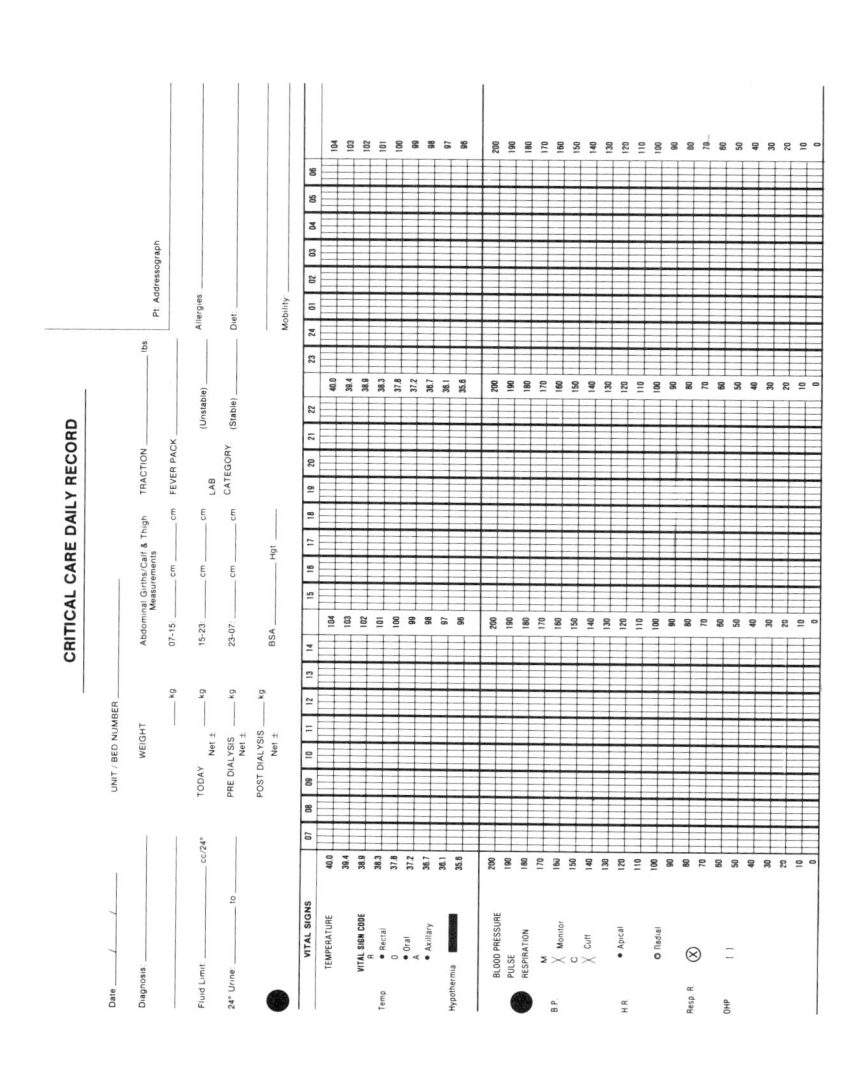

The Trauma Center 267

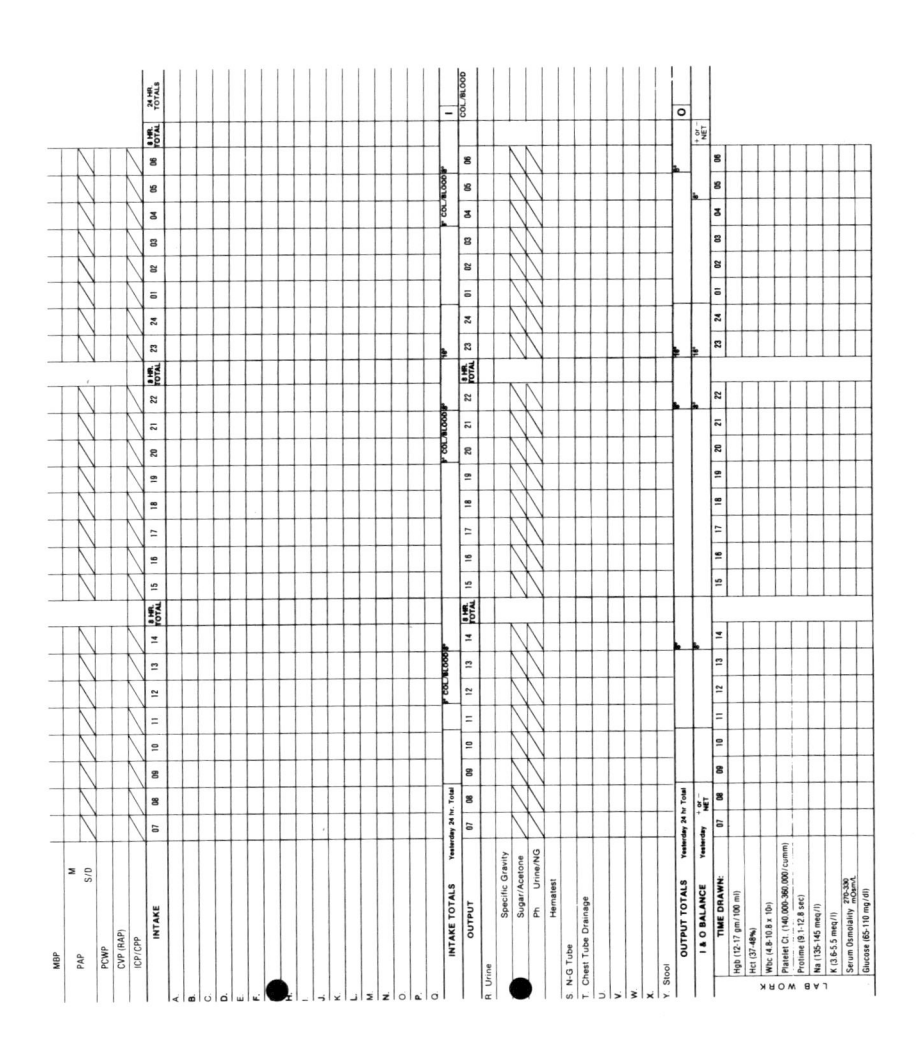

268   PRACTICE OF CRITICAL CARE PHARMACY

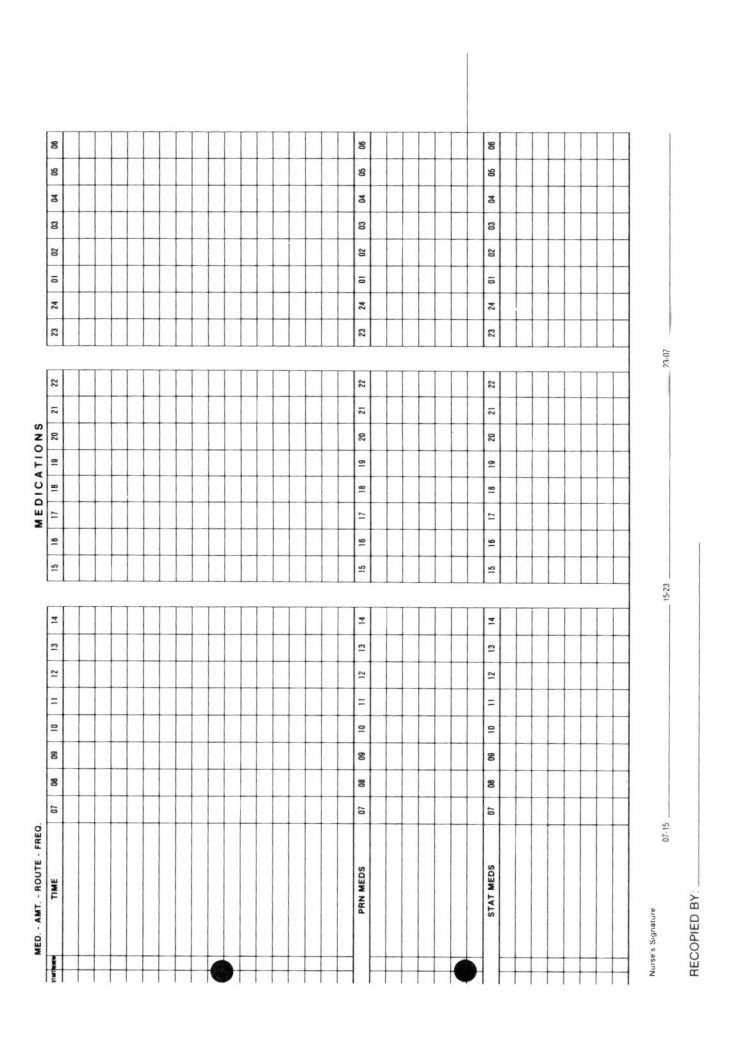

Figure 13–2 continued

ROUTINE TREATMENTS

TIME	07	08	09	10	11	12	13	14	15	16	17	18	19	20	21	22	23	24	01	02	03	04	05	06
TURN (direction)																								
SKIN CARE (area)																								
NG IRRIGS.																								
MOUTH CARE & EYE CARE																								
TRACH CARE																								
FOLEY & PERI. CARE																								
DSSGS. (where)																								
IV TUBINGS (which)																								
BATH & SHAMPOO																								
SUCTION & CHEST PT.																								
CULTURES (which)																								
LAB. STUDIES (which done)																								
X-RAY (Type)																								

TIME	07	08	09	10	11	12	13	14	15	16	17	18	19	20	21	22	23	24	01	02	03	04	05	06

CULTURE REPORTS:

	ORGANISM/SENSITIVITY	DATE CULTURE TAKEN.
Blood:		
Urine:		
Sputum:		
Wound:		
Other:		

PROCEDURES:	TIME	COMMENTS
Daily Chest X-Ray		
Angio		
Ultrasound		
CT-Head		
CT-Body		
Scans-Lung		
Liver/Spleen		
Echo		
Doppler		
EEG		
Dialysis – On/Off		

	LINE	DATE/TIME
LINE CHANGES:		

DRAINAGE:

NG: ____________

CHEST TUBES: ____________

OTHER: ____________

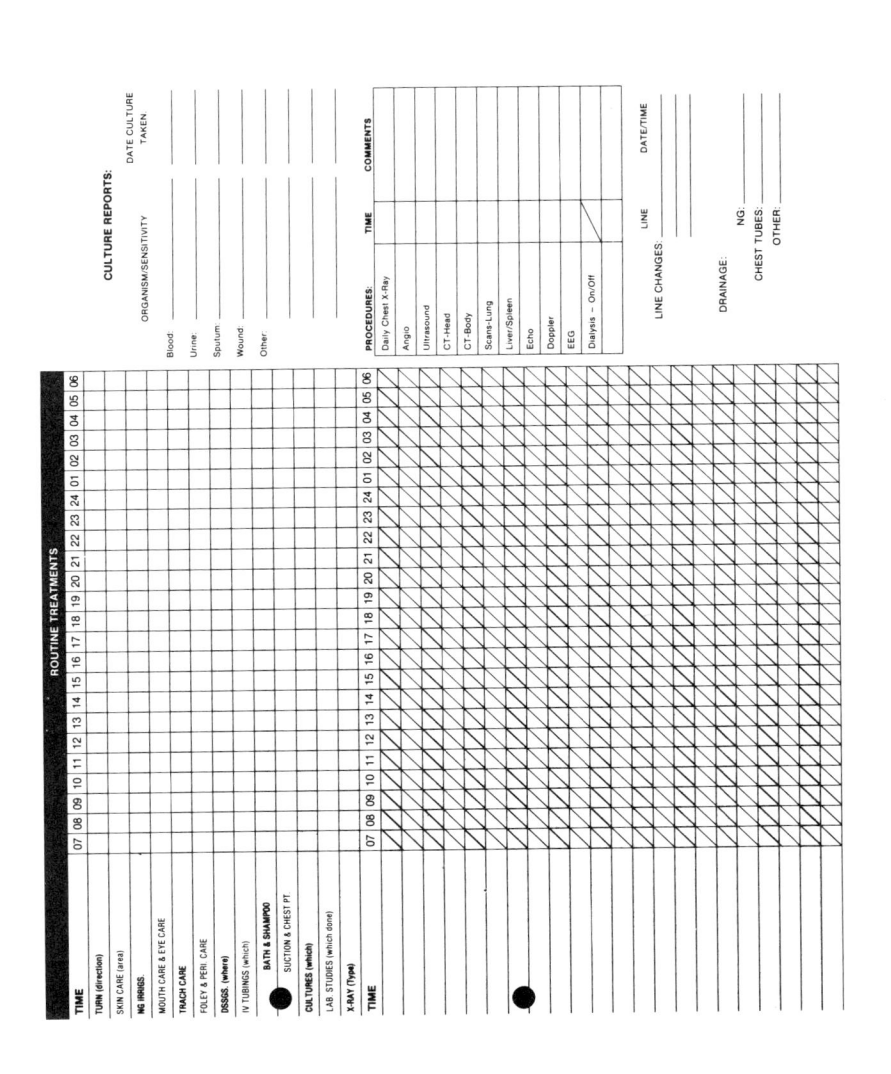

Figure 13-2 continued

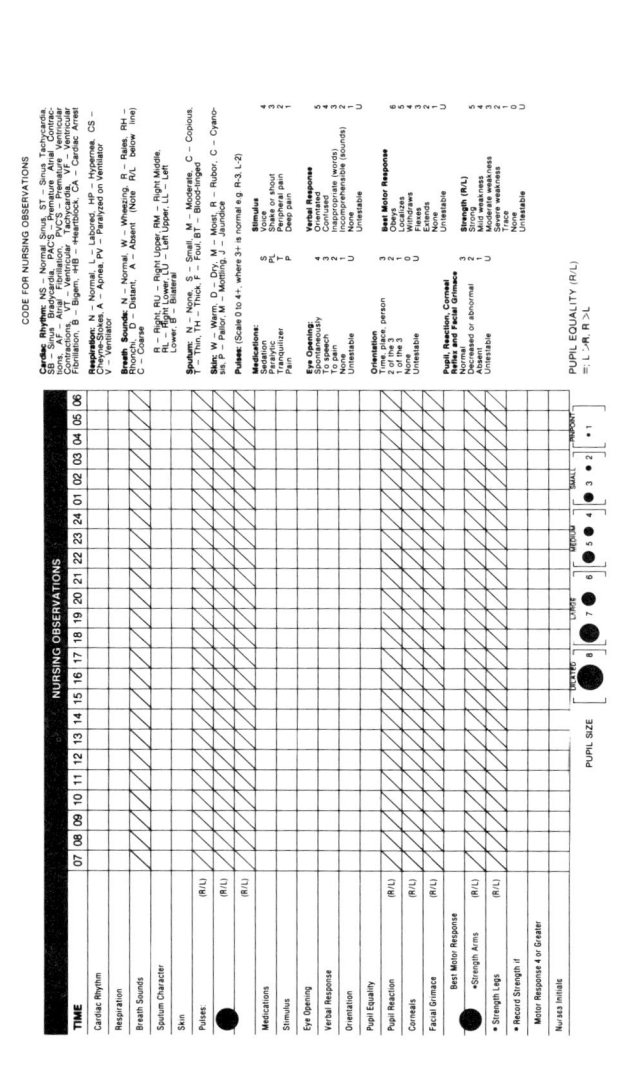

The Trauma Center 271

	PHYSIOLOGIC OBSERVATIONS	CODE FOR VENTILATORS AND O₂ APPARATUS

PHYSIOLOGIC OBSERVATIONS

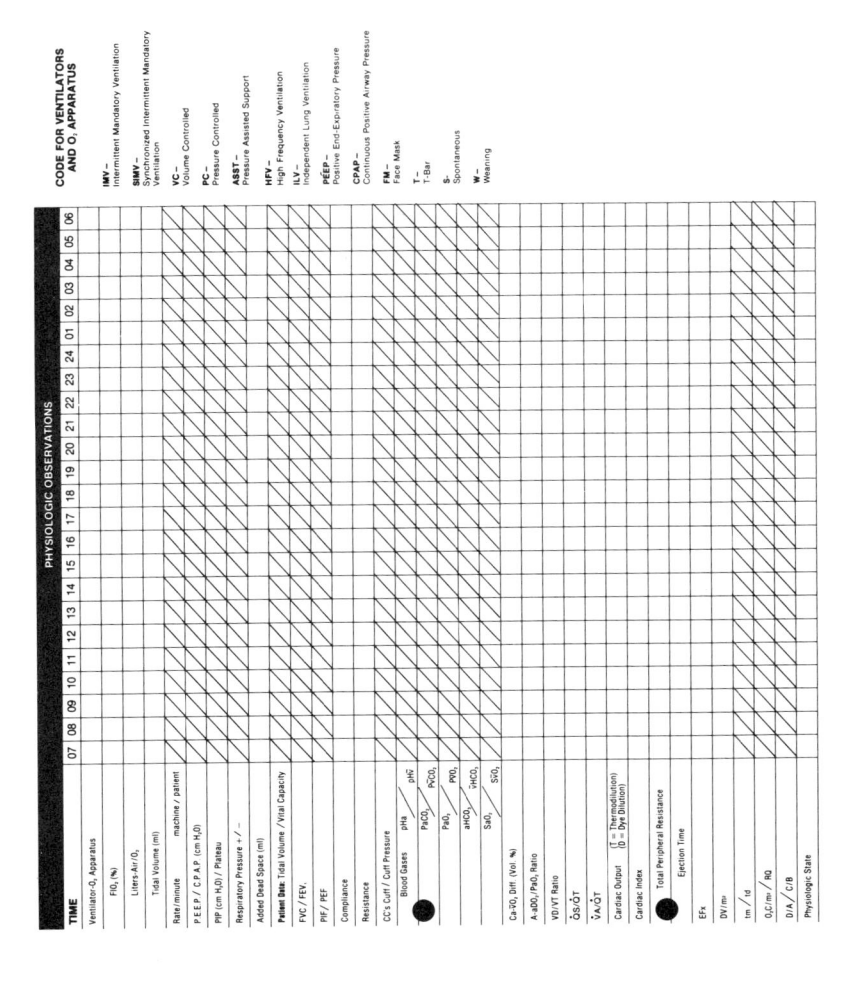

TIME: 07 08 09 10 11 12 13 14 15 16 17 18 19 20 21 22 23 24 01 02 03 04 05 06

- Ventilator-O₂ Apparatus
- FiO₂ (%)
- Liters Air/O₂
- Tidal Volume (ml)
- Rate/minute machine / patient
- P E E P / C P A P (cm H₂O)
- PIP (cm H₂O) / Plateau
- Respiratory Pressure +/−
- Added Dead Space (ml)
- **Patient Data:** Total Volume / Vital Capacity
- FVC / FEV₁
- PIF / PEF
- Compliance
- Resistance
- CC's Cuff / Cuff Pressure
- Blood Gases pHa pHv̄
  - PaCO₂ / PvCO₂
  - PaO₂ / PvO₂
  - aHCO₃ / v̄HCO₃
  - SaO₂ / Sv̄O₂
- Ca-v̄O₂ Diff. (Vol %)
- A-aDO₂/PaO₂ Ratio
- VD/VT Ratio
- Q̇s/Q̇t
- V̇A/Q̇T
- Cardiac Output (T = Thermodilution / D = Dye Dilution)
- Cardiac Index
- Total Peripheral Resistance
- Ejection Time
- EFx
- DV/m
- tm / td
- O₂Ci/m / RQ
- D/A / C/B
- Physiologic State

CODE FOR VENTILATORS AND O₂ APPARATUS

IMV – Intermittent Mandatory Ventilation
SIMV – Synchronized Intermittent Mandatory Ventilation
VC – Volume Controlled
PC – Pressure Controlled
ASST – Pressure Assisted Support
HFV – High Frequency Ventilation
ILV – Independent Lung Ventilation
PEEP – Positive End-Expiratory Pressure
CPAP – Continuous Positive Airway Pressure
FM – Face Mask
T – T-Bar
S – Spontaneous
W – Weaning

Source: The Maryland Institute for Emergency Medical Services Systems.

impact on drug dosing is the use of phenytoin. It has been demonstrated that patients who have decreased plasma protein binding with low total phenytoin serum concentrations may have therapeutic or possibly toxic-free plasma concentrations of phenytoin. This condition may result in therapeutic concentrations, even though total plasma concentrations are low, or in toxicity when total plasma concentrations are in the normally accepted therapeutic range.[8]

The effect of lidocaine binding in trauma patients has been studied.[9] Most importantly, this study—and ones like it—point to the varying pharmacokinetic profiles exhibited by trauma patients and help explain why a drug may have a toxic effect when one is not expected or why therapeutic effects are not seen when logic says that they should be expected.

The shock present in all trauma patients (regardless of the etiology of the shock) alters various pharmacokinetic parameters, particularly the prediction of serum concentrations in patients with rapidly fluctuating compartment volumes. Total body clearance of drugs, including hepatic clearance and renal clearance, is affected, necessitating continuous monitoring for therapeutic and toxic effects and measurement of the serum or plasma concentration. Trauma patients display constant clearance changes of drugs administered to them. Consequently, if these patients reach steady-state serum or plasma levels, they do so longer than one would expect.

NUTRITION SUPPORT

Nutrition support is appropriately aggressive and may be a long-term therapeutic maneuver in the trauma patient. Historically, there has been little evidence to convince clinicians that total parenteral nutritional support is of proven benefit to any patient.[10] Intuitively, however, most clinicians believe that nutrition support is of proven benefit to patients. Nutrition support is a necessary part of the critically ill patient's therapy. Recently, more data are becoming available to show that nutrition support has a definitive impact on the outcome in specific trauma patients.[11]

The purpose of nutrition support for the critically ill patient is essentially the same as that for any patient. In instituting nutrition support, one desires to maintain the visceral and the somatic protein pool. At the very least, one wishes to minimize the possibility of the destruction of these two pools. Starvation, sepsis, and trauma (whether accidental or surgical) result in the degradation of these protein pools. In the case of degradation of protein pools, one can expect an impairment of physiological systems, such as the immunological, hormonal, and metabolic systems. This disruption is felt to predispose the patient to sepsis and to further exacerbate systems dysfunction.

Changes in the biochemistry of patients after injury are becoming more and more open to understanding.[12] The stress of injury is followed by a high degree of metabolic modulation at the cellular level. As the energy production and protein synthesis requirements increase, nutritional substrate delivery is increased to meet these demands. Increased mobilization of fat from fatty acids and triglycerides and of protein from amino acid occurs. Initially, gluconeogenesis increases using glycogen stores, followed by the degradation of somatic protein pools for amino acid and energy requirements. Ketone body production increases, and hepatic protein synthesis causes increases in the concentrations of albumin, acute-phase reactants, and coagulation factors. With increasing stress, glucose requirements diminish, while fatty acid requirements increase. The net result of all the metabolic changes in the stressed patient is a negative nitrogen balance, which increases in severity in proportion to the increases in the stress stimulus. The application of nutrition support for patients with respiratory failure, renal dysfunction, or hepatic dysfunction is different in the case of the trauma patient. Many trauma patients undergo dialysis of varying lengths of time; nutrition requirements in these patients are different. Hand in hand with logical nutritional support of trauma patients goes a usable, fingertip knowledge of acid-base, fluid, and electrolyte balances. Indeed, nutrition support of the trauma patient can become the full-time endeavor of a pharmacist working in the trauma setting.

Another area requiring attention is that of drug-nutrient interactions. Drugs have a definite effect upon the nutritional status and medical processes in the body. It is a well-established fact that drugs and nutrients interact in patients, causing either a deficiency of the nutrient or an altered pharmacokinetic pattern in the drug. Chronic ethanol ingestion, for example, may present as an iron deficiency anemia, a vitamin B_{12} deficiency, or a megaloblastic anemia due to folic acid deficiency. Chronic ethanol ingestion may make phenytoin dosing extremely difficult due to increased phenytoin metabolism.

DRUG DISTRIBUTION

The director of the pharmacy must skillfully integrate the conventional pharmacy services with the developing clinical offerings of the department. Coincident with this maneuvering, the director must ensure that continuous cooperation is maintained among the pharmacists on the staff, regardless of specialties. Pharmacists, even those who devote most of their time to clinical activities, must be concerned with the drug distribution system within the trauma center. Orders are evaluated, and traditional pharmacy activities begin with order transcription, selection of administration times, labeling, and delivery. Unit dose systems are modified, as needed, to ensure timely delivery of medications to the patient. Systems must be instituted for efficiently delivering expensive, infrequently used, or unstable medications to the patient. Many times, medications must be prepared specifically for a given patient. The custom preparation may relate to intravenous piggyback solutions (IVPBs) or to special considerations for fluid, sodium, potassium, or other restrictions in a given patient. Flow rates are monitored for safety and efficacy, and it may become necessary to increase or decrease the concentration of a drug in an infusion to maintain flow. Fluid restrictions in patients may make higher concentrations of cardiotonic and vasoactive agents necessary.

In an effort to control the cost of drug therapy within the trauma center without decreasing therapeutic efficacy or increasing the toxicity of the agents used, ongoing audits are necessary to assess drug utilization. Whenever possible, cost review is done in an effort to decrease costs of expensive items, such as colloid solutions and antibiotics, used in the trauma center. Security of controlled substances is more difficult in a trauma center than in a regular hospital because of the necessity of having larger amounts of controlled medications available in the floor-stock supplies. Overall, the inventory in the pharmacy of a trauma center is different from that of standard hospital pharmacies. The frequency of orders for drugs, the sizes of such orders, and the types of drugs available and needed are different.

THERAPEUTIC MONITORING

As is the case in any area of medicine or surgery in which critically ill patients are cared for, multiple pharmacologic interventions for the trauma patient are the rule. In many ways, drug therapy in the trauma patient presents unique problems, complicating an already difficult situation. Drugs with narrow therapeutic indices and drugs administered by continuous intravenous infusion are the main focus of therapeutic drug monitoring. When a decision or a recommendation is required for a unique therapeutic intervention, such as levodopa in hepatic failure[13] or tolazoline for limb salvage,[14] research of the possibility can assist the pharmacist in making a sound therapeutic decision.

Traditionally, a medication history has been useful in the assessment of drug therapy. However, in the trauma center, with patients arriving immediately from the scene of the accident, a past medical history is seldom available immediately and may not be known even days after admission.

The key to ensuring adequate drug therapy is the ready availability of knowledge of drug therapy and of the pharmacological manipulation of the patient's chemistry and physiology.[2] Although the choice of agents may be made by the physician, it is the pharmacist's expertise in knowing how agents are used and dosed that should guarantee a positive effect on total patient care. The pharmacist is the drug expert in every sense of the word and should become the one source of drug information upon whom the physician and the nursing staff can rely totally.

Drug prescribing by pharmacists is a new topic discussed with increasing frequency. Many pharmacy practitioners, both in and out of critical care, have developed systems designed to expedite proper drug dosing. For example, pharmacists can change antibiotic orders appropriately for changes in renal function. Tube feeding and parenteral nutrition solutions can be modified, as dictated by changes in fluid status or patient response. Protocols outline the dosing of antidysrhythmic agents, aminoglycoside antibiotics, anticonvulsant drugs, and bronchodilators. The clinical pharmacist prescribes the drug, the dose and, if needed, the serum samples. The question about whether such prescribing should be countersigned by a physician and the lack of autonomy if countersigning is required are not important. The involvement of pharmacists in this effort has evolved and is a reality. The ability of our profession to interact with the other health care providers in a positive way to improve patient care is the most valued product of any clinical activity.

At the MIEMSS Shock Trauma Center, full toxicological screens are performed on all patients. Ethanol is the predominant drug present in the initial blood sample drawn, but other recreational drugs frequently are found. These include the cannabinoids, cocaine, phencyclidine, benzodiazepines, and methaqualone.[15] As has been discussed,[16] the utility and the value of general drug screens, or any initial partial drug level testing in a trauma center, is open to evaluation at each institution. However, since most trauma centers work closely with organ procurement centers for transplantation, a general drug screen (qualitative or quantitative) immediately available goes far in assisting the staff to decide on the suitability of organ donation from patients who are potential donors. The cost of various drug screens varies from one institution to another. However, the cost for a quantitative and general drug screen is substantial; so because of this increased cost, careful consideration of the cost-benefit of general drug screens must be made periodically.

DRUG INTERACTIONS IN THE TRAUMA PATIENT

Much has been written about drug interactions with other drugs, as well as with food and nutrients. In evaluating drug-drug or drug-food interactions in the trauma patient, one is able to reduce the long list of these interactions to those most likely to be encountered in a given clinical practice. It has been said that a drug without side effects will have no effects. This broad statement may not necessarily apply to all agents, but it does point out that one must expect some side effects, whether intrinsic or not, and that such side effects may be avoidable. Multiple-drug therapy and fingertip knowledge of where the patient is in his or her course of treatment, what the drug can do, and the therapeutic end-point, allow one to avert most adverse drug effects. The majority of drugs that cause interactions in the trauma patient fall into one of the following categories: (a) antibiotics or antibacterials,

(b) H$_2$-receptor antagonists, (c) digoxin, (d) phenytoin, (e) other anticonvulsants, and (f) corticosteroids.[17]

The following drugs, used in trauma centers, warrant close monitoring and compulsive manipulation of doses because of their high propensity to interact with other agents: sulfonamides, warfarin, chloramphenicol, metronidazole, rifampin, aminoglycoside antibiotics, amphotericin B, cephalosporin antibiotics, semisynthetic penicillins, quinidine, cimetidine (and probably many of the newer H$_2$-receptor antagonists on the horizon), theophylline, benzodiazepines, digoxin, phenytoin, barbiturates, carbamazepine, and corticosteroids.

Treatment procedures for the trauma patient are necessarily sophisticated. With a working knowledge of potential drug interactions and adverse reactions, a pharmacist is able to guarantee that the needed pharmacotherapy will have its expected beneficial effects.

TRAUMA PATIENTS IN A NONTRAUMA HOSPITAL

Trauma patients are best cared for within a network of hospitals dedicated to the care of the patient with blunt or penetrating trauma. There are areas, however, in which a trauma center may not exist, either because one is planned but not yet a reality or because the predicted trauma patient load is insufficient to support a hospital dedicated to the care of such patients. A hospital serving such an area may have a trauma team operating from it.

A trauma team works as a specialized team for traumatized patients in a manner analogous to a nutrition support team or a cardiac arrest team. Each is made up of specialists from required disciplines who are trained to handle any contingency—expected and unexpected—that may occur with a trauma patient. The team leader is a surgeon, preferably one who has experience and training in traumatology. Surgical specialties—neurosurgery, cardiovascular, thoracic, and orthopedic surgery—also are available. Anesthesiologists or certified registered nurse anesthetists are responsible for airway and ventilatory management as well as anesthesia. Protocols must be set up and followed as they would be in a trauma center—that is, with the aim of stabilization and treatment during the short, initial phase of shock.

As in the case of all trauma patients, surgical intervention is the most important of the strategies in the first hour after injury. The roles of the other disciplines are as one would expect. A pharmacist can complement the care the trauma patient receives from a trauma team in the same way as he does in a trauma center. Initially, the presence of the pharmacist is not necessary. Nevertheless, the pharmacist's assistance is required, for example, in cases involving drug overdose or poisoning, general drug screens on patients involved in organ donation, and routine or extraordinary pharmacological manipulations. Remember that the protocol system addresses most courses of action and, until stabilization is completed and the diagnoses are made, most energies are directed toward surgery and ventilatory support. Nevertheless, the pharmacist can be a member of the trauma team and, while not always "in the trenches," he must be present at least on the periphery.

RESEARCH

The single characteristic that allows the practice of critical care pharmacy in the trauma center to be so satisfying, enjoyable, and rewarding is the opportunity the pharmacist has to cross all medical and surgical boundaries. This is true in clinical activities as well as in research endeavors. Drug therapy is applied by all specialists in the trauma center. Research on new therapy and on modifications of existing therapy is a continuous requirement. As the application of nutrition support to trauma patients is expanded and refined, the research horizon in the nutrition of trauma patients is expected to widen tremendously. Fluid therapy, especially its use in the resuscitation of trauma patients, is an area in which there is little universal agreement. Finally, with solid backing by pharmacokineticists, the pharmacist in the trauma center has an almost endless opportunity for pharmacokinetic research.

TEACHING

The teaching responsibilities in a viable clinical pharmacy service are both great and continuous. The turnover of medical and surgical residents is high even in a center that is not a part of a teaching center. Drug therapy is a very large portion of the total care offered to the critically ill patient. The classes of drugs, dosages, and applications of pharmacotherapy are different for such patients. In view of the rapid pace of the center, the pharmacist is charged with reviewing and explaining pharmacotherapy. Indeed, a rotation through the center is incomplete without formal and informal teaching programs addressing drug therapy, nutrition and metabolic support, drug interactions, drug side-effects, and fluid and electrolyte therapy. At MIEMSS, a formal program of core curriculum lectures is given every two months. This program is supplemented by a monthly journal club, a weekly morbidity and mortality conference, and a weekly grand rounds with presentations by staff and visiting lecturers. Training also is provided for the MIEMSS Field Program (cardiac rescue technicians and emergency medical technician-paramedics), Aviation Trauma Training Program, Trauma Training Program, and at the areawide trauma centers.

SERVICE JUSTIFICATION

Justification of pharmacy services in any area of medicine or surgery involves identifying areas in need of refinement, making specific changes, and evaluating outcome to make the contrast apparent. Although the worth of the final result depends on the perspective of the viewer—patient, hospital administrator, or third-party payer—the ultimate recipient is the patient.

Decreasing the cost of hospitalization is the top priority now and for the future. In other areas of patient care, decreased lengths of stay in the hospital may mean fewer patient days and more empty beds. However, an unfortunate fact in trauma medicine is that there is no diminution in the number of patients. Patient loads increase yearly. Indeed, patient disposition to open beds for new admissions is a full-time endeavor at a trauma center.

One must be able to show a lessened incidence of toxicity, like that shown when pharmacokinetic principles are applied to aminoglycoside antibiotic dosing or to anticonvulsant dosing. Appropriate intervention on the part of the pharmacist and the nutrition support team results in rational use of laboratory tests as the apparent justification of services. Evaluation of cost-effectiveness is facilitated when a detailed and programmed analysis of available clinical services is made.

GENERAL CONSIDERATIONS

Any existing system for delivering pharmacy services can be adapted to meet the demands of a fast-moving trauma center. One must assess the drug and poison information capabilities of the hospital, as well as the laboratory support needed to provide premium clinical pharmacy services. Regardless of the organization of the trauma teams, a pharmacist can serve any system well and bring with his or her clinical expertise a valued service. Without a doubt, the profession of pharmacy possesses an advantage in a trauma center (or in any critical care setting for that matter): pharmacists are able to cross all specialty boundaries to provide their services. Although specialty barriers cannot exist, boundaries between professions are a necessary characteristic of any multidisciplinary care setting. Clinical pharmacy can offer the neurosurgeon as much in the care of neurosurgical patients as it can offer other surgeons and internists in the care of their patients.

The success of individual clinical pharmacists in the trauma center is related directly to the effort, the dedication, and the hard work expended by the individual pharmacist. A significant but almost subliminal factor in this success is the relationship of the pharmacy to the hospital. Clinical pharmacy remains a part of the pharmacy profession. Pharmacists, whose practices entail less distributive emphasis, cannot neglect the base from which clinical pharmacy emerged and upon which clinical pharmacy relies. Clinical pharmacy services will succeed in the trauma care setting if the person exercising and providing these services is given the administrative support to function. Without this support, a great deal of additional time will be necessary to make the services in the trauma center a reality.

Finally, knowledge and hard work are necessary for the promise of a successful clinical practice in a trauma center to become a reality. The clinical fraternity of critical care pharmacy and its function in the trauma center is enhanced by the participation of its members in professional societies. Benefits far outweigh the costs of membership in such societies as the Society of Critical Care Medicine, The American Trauma Society, The American Society for Parenteral and Enteral Nutrition, the American Association of Colleges of Pharmacy, and the American Society of Hospital Pharmacists. Pharmacists and nurses have full membership opportunities in medical and surgical societies, and one does not need to be a physician to enjoy the benefits of these organizations.

COMMENCING CRITICAL CARE PHARMACY SERVICES

Before anyone can follow a road map or diagram such a map for others, one must know two pieces of information: the starting point (or the present location) and the destination. The early development of clinical pharmacy is analogous to a revolution that swept the profession into the mainstream of patient care. This change has left pharmacists in clinical positions that were guaranteed to be successful even with minimal enterprising effort. Today, with more and more control being exercised in the cost of health care, it is increasingly difficult to start new clinical services without careful assessment of the value of these services relative to the health care dollar expended. The revolutionary process is over; the time has come to begin the evolutionary process that will ensure the position the profession has taken in critical care.

Therefore, the starting point for critical care pharmacy and the services it renders is the individual hospital pharmacy or, more specifically, the director of the pharmacy. A farsighted director who is in touch with everything affecting the department is able to conduct the necessary value analysis. The director is usually the one person who, while working a reasonable work week, must live the position and think about it almost all the time.

Value analysis is an investigative process in which every element of a material, component, or service in terms of function and associated cost is systematically studied. Value analysis is a problem solving approach that challenges the use and specification of, and the need for, any given product or service. The value analysis of future pharmacy services is similar to that conducted when new equipment for the hospital is evaluated. If a new piece of equipment is needed, the easiest way to procure it is to look at three or four different models and pick the one that will work the best. This process seldom results in a completely satisfactory selection and generally ends up costing more than it should. A list of specifications and needs must be formulated so that an analysis can be made of the value of each proposed product in meeting these specifications.

The value analysis can be done by the director, or it may be delegated to a staff pharmacist who wants involvement in a given clinical area. The best manner in which to conduct the value analysis is through the joint effort of the director and interested personnel. (All too often, a physician working in an area is contacted directly by a pharmacist wanting exposure in a clinical area of the hospital. Although this was the only tenable tactic used during the early developmental stage of critical care pharmacy services, the new, controlled atmosphere dictates a more formal approach.) Through the process, a line must be followed that does not leave open the question of who runs the critical care pharmacy service.

A study of the general critical care atmosphere and services of the hospital serves as the first point in the outline of critical care pharmacy in the institution. Questions need to be asked and answers must be obtained.

The following questions must be asked about therapeutic drug monitoring:

- Does a mechanism exist for pharmacokinetic drug dosing?
- Who orders the serum levels?
- Which laboratory does the testing?
- Who reports the results?
- What is done with the data once they are received?

Clinical pharmacy essentially began with the science of pharmacokinetic dosing of drugs. The care of the trauma patient and subsequent pharmacological therapy are fine-tuned to a tremendous degree through the application of pharmacokinetics. This is especially true for antibiotic therapy in surgical patients and anticonvulsant therapy in patients with CNS trauma. All pharmacists are scientists at heart, and so all of them are comfortable with the mathematical manipulation of serum or plasma drug concentrations. The service is necessary. Indeed, it is the state of the art of drug dosing and may be needed or expanded upon by the pharmacy.

Questions about nutritional support services also must be asked; answers to the following questions are needed:

- Is there a nutrition support team active in the hospital?
- If so, is it viable or is it a paper tiger?
- What is the pharmacist's role on the team?
- Does the team simply count calories or does it do an actual assessment of nutrition support and its impact on patient care?

Even though objective proof of the value of nutrition support is slow in coming, no one can argue logically that nurturing is not beneficial to critically ill or traumatized patients, who are under severe stress. For the critically ill patient, the nutrition support given is drug therapy in every sense of the word because the biochemistry and physiology of these patients are unlike those of other patients. Pharmacists' involvement on nutrition support teams has been defined and the continuous refining of that role transcends the conventional one as "preparer of solutions."

The following questions about the emergency department are some of those that need to be answered in any value analysis.

- What is the description of the patient population entering the emergency room?
- How many poisoning and drug overdose victims are admitted to the hospital through the emergency department?
- Is a poison information center or poison control center needed as a resource?
- Who participates on codes?
- Is there an outpatient pharmacy in or near the emergency department?
- What pharmacy services, such as IV fluid preparation and drug information, could be provided by means of a satellite pharmacy in the emergency department?

A hospital gains many of its admissions through the emergency department. The patient flow is rapid, and the initial patient assessment is most important. Poison information centers exist to serve the community, but their usefulness can be maximized by locating them in the emergency room, where many acute cases are seen. A satellite pharmacy in the emergency department can be the center of drug information resources, as well as the controller of drug distribution for that department.

Outpatient pharmacies in hospitals have existed to serve patients. There are cases in which such pharmacies have been closed because some groups contend that drug delivery is the purview of other types of pharmacy practice. The hardship and the inconvenience imposed on the patient, as well as on the hospital-based physician, are probably much greater than the economic benefit to pharmacies that are not part of the hospital. The benefits of the revenue generated by an outpatient pharmacy are substantial.

Certification as a provider of advanced cardiac life support (ACLS) is a prerequisite for employment as a physician in most hospital emergency departments. Pharmacists have not been a part of this certification process in the past, not because of overt exclusion, but because the initiative has not been taken—either collectively by pharmacists as members of a profession or individually by pharmacists—to take advantage of this training. Pharmacists would benefit immeasurably from the knowledge they would gain from this training, particularly in the area of cardiopulmonary resuscitation pharmacology. The pharmacists in this country who are active in ACLS training can attest to its value.

SUMMARY

Clinical pharmacy services have been established in trauma centers,[2] and the significant involvement and positive impact of these services in the care of the trauma patient will continue to thrive. The efforts needed for the establishment and proliferation of clinical pharmacy services in the trauma center emanate largely from the individual practitioner. Patience in developing and nurturing a clinical pharmacy program in the trauma center is necessary. The professional satisfaction derived from working in this rewarding clinical area can make most efforts and sacrifices worthwhile.

REFERENCES

1. Trunkey DD: Trauma. *Sci Am* 1983;249:28–35.

2. Majerus TC: Shock-trauma: clinical pharmacy in emergency medicine. *Top Hosp Pharm Manage* 1982;2:87–93.

3. Maryland Institute for Emergency Medical Services Systems Annual Report: 1982–1983, Baltimore, 1983.

4. Bond-Lillicropp S, Cowley RA, Boyd DR: Trauma/emergency medical services systems, in Cowley RA, Dunham CM (eds): *Shock Trauma/Critical Care Manual*. Baltimore, University Park Press, 1982, pp 559–569.

5. Conn AK: Prehospital protocols, in Cowley RA, Dunham CM (eds): *Shock Trauma/Critical Care Manual*. Baltimore, University Park Press, 1982, pp 531–532.

6. Cowley RA: Trauma center—a new concept for the delivery of critical care. *J Med Soc NJ* 1977;74:979–986.

7. Holt MR: The ICU pharmacy, in Chernow B, Lake CR (eds): *The Pharmacologic Approach to the Critically Ill Patient*. Baltimore, Williams & Wilkins, 1983, pp 133–139.

8. Bauer LA, Edwards WAD, Dellinger EP, et al: Importance of unbound phenytoin serum levels in head trauma patients. *J Trauma* 1983;23:1058–1060.

9. Edwards DJ, Lalka D, Cerra F, et al: Alpha$_1$-acid glycoprotein concentration and protein binding in trauma. *Clin Pharmacol Ther* 1982;31:62–67.

10. Goodgame JT Jr: A critical assessment of the indications for total parenteral nutrition. *Surg Gynecol Obstet* 1980;151:433–441.

11. Rapp RP, Young B, Twyman D, et al: The favorable effect of early parenteral feeding on survival in head-injured patients. *J Neurosurg* 1983;58:906–912.

12. Majerus TC: Current problems in nutritional support of the critically ill patient, in Cowley RA, Conn AK (eds): *Critical Problems in Trauma Care II. Medical Management*. Philadelphia, JB Lippincott, (In press).

13. Fischer JE: False neurotransmitters and hepatic failure. *Lancet* 1971;2:75–79.

14. Peck JJ, Fitzgibbons TJ, Gaspar MR: Devastating distal arterial trauma and continuous intra-arterial infusion of tolazoline. *Am J Surg* 1983;145:562–566.

15. Majerus TC: Full toxicology screens for all patients, letters. *Drug Intell Clin Pharm* 1983;17:558.

16. Thomas R: Comment on care of the critically ill, letters. *Drug Intell Clin Pharm* 1983;17:558.

17. Majerus TC: Drug interactions in the trauma patient, in Cowley RA (ed): *Proceedings of the Sixth Annual National Trauma Symposium*. Baltimore, Maryland Institute for Emergency Medical Services Systems/National Study Center for Emergency Medical Systems 1983:59–69.

Epilogue

The Future of Critical Care Pharmacy

Thomas C. Majerus

Countless factors can lay claim to a portion of the success the profession of pharmacy is enjoying in critical care. The support of the Schools and Colleges of Pharmacy and that of the national and state professional societies is a significant part of the story. Not to be forgotten are the physicians and the nurses practicing in various areas of the budding practice of intensive and critical care medicine, who recognized a good thing when they saw it. Years ago these professions recognized the largely untapped resource of the pharmacist who was either leaving the protective framework of the hospital pharmacy or spreading his clinical wings in the profession to move into emergency rooms (ERs), intensive care units (ICUs), or coronary care units (CCUs). Yet, the individual pharmacy practitioners remain the fundamental reason for the productivity of the pharmacy as a health profession in critical care at this time.

The fact that critical care pharmacy practice is a reality is evidenced by the experiences recounted in the foregoing chapters. It is unclear whether the profession began its efforts in the care of the critically ill patient at the same time as medicine and nursing did or shortly after the conception of a multiprofessional, multidisciplinary approach to the training in and the practice of critical care medicine (CCM). Through the individual practitioners, the profession of pharmacy has enjoyed the success of the revolution in critical care and has weathered the challenges to the idea. It is now time for the profession of pharmacy to garner its collective forces and to recognize and to support the concept of CCM that was germinated years ago and has been nurtured in an organized way since 1970.

The appeal of critical care pharmacy practice is evident to some practitioners viewing the system from without, but it is very often intimidating. Once a pharmacist enters the mainstream of critical care, initial apprehension is soon replaced by an almost impatient interest in the pathophysiology of the illnesses encountered and the multifaceted approach necessary to reverse the process of severe illness or injury.

The success of the pharmacists in the realm of critical care is a fact. Now the profession of pharmacy must continue the efforts started and must do so in an organized, cooperative way. In spite of differences of opinion and the challenges and setbacks to the basic approach to critical care, the medical profession is persisting in its basic course of action designed to formalize critical care medicine as a specialty. The ordered approach began with the Society of Critical Care Medicine (SCCM) and the formation of the Joint Committee on Critical Care Medicine (JCCCM). Specialty boards such as the American Board of Anesthesiology, the American Board of Internal Medicine, the American Board of Pediatrics, and the American Board of Surgery made joint recommendations to the American Board of Medical Specialties (ABMS). The result was the development of a Task Force on Critical Care Medicine to follow through with the wishes and the recommendations of the society and its members. Although a systematic approach by the pharmacy profession to organize critical care pharmacy as an area of clinical practice is not expected in the near future, most of what must be done to carry critical care pharmacy further along can be accomplished by pharmacists.

Pharmacy managers begin by making the value analysis explained in Chapter 13. They then follow through with the clinical pharmacy staff to provide services such as pharmacokinetic dosing, nutrition support, therapeutic drug monitoring, and teaching. They should begin slowly, methodically, and take one step at a time. The surprising fact realized by anyone now practicing critical care pharmacy is that clinical services become rooted very swiftly. Critical care pharmacy not only quickly became a part of the critical care system but also in a short time has become firmly entrenched. In addition, medical and surgical residents spending time in a critical care rotation want to know whether critical care pharmacy is a regular feature of clinical pharmacy and whether it can be expected wherever they train or go on to establish practices.

The most unexpected reaction that any well-trained clinical pharmacist will notice from the medical, nursing, and surgical staff is that members of the other disciplines display a genuine appreciation of the pharmacist. Possibly, only those who truly understand the dynamic nature of the critical care environment are in a position to value the specialized knowledge the clinical pharmacist brings to the critically ill or injured patient. Anyone who has practiced pharmacy for a decade or more knows that pharmacy practitioners have a history of voicing most of their criticisms to each other. That learned behavior alone may explain the astonishment of clinical pharmacists at their acceptance in intensive care medicine.

The distinctive characteristic of critical care pharmacy practice is that it crosses all specialty boundaries and diligently applies the pharmacology, the biochemistry, and the therapeutic manipulations in appropriate ways. Because the diagnosis will have been made most times, the scientific logic of drug therapy, nutrition support, and patient response can be weighed with clinical judgment in a mutually supportive fashion.

All hospital-based pharmacists know one or more areas in their hospital that are dedicated to critical care. Surgical Intensive Care Units, Neurological Surgery Intensive Care Units, Coronary Care Units, Medical Intensive Care Units, Pediatric and Neonatal Intensive Care Units, Emergency Rooms, and Trauma Centers are already enjoying the skill and the dedication brought to them by critical care pharmacists. The critically ill or injured patient is the ultimate beneficiary of this multidisciplined interaction.

Critical care pharmacy has become and will remain a lively, exciting form of clinical pharmacy practice. The rewards parallel the responsibilities. Nevertheless, it exists for better patient care and complements critical care medicine and critical care nursing.

Cost containment and increased use of outpatient clinics, outpatient surgery, home hyperalimentation and other forms of nutrition support, and home dialysis will decrease the need for traditional hospital beds. Nonetheless, a continuing increase is expected in the numbers of critically ill patients requiring critical care support after herculean medical and surgical measures. Trauma-related injuries become more numerous yearly. Perhaps some of the general hospital beds or entire floors of some hospitals will be converted to allow for the care of the rehabilitation patient or for the patient requiring long-term care too routine for hospitalization but too complicated for discharge home.

Are there any caveats of which a critical care pharmacy practitioner must be mindful? Some may argue that once the service begins, the persons with whom one works will wish to learn all that is possible about drug therapy, its application, and other systems of care addressed by the clinical pharmacist. To carry this to the extreme, one might think that a practitioner could perform so well and teach so completely that his obsolescence would be the result. Such has not been the case since the unofficial birth of critical care pharmacy, and the potential for such an outcome is hypothetical and questionable.

Regardless of the final format of critical care medicine, all professions—medicine, nursing, pharmacy and surgery—will continue to thrive, but planning is crucial. That planning must consider, however, the immediate situation facing each profession as well as the status of health care expected in the future. While flexibility in attitude can ease the course, the key to success is to plan in concert with others—intraprofessionally as well as interprofessionally.

The career satisfaction afforded the practitioner of critical care pharmacy is immediately apparent and is unceasing. The groundwork has been laid by the authors who have told in the preceding chapters of their experiences and the experiences of others around the world. Such efforts will guarantee the profession of pharmacy an advantageous position as changes are made in the health care system of this country.

Appendix A

A Critical Care Bibliography

Joseph F. Dasta

Scientific information relating to critical care has burgeoned enormously in the last five to ten years. This explosion of data parallels the growth of the discipline and the scope of the subject. Because many specialists have a vested interest in caring for the critically ill, information on this subject appears in the literature about pharmacy, internal medicine, surgery, anesthesiology, traumatology, neurosurgery, thoracic surgery, emergency medicine, and pediatrics. The bibliography in this appendix is generated from 55 different journals. In addition, specialty journals devoted solely to critical care (such as *Critical Care Medicine, Intensive Care Medicine, Heart and Lung,* and *Critical Care Quarterly*) are now available. Recently, *Drug Intelligence and Clinical Pharmacy, Archives of Internal Medicine* and *Journal of the American Medical Association* have developed specialty columns on critical care. The sources of information about critical care research and practice are, therefore, immense. Critical care information has also been packaged in textbook form. Since 1980, over 30 books relating to the care of the acutely ill patient have been published. These publications exclude books on drug overdose, which have been available for several years.

Despite this abundance of information, the critical care novice may find it difficult to obtain the latest information on a given topic without the assistance of a computer retrieval system. The purpose of this appendix is to consolidate a vast amount of the information on critical care topics for easy access to those needing information on a selective topic. This bibliography should be useful to practitioners beginning a practice in a given area and also to those who have been practicing in critical care units for some time. The list of references should also help to answer the question about the knowledge base needed to function in a critical care unit. Not every pharmacist should read and digest each of the 204 references listed in this appendix; however, to obtain a fundamental understanding of the scope of the discipline of critical care, pharmacists should at least have read *key* articles pertaining to the population of their critical care unit. In addition, a sound knowledge of information common to any critical care unit—hemodynamic monitoring, stress ulcers, and shock—is needed by anyone monitoring the critically ill.

The first published bibliography on critical care appeared in *Drug Intelligence and Clinical Pharmacy* (1983;17:722–25) under the critical care therapeutics column. The reference list in this appendix is built upon this framework. Since the original list of articles was published, several additional articles and books have appeared. This new information has been incorporated where appropriate. It should be noted, however, that areas such as pediatric emergencies, endocrine emergencies, and acute myocardial infarction have not been covered because the previously published bibliography has provided adequate reference material. (For example, Chapter 11 by Dr. Cupit contains a selected bibliography on pediatric and neonatal intensive care.)

The majority of the papers in this appendix are review articles. This approach was chosen to provide the reader with the maximal amount of information for each subject. The review articles are well-referenced and the reader needing more in-depth information can refer to the primary reference. Also, there may be several review articles on the same topic. The articles, however, are often written at different levels of sophistication and from different viewpoints. This reporting method should provide the maximum benefit for the reader. It is hoped that this bibliography will be a useful tool for clinicians practicing in critical care.

CRITICAL CARE LITERATURE

General Information

Discipline of Critical Care

Abramson NS, Wald KS, Grenvik A, et al: Adverse occurrences in intensive care units. *JAMA* 1980;244:1582–1584.

Cottrell JJ, Pennock BE, Grenvik A, et al: Critical care computing. *JAMA* 1982;248:2289–2291.

NIH consensus development conference on critical care. *Crit Care Med* 1983;11:466–469.

Parrillo JE, Ayres SM: *Major Issues in Critical Care Medicine.* Baltimore, Williams & Wilkins, 1984.

Thibault GE, Mulley AG, Barnett GO, et al. Medical intensive care: Indications, interventions, and outcomes. *N Engl J Med* 1980;302:938–942.

Weil MH, Rackow EC: Critical care medicine—caveat emptor. *Arch Intern Med* 1983; 143:1391–1392.

Critical Care Pharmacy-Pharmacology

Angaran DM: Critical care pharmacy service, in McLeod DC, Miller WA (eds): *The Practice of Pharmacy—Institutional and Ambulatory Pharmaceutical Services.* Cincinnati, Harvey Whitney Books, 1981, pp. 171–181.

Bledsoe B, Bosker G, Papa F: *Prehospital Emergency Pharmacology*. Bowie, Md, Robert J. Brady Co, 1984.

Chernow B: *The Pharmacologic Approach to the Critically Ill Patient*. Baltimore, Williams & Wilkins, 1983.

Civetta JM: *Intensive Care Therapeutics*. New York, Appleton-Century-Crofts, 1980.

Dasta JF: Progress in critical care pharmacy. *Drug Intell Clin Pharm* 1984;18:157–158.

Dasta JF: Pharmacokinetics of drugs in critically ill patients. *Syva Monitor* 1982;11:1–9.

Gangeness D, White R: *Emergency Pharmacology*. Bowie, Md, Robert J. Brady Co, 1984.

Majerus TC: Shock-trauma: Clinical pharmacy in emergency medicine. *Top Hosp Pharm Manag* 1982:2;89–93.

Pentel P, Benowitz N: Pharmacokinetic and pharmacodynamic considerations in drug therapy of cardiac emergencies. *Clin Pharmacokinet* 1984;9:273–308.

Reference Material

Beal JM: *Critical Care for Surgical Patients*. New York, Macmillan, 1982.

Berk JL, Sampliner JE: *Handbook of Critical Care*. Boston, Little, Brown & Company, 1982.

Bone RC. Symposium on critical care medicine. *Med Clin North Am* 1983;67:1177–1402.

Cowley RA, Conn A: *Critical Problems in Trauma Care, I-Surgical Management, II-Medical Management*. Philadelphia, JB Lippincott, 1984.

Cowley RA, Dunham CM: *Shock Trauma/Critical Care Manual—Initial Assessment and Management*. Baltimore, University Park Press, 1982.

Critical Care Editorial Panel: Therapeutic bibliography of critical care. *Drug Intell Clin Pharm* 1983;17:722–725.

Goldman DR, Brown FH, Levy WK et al: *Medical Care of the Surgical Patient*. Philadelphia, JB Lippincott, 1982.

Hechtman HB: Symposium on critical illness. *Surg Clin North Am* 1983;63:1–511.

Neville WE: *Intensive Care of the Surgical Cardiopulmonary Patient*. Chicago, Year Book Medical Publishers, 1983.

Rogers MC: *The 1983 Year Book of Critical Care Medicine*. Chicago, Year Book Medical Publishers, 1983.

Shoemaker WC, Thompson WL: *Critical Care—State of the Art*. Fullerton, Calif., Society of Critical Care Medicine, 1980–1983, vol 1–4.

Shoemaker WC, Thompson WL, Holbrook PR: *The Society of Critical Care Medicine, Textbook of Critical Care*. Philadelphia, WR Saunders, 1983.

Sibbald WJ: *Synopsis of Critical Care*. Baltimore, Williams & Wilkins, 1983.

Wilson RF: *Principles and Techniques of Critical Care*. Philadelphia, FA Davis, 1984.

Worth MH: *Principles and Practice of Trauma Care*. Baltimore, Williams & Wilkins, 1982.

Hemodynamic Monitoring

Adams NR: Hemodynamic monitoring *Crit Care Q* 1979;2:1–86.

Baele PL, McMichan JC, Marsh HM, et al: Continuous monitoring of mixed venous oxygen saturation in critically ill patients. *Anesth Analg* (Cleve) 1982;61:513–517.

Calvin JE, Driedger AA, Sibbald WJ: Does the pulmonary capillary wedge pressure predict left ventricular preload in critically ill patients. *Crit Care Med* 1981;9:437–443.

Connors AF, McCaffree DR, Ceray BA: Evaluation of right-heart catheterization in the critically ill patient without acute myocardial infarction. *N Engl J Med* 1983;308:263–267.

Daily EK, Schroeder JS: *Techniques in Bedside Hemodynamic Monitoring*. Saint Louis, CV Mosby, 1980.

Hoffman EW: Basics of hemodynamic monitoring. *Drug Intell Clin Pharm* 1982;16:657–664.

Kandel G, Aberman A: Mixed venous oxygen saturation—Its role in the assessment of the critically ill patient. *Arch Intern Med* 1983;143:1400–1402.

Sprong C: *The Pulmonary Artery Catheter—Methodology and Clinical Applications*. Baltimore, University Park Press, 1983.

Swan HJC, Ganz W, Forrester J, et al: Catheterization of the heart in man with use of a flow-directed balloon-tipped catheter. *N Engl J Med* 1970;283:447–451.

Understanding Hemodynamic Measurements Made With the Swan-Ganz Catheter. American Edwards Laboratories, Santa Ana, Calif, 1982.

Wiedemann HP, Matthay MA, Matthay RA: Cardiovascular-pulmonary monitoring in the intensive care unit. *Chest* 1984;85: Part I, 537–549 Part II, 656–668.

Arterial Blood Gas Analysis/Acid-Base Balance

Ackerman GL, Arruda JA: Acid-base and electrolyte imbalance in respiratory failure. *Med Clin North Am* 1983;67:645–656.

Broughton JO: *Understanding Blood Gases*. Madison, Wis, Ohio Medical Products, 1979.

Emmett M, Narins RG: Clinical use of the anion gap. *Medicine* (Baltimore) 1977;56:38–54.

Martin WJ, Matzke GR: Treating severe metabolic alkalosis. *Clin Pharm* 1982;1:42–48.

Narins RG, Emmett M: Simple and mixed acid-base disorders: A practical approach. *Medicine* (Baltimore) 1980;59:161–187.

Schade DS: Metabolic acidosis. *Clin Endocrinol Metab* 1983;12:265–465.

Schaer M: A practical review of simple acid-base disorders. *Vet Clin North Am* 1982;12:439–452.

Shapiro BA, Harrison RA, Walton JR: *Clinical Application of Blood Gases*. Chicago, Year Book Medical Publishers, 1982.

Fluid and Electrolyte Therapy

Defronzo RA, Thier SO: Pathophysiologic approach to hyponatremia. *Arch Intern Med* 1980;140:897–902.

DeVenuto F: Acellular oxygen-delivering resuscitation fluids. *Crit Care Med* 1982;10:237–293.

Elliott GT, McKenzie MW: Treatment of hypercalcemia. *Drug Intell Clin Pharm* 1983;17:12–22.

Feig DV: Hypernatremia and hypertonic syndromes. *Med Clin North Am* 1981;65:271–290.

Gorbea HF, Snydman DR, Delaney A, et al: Intravenous tubing with burettes can be safely changed at 48-hour intervals. *JAMA* 1984;251:2112–2115.

Juan D: Clinical review: The clinical importance of hypomagnesemia. *Surgery* 1982;91:510–517.

Kee JL: *Fluid and Electrolytes With Clinical Applications: A Programmed Approach*. New York, John Wiley & Sons, 1982.

Lentz RD, Brown DM, Kjellstrand CM: Treatment of severe hypophosphatemia. *Ann Intern Med* 1978;89:941–944.

Lucas CE, Ledgerwood AM: The fluid problem in the critically ill. *Surg Clin North Am* 1983;63:439–454.

Majerus TC: *Electrolyte Imbalance: Potassium, Calcium, and Phosphorus.* Therapeutics—Drug Monographs for the Pharmacist, Philadelphia, Smith Kline & French Laboratories, 1977.

Massry SG, Seelig MS: Hypomagnesemia and hypermagnesemia. *Clin Nephrol* 1977;7:147–153.

Nanji AA. Drug-induced electrolyte disorders. *Drug Intell Clin Pharm* 1983;17:175–185.

Sherman RA, Eisinger RP: The use (and misuse) of urinary sodium and chloride measurements. *JAMA* 1982;247:3121–3124.

Singer FR, Beherne JE, Massry SG: Hypercalcemia and hypocalcemia. *Clin Nephrol* 1977;7:154–162.

Slatopolsky E, Rutherford WE, Rosenbaum R, et al: Hyperphosphatemia. *Clin Nephrol* 1977;7:138–146.

Colloid-Crystalloid Controversy

Dodge C, Glass DD: Crystalloid and colloid therapy. *Sem Anesth* 1982;1:293–301.

Lewis RT: Albumin: Role and discriminative use in surgery. *Can J Surg* 1980;23:322–328.

Nakasato SK: Evaluation of hetastarch. *Clin Pharm* 1982;1:509–514.

Poole GV, Meredith JW, Pennell T, et al: Comparison of colloids and crystalloids in resuscitation from hemorrhagic shock. *Surg Gynecol Obstet* 1982;154:577–586.

Ross AD, Angaran DM: Colloids versus crystalloids: A continuing controversy. *Drug Intell Clin Pharm* 1984;18:202–212.

Cardiovascular Emergencies

Cardiopulmonary Resuscitation

Donegan JH: New concepts in cardiopulmonary resuscitation. *Anesth Analg* 1981;60:100–108.

Kroboth PD, Kroboth FJ: Pharmacological therapy in CPR. *US Pharm* 1982;7:H1–16.

National conference on CPR and emergency cardiac care. Standards and guidelines for cardiopulmonary resuscitation and emergency cardiac care. *JAMA* 1980;244:453–509.

Nowak RM: Cardiopulonary-cerebral resuscitation: State of the art. *Ann Emer Med* 1984;13:755–875.

Redding JS: 2nd Wolf Creek conference on CPR. *Crit Care Med* 1981;9:357–435.

Roberts JR, Greenberg MI, Baskin SI: Endotrachael epinephrine in cardiorespiratory collapse. *JACEP* 1979;8:515–519.

Safar P: *Cardiopulmonary Cerebral Resuscitation.* Philadelphia, WB Saunders, 1981.

Shapter, RK: Cardiopulmonary resuscitation: Basic life support. *Ciba Clinical Symposium* 1974;26:4–31.

Weisfeldt ML, Chandra N: Key references—Cardiopulmonary resuscitation. *Circulation* 1982;66:898–900, 1133–1135.

Life-Threatening Arrhythmias

Brown JE, Shand DG: Therapeutic drug monitoring of antiarrhythmic agents. *Clin Pharmacokinet* 1982;7:125–148.

Gabor G: Management of cardiac arrhythmias occurring in myocardial infarction. *Pharmacol Ther* 1979;6:513–550.

Gunnar RM, Lambrew CT, Abrams W, et al: Task force IV: Pharmacologic interventions. *Am J Cardiol* 1982;50:393–408.

Harrison DC: Symposium on perspectives on the treatment of ventricular arrhythmias *Am J Cardiol* 1983;52:1c–59c.

Lucchesi BR: Key references—Antiarrhythmic drugs. *Circulation* 1979;59:1976–1978.

Pittman AW, Patterson JH, Willis PW: Basic concepts of electrocardiography. *US Pharm* 1983; 8:34–52.

Schwartz KM, MacLean WAH, Waldo AL: Treatment of life-threatening cardiac arrhythmias, in Rackley C: *Critical Care Cardiology*. Philadelphia, FA Davis, 1981, pp 25–48.

Acute Congestive Heart Failure

Carlet J, Francoual M, Lhoste F, et al: Pharmacological treatment of pulmonary edema. *Intens Care Med* 1980;6:113–122.

Forrester JS, Waters DD: Hospital treatment of congestive heart failure. *Am J Med* 1978;65:173–180.

Taylor SH, Silke B, Nelson GIC: Principles of treatment of left ventricular failure. *Eur Heart J* 1982;3suppl D:19–43.

Respiratory Emergencies

Ventilator Therapy

Bone RC, Stober G: Mechanical ventilation in respiratory failure. *Med Clin North Am* 1983; 67:599–619.

Gallagher TJ: High-frequency ventilation. *Med Clin North Am* 1983;67:633–643.

Hotchkiss RS, Wilson RS: Mechanical ventilatory support. *Surg Clin North Am* 1983;63:417–438.

Petty TL: Intermittent mandatory ventilation—reconsidered. *Crit Care Med* 1981;9:620–621.

Tyler DC: Positive end-expiratory pressure: A review. *Crit Care Med* 1983;11:300–308.

Adult Respiratory Distress Syndrome

Balk R, Bone RC: The adult respiratory distress syndrome. *Med Clin North Am* 1983;67:685–700.

Flick MR, Murray JF: High-dose corticosteroid therapy in the adult respiratory distress syndrome. *JAMA* 1984;251:1054–1056.

Loyd JE, Newman JH, Brigham KL: Permeability pulmonary edema: diagnosis and management. *Arch Intern Med* 1984;144:143–147.

Nicholson DP: Corticosteroids in the treatment of septic shock and the adult respiratory distress syndrome. *Med Clin North Am* 1983;67:717–723.

Weisman IM, Rinaldo JE, Rogers RM: Positive end-expiratory pressure in adult respiratory failure. *N Engl J Med* 1982;307:1381–1384.

Acute Respiratory Failure/Pulmonary Edema

Bone RC: Treatment of respiratory failure due to advanced chronic obstructive lung disease. *Arch Intern Med* 1980;140:1018–1021.

Gallagher TJ, Civetta JM: Goal-directed therapy of acute respiratory failure. *Anesth Analg* 1980;59:831–834.

Martin L: Respiratory failure. *Med Clin North Am* 1977;61:1369–1396.

Yu PN: Key references—Pulmonary edema. *Circulation* 1981;63:724–728.

Pulmonary Aspiration

Broe PJ, Toung TJK, Cameron JL: Aspiration pneumonia. *Surg Clin North Am* 1980;60:1551–1564.

Johanson WG, Harris GD: Aspiration pneumonia, anaerobic infections, and lung abscess. *Med Clin North Am* 1980;64:385–394.

Acute Asthma

Fanta CH, Rossing TH, McFadden ER: Glucocorticoids in acute asthma—A controlled clinical trial. *Am J Med* 1983;74:845–851.

Hiller FC, Wilson FJ: Evaluation and management of acute asthma. *Med Clin North Am* 1983;67:669–684.

Leffert F: Management of acute severe asthma. *J Pediatr* 1980;96:1–12.

Mansmann HC: A 25-year perspective of status asthmaticus. *Clin Rev Allerg* 1983;1:147–162.

Raffin T, Roberts P: The prevention and treatment of status asthmaticus. *Hosp Pract* 1982;17:80A–80Z6.

Rossing TH, Fanta CH, Goldstein DH, et al: Emergency therapy of asthma: Comparison of the acute effects of parenteral and inhaled sympathomimetics and infused aminophylline. *Am Rev Respir Dis* 1980;122:365–371.

Stiell, IG: Adrenergic agents in acute asthma: Valuable new alternatives. *Ann Emerg Med* 1983;12:493–500.

Pulmonary Embolism

Russell JC: Prophylaxis of postoperative deep vein thrombosis and pulmonary embolism. *Surg Gynecol Obstet* 1983;157:89–104.

Rutkowski DM, Burkle WS: Advances in thrombolytic therapy. *Drug Intell Clin Pharm* 1982;16:115–121.

Sasahara AA, Sharma GVRK, Barsamian EM, et al: Pulmonary thromboembolism—Diagnosis and treatment. *JAMA* 1983;249:2945–2950.

Shock

General Reviews

Faden AI: Opiate antagonists and thyrotropin-releasing hormone—Potential role in the treatment of shock. *JAMA* 1984;252:1177–1180.

Kreisberg RA: Lactate homeostasis and lactic acidosis. *Ann Intern Med* 1980;92:227–237.

Makabali CG, Weil MH, Rackow EC: New concepts of circulatory shock. *J Cardiovasc Med* 1983;8:1285–93.

Rosenthal MH: Physiologic approach to the management of shock. *Sem Anesth* 1982;1:285–292.

Schwartz RA, Cerra FB: Shock: A practical approach. *Urol Clin North Am* 1983;10:89–100.

Shine KI: Aspects of the management of shock. *Ann Intern Med* 1980;93:723–734.

Cardiogenic

Resnekov L: Cardiogenic shock. *Chest* 1983;83:893–898.

Rude RE: Pharmacologic support in cardiogenic shock. *Adv Shock Res* 1983;10:35–49.

Scheidt S, Collins M, Goldstein J, et al: Mechanical circulatory assistance with the intraaortic balloon pump and other counterpulsation devices. *Prog Cardiovasc Dis* 1982;25:55–76.

Septic

Gleckman R, Esposito A: Gram-negative bacteremic shock: Pathophysiology, clinical features, and treatment. *South Med J* 1981;74:335–341.

Hess ML, Hastillo A, Greenfield LJ: Spectrum of cardiovascular function during gram-negative sepsis. *Prog Cardiovasc Dis* 1981;23:279–298.

Nicholson DP: Glucocorticoids in the treatment of shock and the adult respiratory distress syndrome. *Clin Chest Med* 1982;3:121–132.

Sheagren JN: Septic shock and corticosteroids. *N Engl J Med* 1981;305:456–457.

Hypovolemic/Hemorrhagic

Blajchman MA, Perrault RA: Blood component therapy in anesthetic practice. *Can Anesth Soc J* 1983;30:382–389.

Buchanan EC: Blood and blood substitutes for treating hemorrhagic shock. *Am J Hosp Pharm* 1977;34:631–636.

DeFelippe J, Timoner J, Velasco IT, et al: Treatment of refractory hypovolemic shock by 7.5% sodium chloride injections. *Lancet* 1980;2:1002–1004.

Gurll NL, Vargish T, Reynolds DG, et al: Opiate receptors and the endorphins in the pathophysiology of hemorrhagic shock. *Surgery* 1981;89:364–369.

Offenstadt G, Pinta P: Hemorrhagic shock. *Resuscitation* 1982;10:1–11.

Rothstein RJ: Hemorrhagic shock in multiple trauma, in Meislin HW: *Priorities in Multiple Trauma.* Germantown, Aspen Systems, 1980, pp. 29–40.

Anaphylactic

Barach EM, Nowak RM, Leet G, et al: Epinephrine for treatment of anaphylactic shock. *JAMA* 1984;251:2118–2122.

Fath JJ, Cerra FB: The therapy of anaphylactic shock. *Drug Intell Clin Pharm* 1984;18:14–21.

Acute Renal Failure

Brenner BM, Lazarus JM: *Acute Renal Failure,* Philadelphia, WB Saunders, 1983.

Tiller DJ, Mudge GH: Pharmacologic agents in the management of acute renal failure. *Kidney Int* 1980;18:700–711.

Tilney NL, Lazarus JM: Acute renal failure in surgical patients. *Surg Clin North Am* 1983; 63:357–377.

Sladen RN: Renal function and critical care. *Sem Anesth* 1982;4:323–332.

Head Trauma/Cerebral Edema

Becker AH: *Head Injury*. Philadelphia, WB Saunders, 1983.

Braakman, R, Schouten HJA, Blaauw-vanDishoeck M, et al: Megadose steroids in severe head injury. *J Neurosurg* 1983;58:326–330.

Earnest MP: *Neurologic Emergencies*. New York, Churchill Livingstone, 1983.

Frost EAM: Brain preservation. *Anesth Analg* 1981;60:821–832.

Frost EAM: The intensive care of the neurosurgical patient. *Sem Anesth* 1982;1:340–353.

Grenvik A, Safar P: *Brain Failure and Resuscitation*. New York, Churchill Livingstone, 1981.

Hamilton GC: Brain resuscitation. *Crit Care Q* 1983;5:1–98.

North JB, Penhall RK, Hanieh A, et al: Phenytoin and post operative epilepsy. *J Neurosurg* 1983;58:672–677.

Quandt CM, de los Reyes RA: Pharmacologic management of acute intracranial hypertension. *Drug Intell Clin Pharm* 1984;18:105–112.

Quandt CM, de los Reyes RA, Diaz FG, et al: Pharmacologic management of subarachnoid hemorrhage. *Drug Intell Clin Pharm* 1982;16:909–915.

Ropper AH, Kennedy SK, Zervas NT: *Neurological and Neurosurgical Intensive Care*. Baltimore, University Park Press, 1983.

White BC, Winegar CD, Wilson RF, et al: Possible role of calcium blockers in cerebral resuscitation: A review of the literature and synthesis for future studies. *Crit Care Med* 1983;11:202–207.

Young B, Rapp RP, Norton JA, et al: Failure of prophylactically administered phenytoin to prevent early posttraumatic seizures. *J Neurosurg* 1983;58:231–241.

GI Bleeding, Stress Ulceration, Hepatic Failure

Barer D, Ogilvie A, Henry D, et al: Cimetidine and tranexamic acid in the treatment of acute upper-gastrointestinal tract bleeding. *N Engl J Med* 1983;308:1571–1575.

Cerra FB, Schentag JJ, McMillen M, et al: Mental status, the intensive care unit, and cimetidine. *Ann Surg* 1982;196:565–570.

Fogel MR, Knaver M, Andres LL, et al: Continuous intravenous vasopressin in active upper gastrointestinal bleeding—A placebo-controlled trial. *Ann Intern Med* 1982;96:565–569.

Hallemans R, Naeye R, Mols P, et al: Treatment of portal hypertension with isosorbide dinitrate alone and in combination with vasopressin. *Crit Care Med* 1983;11:536–540.

Hanna SS, Warren WD, Galambos JT, et al: Bleeding varices: Emergency management. *CMA Journal* 1981;124:29–41.

Lebrec D, Poynard T, Hillon P, et al: Propranolol for prevention of recurrent gastrointestinal bleeding in patients with cirrhosis. *N Engl J Med* 1981;305:1371–1374.

Lucas CE: Stress ulceration: The clinical problem. *World J Surg* 1981;5:139–151.

Nachbauer CA, Fischer JE: The failing liver. *Surg Clin North Am* 1981;61:221–230.

Nord HJ, Brady PG: *Critical Care Gastroenterology*. New York, Churchill Livingstone, 1982.

Priebe H-J, Skillman JJ: Methods of prophylaxis in stress ulcer disease. *World J Surg* 1981;5:223–233.

Schweitzer EJ, Kerr JC, Swan KG: Clinical use of vasopressin in the management of bleeding esophageal varices. *Am Surg* 1982;48:558–562.

Silen W, Merhav A, Simson JNL: Pathophysiology of stress ulcer disease. *World J Surg* 1981;5:165–174.

Torsoli A: Gastrointestinal emergencies. *Clin Gastroenterol* 1981;10:1–254.

Wong PY, McCoy GC, Spielberg A, et al: Hepatorenal syndrome. *Gastroenterology* 1979; 77:1326–1334.

Nutrition

Apelgren KN, Wilmore DW: Nutritional care of the critically ill patient. *Surg Clin North Am* 1983;63:497–507.

Gadisseux P, Ward JD, Young HF, et al: Nutrition and the neurosurgical patient. *J Neurosurg* 1984;60:219–232.

Homsy FN, Blackburn GL: Modern parenteral and enteral nutrition in critical care. *J Am Coll Nutr* 1983;2:75–95.

Jarnberg P-O, Lindholm M, Eklund J: Lipid infusion in critically ill patients. *Crit Care Med* 1981;9:27–31.

Kudsk KA, Mirtallo JM: Nutritional support of the critically ill patient. *Drug Intell Clin Pharm* 1983;17:501–506.

Gynecologic Emergencies

Berkowitz RL: *Critical Care of the Obstetric Patient.* New York, Churchill Livingstone, 1983.

Queenan JT: *Managing Ob/Gyn Emergencies.* Oradell, New Jersey, Medical Economics Books, 1983.

Taber B-Z: *Manual of Gynecologic and Obstetric Emergencies.* Philadelphia, WB Saunders, 1984.

Sympathomimetic Drugs

Chatterjee K, Bendersky R, Parmley WW: Dobutamine in heart failure. *Eur Heart J* 1982; 3(suppl D):107–114.

Chernow B, Rainey TG, Lake R: Endogenous and exogenous catecholamines in critical care medicine. *Crit Care Med* 1982;10:409–416.

Parker S, Carlon GC, Isaacs M, et al: Dopamine administration in oliguria and oliguric renal failure. *Crit Care Med* 1981;9:630–632.

Rajfer SI, Goldberg LI: Dopamine in the treatment of heart failure. *Eur Heart J* 1982; 3(suppl D):103–106.

Regner B, Safran D, Carlet J, et al: Comparative hemodynamic effects of dopamine and dobutamine in sepctic shock. *Intensive Care Med* 1979;5:115–120.

Richard C, Ricome JL, Rimailho A, et al: Combined hemodynamic effects of dopamine and dobutamine in cardiogenic shock. *Circulation* 1983;67:620–626.

Ward DS, Bellville JW: Reduction of hypoxic ventilatory drive by dopamine. *Anesth Analg* 1982;61:333–337.

Vasodilators

Blakeley C, Tinker J: Vasodilators in acute circulatory failure. *Intensive Care Med* 1983;9:5–11.

Cohn JN, Burke LP: Nitroprusside. *Ann Intern Med* 1979;91:752–757.

Flaherty JT, Magee PA, Gardner TL, et al: Comparison of intravenous nitroglycerin and sodium nitroprusside for treatment of acute hypertension developing after coronary artery bypass surgery. *Circulation* 1982;65:1072–1077.

Ivankovich AD, Braverman B, Stephens TS, et al: Sodium thiosulfate disposition in humans: Relation to sodium nitroprusside toxicity. *Anesthesiology* 1983;58:11–17.

Jaffe AS, Roberts R: The use of intravenous nitroglycerin in cardiovascular disease. *Pharmacotherapy* 1982;2:273–280.

Massie BN, Chatterjee K: Vasodilator therapy of pump failure complicating acute myocardial infarction. *Med Clin North Am* 1979;63:25–51.

Proceedings, 28th annual meeting, American College of Angiology. Intravenous nitroglycerin: A new clinical entity. *Angiology* 1982;33:287–324.

Ribner HS, Bresnahan D, Hsieh A-M, et al: Acute hemodynamic responses to vasodilator therapy in congestive heart failure. *Prog Cardiovasc Dis* 1982;25:1–42.

Sorkin EM, Brogden RN, Romankiewicz JA: Intravenous glyceryl trinitrate. *Drugs* 1984;27:45–80.

Infections in Critical Care

Alexander JW: Prophylactic antibiotics in trauma. *Am Surg* 1982;48:45–48.

Bartlett JG: New developments in infectious diseases for the critical care physician. *Crit Care Med* 1983;11:563–573.

Guglielmo BJ, Hohn DC, Koo PJ, et al: Antibiotic prophylaxis in surgical procedures. *Arch Surg* 1983;118:943–955.

Roderick M: Infection control in critical care. *Crit Care Q* 1980;3:1–108.

Simmons RL, Howard RJ: *Surgical Infectious Disease*. New York, Appleton-Century-Crofts, 1982.

Snyder SK, Hahn HH: Diagnosis and treatment of intraabdominal abscess in critically ill patients. *Surg Clin North Am* 1982;62:229–239.

Drug Overdose

Berg MJ, Berlinger WG, Goldberg MJ, et al: Acceleration of the body clearance of phenobarbital by oral activated charcoal. *N Engl J Med* 1982;307:642–644.

Curtis RA, Barone J, Giacona N: Efficacy of ipecac and activated charcoal/cathartic. *Arch Intern Med* 1984;144:48–52.

Elenbaas RM: Poisonings and overdose. *Crit Care Q* 1982;4:1–104.

Haddad LN, Winchester JF: *Clinical Management of Poisoning and Drug Overdose*. Philadelphia, WB Saunders, 1983.

Handal KA, Shauben JL, Salamone FR: Naloxone. *Ann Emerg Med* 1983;12:438–445.

Rosenberg J, Benowitz NL, Pond S: Pharmacokinetics of drug overdose. *Clin Pharmacokinet* 1981;6:161–192.

Teat DW, Stramoski EJ, Green HM: Common household poisons. *US Pharm* 1979;6:50–64.

Index

A

AACN. *See* American Association of Critical Care Nurses
AACN Certification Corporation, 82, 95, 98
AACN Core Curriculum for Critical Care Nurses, 87
Abdominal sepsis. *See* Sepsis
Abdominal trauma, 51
Abrahamson, N.S., 14
Accreditation Standards and Guidelines for Professional Degree Programs of Colleges and Schools of Pharmacy, 40
Acetaminophen, 52
Acid-base disorders, 51
  selected bibliography, 292
Acidosis, 57
Administration techniques, 89
Administrative support, critical care pharmacy and, 16-17
Adult Clinical Pharmacy Practice ASHP SIGs on, 74
Adverse reactions, 52
Agitation, 213
Airway maintenance, 51, 169
Alimentation, 52
Alkalosis, 57
American Association of Colleges of Pharmacy (AACP), 30, 35, 279
American Association of Critical Care Nurses (AACN), 79, 81, 91, 95-97
American Board of Anesthesiology, 286
American Board of Internal Medicine, 286
American Board of Medical Specialties (ABMS), 37, 286
American Board of Pediatrics, 286
American Board of Surgery, 286
American-College of Clinical Pharmacy (AACP), 38, 39, 149
American Council on Pharmaceutical Education, 70
American Heart Association, 254
American Heritage Dictionary, 3
American Journal of Nursing, 86
American Medical Association (AMA), 36

Note: Pages appearing in italics indicate entries found in artwork.

American Nurses' Association (ANA), 78, 81
American Pharmaceutical Association (APhA), 38
American Society of Hospital Pharmacists (ASHP), 35, 39, 59, 89
American Society for Parenteral and Enteral Nutrition, 279
American Trauma Society, 279
Amikacin, 150
Aminocaproic acid, 171, 172, 173
Aminoglycosides, 6, 137, 139, 153, 199
Aminophylline, 146
Ampicillin, 155
Anaphylactic shock
  selected bibliography, 296
Anesthesiology, pharmacist's role in. *See* Surgical intensive care
Aneurysm, 164, 179, 188
Antiarrhythmics, 5, 84
Antibiotics, 7, 26, 52
  intraoperative, 9
  See also Aminoglycosides; Chloramphenicol
Anticholinergics, 165
Anticoagulation, 53, 204
Anticonvulsants, 237
Antineoplastic agents, 199
  See also Cytotoxic preparations
Applicants, qualifications of, 21-22
Archives of Internal Medicine, 9
Arrhythmia, 9, 50, 150, 188, 204
  selected bibliography, 293-294
Arterial blood gases, 7
  selected bibliography, 292
ASHP Minimum Standard for Pharmacies in Institutions, 70
ASHP Research and Education Foundation, 59, 60, *62*, 66, 67, 74
  funded by, 69
Asthma, 237
  acute, selected bibliography, 295
  See also Status asthmaticus
Atropine, 142, 146, 165

B

Bachelor of Science in Pharmacy, 30, *45*
Barbiturates, 52, 165, 168, 176, 177
  in cerebral edema, 233
  in cerebral ischemia, 178-179
  monitoring effects of, 174-175
Beaty, S., 256
Biochemistry, 4
Bioengineering, 4, 51, 57
Biopharmaceutics, 32-33, 40, 44
Biostatistics, 51
Blood chemistry, 7
Blood component, 53
Blood pressure, 7, 128
Blood pressure monitoring, 7
Blood sampling, 56
Board of Pharmaceutical Specialties (BPS), 38
Boards
  medical specialty, 36-37, *37*, 286
  national specialty, *36*
  state, 18
Brain empyema, 177-178
Brain monitoring, 54
Breathing ventilation, 56
Bretylium, 142, 146, 215
Brodie, D., 134
Bronchodilators, 5
Budget
  library equipment, 23
  preparation of, 19-21
Burkholder, 32
Burn intensive care, *46*
  burns, 5, 51
Burn unit, 55
Burnout, 9-10

C

Calcium chloride, 142, 146
California, University of, 42-44
Campos, R.A., 14
Cardiac arrest, 8, 141

Index 303

Cardiac arrest team, 256
Cardiac catheterization laboratory, 55
Cardiac disorders, selected bibliography, 239
Cardiac life support certification (ACLS), 281-282
Cardiac output, 7
Cardiac tamponade, 50
Cardio-Green Techniques, 56
Cardiogenic shock, selected bibliography, 296
Cardiology, *46*
Cardiopulmonary resuscitation (CPR), 8, 50
Cardiovascular emergencies, selected bibliography, 293-294
Cardiovascular surgery unit, 188
  drug distribution systems, 189, 196, 198
  drug records and data collection, 189, *190, 191-192, 193, 194-197*
  educational activities, 202-203
  learning objectives, 110-111
  literature, 293-296
  research activities, 203-205
  therapy planning activities, 202
Case study exercises, 119-120
Case-Western Reserve University, 81
Catheters, 4
  arterial, 7
  central venous, 7, 209
  femoral, 209
  pulmonary artery, 6, 7, 56, 137, 149, 165
  Swan-Ganz, 149, 209, 237
CCRN Certification Program, 98-99
Cefamandole, 155
Cefazolin, 156
Cefotaxime, 156
Cefoxitin, 156-157
Cephalothin, 157
Cephapirin, 157
Central nervous system, 50, 51, 56
  ventilation, in patients with disorders at, 169
Cerebral blood flow, 169

Cerebral edema, 171, 178, 233
Cerebral ischemia, 178, 179
Cerebral vasospasm, 179
Certification, 50-55, 281-282
  CCRN Certification Program, 98-99
  of nurses, 82
  See also Licensure
Charge Nurse Handbook, 115
Chartin. *See* Charts; Documentation
Charts
  clinical data sheet, *266-271*
  for determining dosage, 215-216, *216*
  drug compatibility, *146*
  emergency department, treatment in, *247*
  medical, 32, *247*
  pediatric intensive care daily record sheet, *234-236*
  pharmacology lectures, *251-252*
  pharmacy patient medication profile record, *226-227*
Children's Hospital of Philadelphia, 219-242
  description of, 219, 221
  neonatal intensive care unit, floorplan for, *220*
  pediatric description of, 230-231
  pediatric ICU, floor plan for, *232*
  medical admission, causes for, *231*
  staffing, 231, 233
Chloramphenicol, 6, 157
Circulation, 56
Civetta, J., 15
Clerkships, 31, 41-42, 47, 188
Clinical pharmacist
  expectations of, 25, 248
Clinical pharmacy movement, 29-31, 39
  roles of, 31-35
Clinical pharmacy service, 13-17, 19, 23, 44, 199
  activities of, 135-141, 233
  concepts of, 39
  support of, 15-17
Colitis. *See* Enterocolitis

Collaboration, between nurses and
 pharmacists, 90-93
Colleges of pharmacy
 six-year first degree, 30-31, *44*
 offering the B.S., *45*
 role of, 35, 47, 48
Colloids
 crystalloids vs., 7
 selected bibliography, 293
Coma, 51, 178
 barbiturate-induced, 178-179, 233
Commission on Credentialing, 60
Committee support process, *17*
Communication, 205, 215, 260
Community health center, 8
Compatibility. *See* Drugs
Comprehensive Structure Standard XI, 92
Computer, 4, 54, 56, 104, 147, 169, 289
 hospital information system, 91
 telex system, 189
Condition Critical: The Nurse Makes a Difference (videotape), 96
Congestive heart failure, selected bibliography, 294
Connecticut, University of. *See* Hartford Hospital
Consensus Development Conference, 3
Contract, learning. *See* Learning contract
Coronary care unit, 55, 188, 285, 287
 See also Cardiovascular surgery unit; Coronary intensive care
Coronary intensive care, 46
Cost, 4, 93, 169, 259
 syringes v. minibags, 145
Cost-containment, 9, 20, 127, 150, 287
Cost-effectiveness, 15, 128
 approach, 91
 justification for, 257, 278
 program for, 48
Cost-savings data, 25-26
 See also Evaluation
Creatinine clearance, 5, 56
Critical care
 curriculum, 45
 definition of, 3
 development of, 4
 environment, 79
 explanation of, 3-4, 9-10
 drugs in, 4
 literature on, 9
 medical skills, 55
 objectives of, 13
 pharmacists and, 7-8
 pharmacy and, 7, 9-10, 13, 47
 pharmacy, practice of, 7, 9-10, 47
 See also Evaluation, of program; Literature
Critical care medicine (CCM)
 certification, 50-55
 explanation of, 3
 practice of, 285-287
 skills, 55
"Critical Care Medicine," 9
Critical care nursing, 103-104
 scope of, 79
Critical care pharmacy, justification of
 clinical pharmacy service, 8, 13, 15, 279-282
 hospital's need, 15, 26
 nurse's need, 14-15, 26
 patient's need, 13, 26
 physician's need, 14, 26
"Critical Care Therapeutics," 9
Critical care unit, 3, 13, 14, 18
 need for, 3
 See also Intensive care unit
Crystalloids, 103
 colloids vs., 7
 selected bibliography, 293
Curriculum, 40-43, 50-55, 80, 87
 vitae, 71, 72
Cyr, D.A., 59
Cytotoxic preparations, 89
 See also Antineoplastic agents

D

Dasta, J.F., 46
Data collection, 7, 139, 144, 178, 203
 concentrated intravenous drugs, on, 155-160

Decentralization. *See* Distribution system
Decentralized pharmacist, 19, 187, 189, 198, 200, 202
Delivery, drug, 5-6, 137
Dexamethasone, 171-172, 173
Diabetic ketoacidosis, 207
Diabetes mellitus, 52
Diagnosis related groups (DRGs), 19, 26
Dialysis unit, 55
Diarrhea/dehydration, selected bibliography, 241
Diazepam, 6, 175, 213
Digoxin, 146
Dimethyl sulfoxide. *See* DMSO
Discharge medications and prescriptions, system for, 254-255
DMSO, 179
Dobutamine, 129, 134-135, 142, 146, 158, 215, *216*
Doctor of Pharmacy, 31
See also Pharm. D.
Documentation
  medical administration record, example of, *190*
  therapy sheet, example of, *191-193*
  hemodynamic information, example of, *194-197*
  See also Evaluation
Dopamine, 129, 142, 146, 150, 165, 215
Dosing, 8, 88-89, 102-104, 141, 170, 187, 237, 264, 286
  charts on, 129, *142-143*, 145, *146*, 215-216, *216*
  unit-dose, 32, 89, 134, 145, 189, 198, 205, 209, 245, 273-274
Drugs, 5, 134-135
  administration of, 5, 83-84, 89, 172, 189, 198, 265
  clinical effects, 90
  compatability, 5, 87, 88, 103, 137, 146, *147*
  distribution, 19, 20, 22, 23, 127, 129, 141, 144-145, 147, 187, 189-198, 225, 253-254

information, 32, 84-90
intravenous, 5-6, 88
list for NICU patients, *173*
literature, 298, 299
questions asked by nurses about, 87-90, 103-104
serum levels, interpretation of, 90
stability, 155-161
therapy, effective use of, 87-88, 93
See also Drug questionnaire; Inventory; Pharmacokinetics; Order turn around time
Drug assay laboratory, 204
Drug distribution system, 22, 23, 129, 141, 145, 169, 225, 253-254, 273-274
Drug Intelligence and Clinical Pharmacy, 9
Drug questionnaire, 122-123

E

Education, 91-92, 101-103, 175, 245, 248, 286
  evolution of, 29-31
  graduate study, 82-83, 187
  learning contract, 106-117
  neonatal intensive care unit, 230
  pharmacy, related to, 34-35, 187, 202-203, 237
  teaching responsibilities, 277
  See also Program; Doctor of Pharmacy; Program, for nurses
Electrocardiogram, 7, 128
Electroencephalography, 169
Electrolyte alterations, 51, 56
Elenbaas, R., 8
Elliott, E.C., 29
Embolization, 56
Emergency drug box, 117, 141
Emergency drug dosing chart, 142-143
Emergency medical service (EMS) government, support of, 243
"Emergency Medicine in Critical Care," 9

Emergency room medicine, 46,
243-258, 285, 287
  clinical pharmacy in, 245, 248
  conditions treated in, 247
  cost justification, 257
  crash cart content, 254, 255
  distribution of drugs in, 253-256
  drugs given in, 244
  education, 248, 251-252, 256
  floor plan, 246
  formulary, 254
  inventory control, 257
  research, 252-253
  See also Trauma Center
Endocrine system
  critical illness, effects of, 52
Entercolitis, necrotizing
  selected bibliography, 240
Epidemiological data, 4
Epidural administration, 176, 180
Epiglottis/croup, selected bibliography, 241
Epinephrine, 129, 142, 146
Ethacrynic acid, 172
Ethical aspects, 55
Evaluation
  drug distribution system, 144-145
  drug literature, 41
  critical care pharmacy satellites, 9
  program, 23-26, 27

F

Federal laws, 18
Fellowships, 47
  ASHP Research and Education Foundation, 61, 67-68, 69
  application, 61, 61-63, 70
  application procedure, applicants, 70-71
  application procedure, preceptor, 64-65, 72-73
  critical care pharmacy, in, 59, 60, 61, 67-70, 72-78

  funding, 75
  preceptor-institution application, example of, 64-65, 72-73
  programs, 67-68, 69, 75, 149
  promotion, 74-75
  qualifications of applicant, 70
  qualifications of institution, 70
  qualifications of preceptor, 71
  residencies vs., 59-60, 67-68
  selection procedure, 73, 74
Fetal circulation, 51
Flail chest, 51
Floor stock, 127, 134, 135, 147
Florence Nightingale, 78
Flowsheets, 217, 265
  clinical data sheet, 266-271
  hemodynamic, in cardiovascular unit, 194-197
  neurologic intensive care, example of, 176
  pediatric intensive care unit, 234-236
  surgical intensive care unit, 129, 130-133, 140
  trauma center, 265, 266-271
Fluid and electrolyte therapy, selected bibliography, 292-293
  NICU, example of, 167
Fluosal-DA, 179-180
Focus on Critical Care, 96
Foundation. See ASHP Research and Education Foundation
Francke, D.E., 31
Furosemide, 172

G

Gastric pH, 7
Gastrointestinal disorders, 53, 57
  bleeding, 174, 207
  learning objectives, 111-112
  literature, 297-298
Genitourinary tract
  disorders, 53
  learning objectives, 112-113

Index 307

Gentamycin, 178, 199
Glasgow Coma Scale, 165
Glutethimide, 165
Glycerol, 171 ff
Government
 administration, 260
 hospital, 8
 insurers, 20
Gram-negative, 178
 organism, 177
 rods, 138
Gynecological disorders, 51
Gynecologic emergencies, selected bibliography, 298

H

Haloperidol, 150
Hartford Hospital, 207-218
 description of, *208*
 University of Connecticut Medical School, 207
Head injury, acute, *172*
Head trauma, selected bibliography, 297
Heart & Lung, 96
Heart rate, 7, 128
Heavy metals, 52
Helicopters. See Med-Evac helicopter
Hematology, 57
 disorders, 53
Hemodynamic information, flowsheet of, *194-197*
Hemodynamics, 51
 parameters of, 51
 profile flowsheet, example of, *138, 194-197*
Hemodialysis, 51, 200
Henderson, Virginia, *78*
Henry Ford Hospital, 169 ff
Heparin, 123
Hepatic clearance, 5
Hepatic failure, selected bibliography, 297-298
Herraez, F.X.V., 14

Holistic medicine, 85, 92
Hospitals
 community health center, 7, 8
 critical care pharmacy and, 15
 government, 8
 Ohio State University, 128
 pharmacy practice, 31
 private, 19, 187-188, 206
 residency training in, 47-48
 teaching, 7, 47, 237
 tertiary care, 163
 university medical center, 8
H_2-receptors, 7
Hubbard, W.N., Jr., 33-34
Human Research Committee, 178
Hyperbilirubinemia, selected bibliography, 241
Hypovolemic/hemorrhagic shock, selected bibliography, 296

I

ICP measurement, 165, 168
Implementation
 clinical pharmacy service, 22-23, 27, 198-201, 253
 drug distribution system, 22-23, 144, 202
 satellite pharmacy (SICU), 145, 147
Incompatibility. See Drugs
Infant intensive care flowsheet, example of, *222-224*
Infant, over/under medication, 225
Infection, 57, 139, 164, 175
 learning objectives, 113
 literature, 299
Infection control for special care units, 52
Infection Control Manual, 113
Infectious disease, 52, 209
Information, 32, 84-85, 87-90, 91
 poison, 256
Ingestion, selected bibliography, 241
Inotropes, 237
Insulin, 6

Insurers
    government, 20
    private, 20
Intensive care medicine, 285
Intensive care unit, 4, 55, 150, 285
    See also Burn intensive care; Critical care unit; Cardiovascular surgery unit; Medical intensive care unit; Neonatal intensive care unit; Neurosurgery intensive care; Pediatric intensive care unit; Surgical intensive care unit
Intensive care unit laboratory, 57
Interactions, surveillance, 104, 199
Interdisciplinary activities, 92-93
Internal medicine, 46
Intracranial pressure, 7, 128, 165, *168*, 171, 177, 180, 233
Intrathecal administration, 176, 180
Intravenous administration, 6, 88
    See also IV therapy
Intravenous therapy sheet, 191-192
Intravenous Therapy Practice, 74
Intraventricular administration, 178, 180
Intubation, 4, 56
Inventory, floor stock, 9
Ischemia, 179, 180
Isoproterenol, 142, 146, 158
IV therapy, 191-192
    See also Intravenous therapy
IVAC Corporation, 75

J

Johnson, Dorothy E., *78*
Joint Commission on Accreditation of Hospitals (JCAH), 18, 77, 129, 134, 135
    Standards for Pharmaceutical Services, 135
Joint Committee on Critical Care Medicine (JCCCM), 37, 77, 253, 286

K

Karl, A.F., 59
Kennedy, J.F., 219
Kentucky, University of, 31
Kirking, D.M., 36

L

Laboratory, ICU, 57
Learning contract questions, 106-117
Legal aspects, 55, 79-80
Legislative and political issues, 97
Levy, G., 32-33
Libraries, 87
    for critical care unit, 23
Licensed practical/vocational nurses, 77
    See also Nurses
Licensure, of nurses, 80, 81-82, 104
Lidocaine, 105, 137, 142, 146, 180, 188, 215, 254, 272
Life-support machine, 4, 5
Literature, 9, 265, 289
    critical care, 9, 290-299
    drug reference book, 104
LPN/LVN. *See* Licensed practical/vocational nurses

M

McLeod, D.C., 46
Major organ systems
    cardiovascular, 70
    pulmonary, 70
    renal, 70
    metabolic-endocrine-nutritional, 70
    neurological-neurosurgical, 70
Mannitol, 171ff
Maryland Institute for Emergency Medical Services Systems — Neurotrauma Center (MIEMSS-NTC), 102-103, 104, 260ff
    case studies, 119-120
    drug questionnaire, 122-123

learning contract, 106-117
most widely used drugs in, 105
unit questions, 121
Master of Science in Pharmacy, 70
Meconium aspiration, selected bibliography, 240
Med-Evac helicopter, 261
Medical Administration Record, 22
Medical centers
university, 8
Medical intensive care, *46*, 207-218
Medical intensive care unit, 287
demographics, 207-208
pharmacist's daily activities, 211, *212*
position development in, 208-210
problem solving in, 214-217
procedure and medications for, *209*
research in, 217
service development in, 211-217
Medical societies, 285
national specialty, *36*
Medical staff committee, 21
See also P&T Committee
Medication Administration Record, 189, *190*, 198
Medication administration service, 18
Medication Order Form, 169
Medication Profile Book, 170
Medication Profile Record, 226-227
Metabolic effects of critical illnesses, 52
Metabolism, 5, 57
Methyldopa, 165
Methylprednisolone, 123
Michigan, University of, 31, 33
MIEMSS. *See* Maryland Institute for Emergency Medical Services Systems
Minnesota, University of. *See* University of Minnesota College of Pharmacy; University of Minnesota Family Practice Program; University of Minnesota Surgical Program
Missouri, University of. *See* University of Missouri-Kansas City, 245
Morphine, 176, 213
intrathecal or intraventricular, 180
epidural, 180
Motivation, 22
Monitoring, 4, 15, 24, 51, 54, 56, 57, 128, 137, 147, 149, 170-171, 181, 199, 203, 211, 218, 264, 286, 291-292
bioengineering, 57
blood pressure, 7
drug, 5, 163, 170, 174-175, 201, 229, 280
metabolic, 54
neurological, 165-169
therapeutic, 274-275
Moxalactam, 158
Multidisciplinary committee, 21
Multiple systems, 87, 98, 177
drug, 5
involvement of, 6
Multiple organ system
dysfunction of, 5
failure of, 3, 137, 177

N

Nafcillin, 158
Narcotic box, 145
Narcotics, 52
National Institutes of Health (NIH), 3
conference on critical care, 8
National Federation for Specialty Nursing Organizations, 97
National Teaching Institute, 96-97
Nebraska, University of. *See* University of Nebraska Medical Center
Necrotizing enterocolitis, selected bibliography, 240
Need
fellowship of, 59
See also Critical care pharmacy, justification of; Problem solving
Neonatal intensive care (NICU), *46*, 55, 219-230
clinical activities, 225, 228
description, 219, *220*, 221
development skills in, 228-230

drug distribution services, 225
educational activities, 230
flowsheet, *222-224*
Pharmacy Patient Medication Profile Record, *226-227*
recommended journals for, *229*
research, 230
residencies in, 228
staffing, 221, 225
Neonatology, selected bibliography, 239
Neurologic assessment sheet, 165
example of, *166*
Neurology
learning objectives, 107-109
Neuromuscular blockers, 165
Neurosurgery intensive care, 55, 128, 163-170, 287
admission-discharge guidelines, 161
education in, 175
monitoring CNS in, 165, 168-169, 174-175
neurological assessment, 164-165, *166*
nurse-patient ratio, 164
nutrition support, 175
problem solving, 176-178
research, 178-180
stock list of drugs for, 171-172, 173
Neurotrauma
nursing in, 101-104
Nuerotrauma center, 101-104
drug questionnaire, 122-123
drugs used, 105
learning contract for, 106-117
orientation guidelines, *102*
unit questions, 121
New England Journal of Medicine, 8
NFSNO. *See* National Federation for Specialty Nursing Organization
Nitroglycerin, 6, 129, 146, 149, 215
Nitroprusside, 129, 158, 165, 215
See also Sodium nitroprusside
Norepinephrine, 142, 146, 215
Nurses, 77-99
certification, 82

critical care, 79, 90-93, 98-99, 101, 103-104
critical care pharmacy and, 14-15
drug administration, 83-84
drug information for, 84-90
drug therapy, role in, 83-84
head, 16
licensed practical/vocational nurses, 77
pharmacist's relation to, 213-214, 215
problems, 215
professional, 81
program for, 80-81
registered, 77
supporting critical care pharmacy, 16
technical, 81
See also Nursing
Nurses' Drug Alert, 86
Nursing, 77-83
administration, 16
certification, 82
continuing education programs, 91
definition of, 77-79
flowsheet, example of, *130-133*
education and credentials in, 80-81
entry into practice issue, 81
graduate study in, 82-83
learning objectives, 114-115
legal definition of, 79-80
licensure, 81, 82
primary, 114
See also Flowsheets
Nursing: A Social Policy Statement, 79
Nursing 84, 86
Nutrition, 57, 137, 245
literature, 298
Nutritional support, *46*, 137, 175, 219-220, 272-273, 280-281, 286, 287
TPN therapy sheet, *193*

O

Obstetrics, 51
Ohio State University, 46
surgical intensive care unit, 128-150

Index 311

Ommaya reservoir, 180
Operating room pharmacy, 9
Order turnaround time, 9
Organophosphates, 52
Overdose, 5, 217, 256
  selected bibliography, 299
Oxygen therapy, 51, 56

P

P&T Committee. *See* Pharmacy and Therapeutics Committee
Pace University, 81
Pacemaker insertion, 56
Pain relief, research in, 150
Pancuronium bromide, 122
Paraldehyde, 175
Patient, 14
  comatose, 165, 176
  critical care pharmacy and, 13
  critically ill, definition of, 79
  documentation of, 23-25
  fluid restricted, 6
  handicapped, 55
  mentally retarded, 55
  physiological parameters of, 7
Patient-to-pharmacist ratio, 7
Pediatric intensive care unit (PICU), 230-237, 241, 287
  causes for admission, *231*
  daily record sheet, *234-236*
  developing skills in, 233
  educational activities, 237
  floor plan, *232*
  research, 237
  staffing, 231, 233
Pediatric Pharmacy Practice, 75
  conditions of, 54
Pediatrics, selected bibliography, 241-242
Penicillin GK, 159
Penicillin G Sodium, 159
Pentobarbital, 122, 172, 174, 176, 177, 233
Peplau, Hildegard, E., *78*

Pericardial diseases, 50
Peptides, 180
Pericardiocentesis, 56
Peripheral vascular surgery, *46*
Peritoneal dialysis, 51
Petitions
  practitioner group, by, 38-39
Petroleum distillates, 52
Pharm. D., 8, 35, 39-44, 48, 61, 70, 147-149, 200
  programs, 42-44, *148*
  See also Doctor of Pharmacy
Pharmaceutical Survey of 1948, 29
Pharmacists
  ability to identify needs, 214-215
  activities of, 8, 176-178, 200-205, 211-214, 228-230, 246, 248, 256, 264
  centralized, 198
  critical care nurses and, 91-94
  poison information, role in, 256
  problems, 215-217
Pharmacokinetics, 5, 15, 32-33, 40, 44, 54, 70, 137-139, 171, 237, 264, 272
  dosing service, 152-154, 201
  flowsheet, example of, *140, 266-271*
  response to drugs, 6
  shock, effect on, 272
Pharmacology, 4, 5, 15, 70, 85, 103-104
Pharmacy
  decentralized/satellite, 19, 127-128, 134-135, 144-145, 147, 169, 225, 257, 281
  justification for, 13
  oncology, 59
  service development, 8-9, 15-16, 127-128, 211, 218, 278-282
Pharmacy and Therapeutics Committee, 16, 254
Pharmacy-Medicine-Nursing Conference on Health Education, 33
Pharmacy residency
  critical care, 21, 47-48
  Ohio State University, 46, *46*, 147, 149
Phenylephrine, 142-146

Phenytoin, 105, 122, 137, 165, 171, 172, 173, 174, 175, 272
  IV infusion of, 139-141
Physicians
  critical care medicine and, 14, 16, 54
  pharmacists and, 214-215
Physicians' Desk Reference, 85, 88, 104
Physiology, 4
Piperacillin, 159
Pitressin, 122
Pneumothorax, 56
Poliomyelitis, 4
Polypharmacy
  in critical care unit, 14
Poison information, 256
Poison control program, 187, 261
Postcardiac surgery patients, 51
Postgraduate training, 44-45
Potassium, 123, 146
Powell, S.H., 59
Preceptor, 71
Preceptor-Institution
  application, *64-65*, 72
Problem solving, 176-178, 201, 205, 210
  approach to, 79
  pharmacist, role of, 202, 214-217, 218
Porcainamide, 137, 143, 146, 215
Prochlorperazine, 159
Program
  residency and fellowship programs, 32, 149
  nurses, for, 80-81, 82-83, 91
  See Implementation, Evaluation
Program, Doctor of Pharmacy, 39-44
  Ohio State University, 147-149
  University of Kentucky, 31
  University of Michigan, 31
  University of California at San Francisco, 31, 42, *43*
  University of Southern California, 31
  See also Curriculum
Prophylaxis, 7
Proposal, writing of, 17-19, 27, 97
Propranolol, 143, 165, 217

Prospective Payment System (PPS), 26
Prospective payments, 15, 19, 127
Prostacyclin, 179
Protocol and guidelines, 60-61, 69-75, 171-173, 216, 217, 262-263
  standardization of treatment, 263
Psychiatric emergencies, 52
Publications
  critical care, 289-290
  nursing, 96
Puckett, W., 256
Pulmonary artery catheter, 6, 7, 137, 149, 168
Pulmonary artery pressure monitoring, 51
Pulmonary aspiration, selected bibliography, 295
Pulmonary edema, 50
  selected bibliography, 294
Pulmonary embolism, 50
  selected bibliography, 295
Pulmonary function laboratory, 55
  tests, 56
Pumps, 6, 104

R

Reanimation, 3
Record keeping, 54, 29, 54
  See also Flowsheets
Registered nurses, 77
Reinforcement
  positive, 25
Regulations, 18
Renal disorders, 51, 56, 150, 237
  selected bibliography, 296
Research, emphasis in, 178-180, 217, 230, 252-253, 277
  drug-related, 6-7
  fellowships, 67, 68
  pain control, 180
Reserpine, 165
Residencies, 3, 59-60, 67-68, 228, 245
  definition of, 60
  fellowships vs., 59-60, 67-68

See also Fellowships; Pharmacy residency; Program
Respiratory disorders
 failure, acute, 51, 207
 learning objectives, 109-110
 monitoring, 54
 therapy, 55
 See also Respiratory distress syndrome; Respiratory emergencies; Respiratory therapy quiz
Respiratory distress syndrome, selected bibliography, 239
Respiratory emergencies, selected bibliography, 294-295
Respiratory therapy quiz, 118
Resuscitation, 3
 cardiopulmonary, 2, 188
 central nervous system, 50
 See also Reanimation
Reye's syndrome, 54, 233, 242
 selected bibliography, 242
Richmond screw, 116, 119
Robin, E., 14
Rogers, Martha E., 78
RN. *See* Registered nurses

S

Safer, P., 3
Salicylate, 52
Satellite pharmacy, 9, 135, 144, 145, 147, 169-170, 281
Schools and Colleges of Pharmacy, 285
Scholarships, 97
Schondelmeyer, S.W., 36
Scopolamine, 165
Sepsis
 abdominal, 137-138
 selected bibliography, 240
Seizures
 management of, 175
 selected bibliography, 241
 See also Status epilepticus
Septic shock, selected bibliography, 296
Serum drug levels, 26, 90, 152-154

Shock
 selected bibliography, 295-296
 See also Trauma
Shock-trauma unit, 4, 55
SICU. *See* Surgical intensive care unit
SIGs. *See* Special interest groups
Smoke inhalation, 51
Society of Critical Care Medicine (SCCM), 7, 9, 44, 45, 96, 279, 286
Sodium bicarbonate, 143, 146
Sodium nitroprusside, 89, 104
 See also Nitroprusside
Special interest groups (SIGs), 39, 61
Specialists, 187, 205
Specialization, pharmacy, 35-39
Stability data on intravenous drugs, 155-161
Staffing, 19, 21
 notification, 22
Standards for Nursing Care of the Critically Ill, 95
Status asthmaticus, 51
 See also Asthma
Status epilepticus, 175
 See also Seizures
Sterile Products Department, 176
Sterility techniques, 57
Strategy, 26
 development of, 7
"Street" drugs, 52
Stress ulceration, selected bibliography, 297
Stryker frame, 107
Subarachnoid hemorrhage, 171, 179
Support, 15-16, *17*, 253
 administrative, 16-17
 data, 18
 interdisciplinary, 33-35
 medical, 16
 nursing, 16
Surgical intensive care, *46*
Surgical intensive care unit (SICU), 127, 149, 287
 admission/discharge data, *129*
 nursing flowsheet in, *130-133*
 pharmacy development of, 135-136

pharmacy services in, 127-128
Surveillance, drug, 104
Swan-Ganz catheters, 149, 237
Sympathomimetic drugs, selected bibliography, 298
Syringes, prepacking, 145
Systemic sepsis, 52
Systems Communication Center (SYSCOM), 260

T

Task Force on Critical Care Medicine, 286
TDX equipment, 204
Teaching
  one-on-one, 203
  one-on-two, 203
Teaching program, affiliation with, 19
Theophylline, 9, 137
Therapeutics, 15
Therapy, 50
Thermodilution techniques, 56
Thiopental, 171, 172, 174, 176, 177
Third-party payers, 243
Thora-Drain III, 116
Thoracic and neurosurgical intensive care, 46
Thoracic care unit, 4
Tobramycin, 137, 139, 149-150, 152-154, 160, 199
Toxicology, 4
Thoracic surgery, 46
Ticarcillin, 159
TPN therapy sheet, *193*
Training. *See* Education
Tranquilizers, 52
Transcutaneous pO_2, 230
"Transport Conference," 237
Trauma, 9, 50, 51, 57
  care, echelons of, 261, *262*
  drug interaction in, 275-277
  literature, 297
  treatment in nontrauma hospital, 276-277

Trauma center, 8, 259-283,287
  clinical pharmacist in, 264
  clinical system, 263
  distinguished from emergency department, 259-260
  distribution of drugs in, 273-274
  monitoring, 274-275
  nutrition support in, 272-273
  prehospital care, 261-262
  organization of, 260-262
  pharmacokinetic applications, 264-266
  research, 277
  service justification, 278
  teaching, 277
Trimethobenzamide, 160
Truman Medical Center, 8, 245-258
  crash cart drug contents, *255*
  drug items in emergency department, *249*
  floor plan of, *246*
  general implementation of program, 253-258

U

Ulcer, stress, 7
Unit-dose. *See* Dosing
Unit questions, 121
United Hospitals and Children's, Incorporated, 187-206
US Health Resources Administration – Division of Nursing, 95
University of Minnesota College of Pharmacy, 188
University of Minnesota Family Practice Program, 187
University of Minnesota Surgical Program, 187
University of Missouri-Kansas City (UMKC), 245
University of Nebraska Medical Center, 255
University medical center, 8
  See also Hospitals

Urinary tract. *See* Genitourinary tract
Urine output, 4

V

Value analysis, 279-282
Vancomycin, 160
Vasoactive compounds, 5
Vasodilator therapy, 51
  selected bibliography, 298-299
Vasopressin, 216-217
Vasopressor therapy, 51, 179
Venipuncture, 7
Ventilation, in patients with CNS
  disorders, 169
Ventilator, 3, 5, 22, 51, 128, 169,
  209, 213, 221
  selected bibliography, 294

Verapamil, 143, 146, 150, 178, 179, 217

W

Waisbren, B., 15
Wald, K.S., 14
Walton, C.A., 32
Warfarin, 123
Weaning techniques, 56
Weaver, Larry, 200
White, E., 29

Y

Yale University, 81

Editors

Thomas C. Majerus, Pharm.D.
Clinical Pharmacist
The Maryland Institute for Emergency
Medical Services Systems
University of Maryland

Joseph F. Dasta, M.Sc.
Assistant Professor
College of Pharmacy, College of
Medicine
Ohio State University

Contributors

David Angaran, M.Sc.
Associate Professor
University of Minnesota,
Clinical Pharmacist
United and Children's Hospitals
St. Paul, Minnesota

Deborah K. Armstrong, Pharm.D.
Clinical Pharmacist and Clinical
Instructor
Ohio State University

Jane E. Aumick, R.N.
Unit Teacher
Neurotrauma Center
The Maryland Institute for Emergency
Medical Services Systems
University of Maryland

Henry Blissenbach, Pharm.D.
Assistant Director of Pharmacy
United and Children's Hospitals
St. Paul, Minnesota,
Clinical Associate Professor
University of Minnesota

Joyce B. Comer, Pharm.D.
Associate Professor
University of Connecticut

R Adams Cowley, M.D.
Professor of Cardiovascular and
Thoracic Surgery,
Director
The Maryland Institute for Emergency
Medical Services Systems
University of Maryland

Gary C. Cupit, Pharm.D.
Associate Professor and Vice-
Chairman for Academic Affairs
College of Pharmacy
University of Tennessee
Center for the Health Sciences
Memphis

Robert M. Elenbaas, Pharm.D.
Associate Professor of Clinical
Pharmacy
University of Missouri-Kansas City,
Clinical Pharmacist
Truman Medical Center
Kansas City, Missouri

Contributors continued

Ramón Lavandero, R.N., M.A., M.S.N., C.C.R.N.
Senior Level Coordinator and Assistant Professor of Nursing
Thomas Jefferson University
Philadelphia, Pennsylvania

Warren E. McConnell, Ph.D.
American Society of Hospital Pharmacists
Bethesda, Maryland

Donald C. McLeod, M.Sc.
Associate Professor
Ohio State University

Christine M. Quandt, B.Sc.
Doctoral candidate
University of Texas

Therese S. Richmond, R.N., M.S.N., C.C.R.N.
Clinical Nurse Specialist
Thomas Jefferson University
Philadelphia, Pennsylvania

Susan T. Roberts, R.N.
Primary Nurse
The Maryland Institute for Emergency Medical Services Systems
University of Maryland

Philip J. Schneider, M.Sc.
Associate Director
Department of Pharmacy,
Clinical Associate Professor
Ohio State University

Michael Schobelock, Pharm.D.
Clinical Pharmacist and Clinical Instructor
Ohio State University